CORPVS MEDICORVM GRAECORVM

EDIDERVNT

ACADEMIAE BEROLINENSIS HAVNIENSIS LIPSIENSIS

V 8, 1

GALENI

DE PRAECOGNITIONE

EDIDIT, IN LINGVAM ANGLICAM VERTIT, COMMENTATVS EST

VIVIAN NUTTON

BEROLINI IN AEDIBVS ACADEMIAE SCIENTIARVM MCMLXXIX

GALEN

ON PROGNOSIS

EDITION, TRANSLATION, AND COMMENTARY

BY

VIVIAN NUTTON

AKADEMIE-VERLAG · BERLIN 1979

Erschienen im Akademie-Verlag, DDR – 108 Berlin, Leipziger Straße 3–4

Lizenznummer: 202 · 100/219/79
Herstellung: IV/2/14 VEB Druckerei »Gottfried Wilhelm Leibniz«,
445 Gräfenhainichen · 4831
Bestellnummer: 753 095 7 (2028/22) · LSV 2006
Printed in GDR
DDR 78,– M

VORWORT

Die Galenschrift mit dem Titel De praecognitione, die den Gegenstand der vorliegenden Edition bildet, ist kein Lehrbuch zu dem für die antike Medizin außerordentlich wichtigen Thema „Prognose“, wie man es zunächst von der Überschrift her erwarten würde. In ihr schildert Galen vielmehr einige Fälle aus seiner ärztlichen Praxis, die deutlich machen sollen, daß die Prognose ein unentbehrliches Hilfsmittel des Arztes ist und, sachkundig angewandt, in schwierigen Fällen entscheidende Hinweise für eine erfolgreiche Therapie zu geben vermag.

Galen hat seine Schrift Über die Prognose aus ganz persönlichen Gründen abgefaßt, und das erklärt den besonderen Charakter dieser Abhandlung, die sich sowohl inhaltlich durch eine Fülle autobiographischer und zeitgeschichtlicher Nachrichten wie formal durch die souveräne Handhabung des literarischen und stilistischen Rüstzeugs der Zweiten Sophistik auffällig von seinen sonstigen medizinischen Werken unterscheidet und deswegen ein besonderes Interesse für sich beanspruchen darf. Mit ihr wollte der Pergamener sich gegen Verleumdungen von seiten seiner ärztlichen Kollegen verteidigen, die ihm, wie er glaubte, aus Konkurrenzneid unterstellten, er benutze die Prognose lediglich zu dem Zweck, sich in den Ruf divinatorischer Fähigkeiten zu bringen und auf diese Weise einen größeren Patientenkreis anzulocken. Um die Lauterkeit seiner eigenen Person und seine eigenen wissenschaftlichen Leistungen um so mehr zur Geltung kommen zu lassen, gibt Galen zunächst einen Bericht über die Unbildung und Korruption, die nach seiner Meinung unter den Ärzten seiner Zeit, speziell in der Großstadt Rom, besonders weit verbreitet waren und von ihm als Ursache für die Mißgunst der Ärzte gegenüber denen angesehen wurden, die sich in ihrem Auftreten und Handeln eines Hippokrates für würdig erwiesen. Diesen Ausführungen läßt er dann die detaillierte Schilderung einiger Fälle aus seiner römischen Praxis folgen, die zeigen sollen, daß prognostisches Vorgehen in der von ihm betriebenen Art wissenschaftlich begründet und für den Arzt gerade in medizinisch schwierigen Fällen unerläßlich ist, wenn er therapeutische Erfolge erzielen will.

Für die Herstellung der vorliegenden ersten kritischen Edition der Schrift Über die Prognose (zuletzt erschienen Leipzig 1827), die eine den Anforderungen der modernen Textkritik entsprechende Ausgabe darstellt, wurde die gesamte heute verfügbare Primär- und Sekundärüberlieferung, einschließlich der zahlreichen arabischen Testimonien zu dieser Abhandlung, ausgewertet. Die englische Übersetzung – es ist dies die erste modernsprachige Übersetzung dieses Textes – und der ausführliche, vor allem auf die Klärung inhaltlicher Probleme ausgerichtete Kommentar machen diese auch in historischer und kulturgeschichtlicher Hinsicht interessante Schrift, die für uns zudem ein wertvolles Zeugnis für Galens Fähigkeiten und Ambitionen auf literarischem Gebiet ist, zum erstenmal auch dem Nichtphilologen zugänglich.

Die Redaktion des
Corpus Medicorum Graecorum
Jutta Kollesch

TABLE OF CONTENTS

BIBLIOGRAPHY[1]

Artemidori Daldiani Onirocriticon libri V, ed. R. A. Pack, Leipzig 1963

K. Bardong, Beiträge zur Hippokrates- und Galenforschung, Nachrichten d. Akademie d. Wiss. in Göttingen, phil.-hist. Kl. 1942, pp. 577–640

T. D. Barnes, Hadrian and Lucius Verus, Journal of Roman Studies 57, 1967, pp. 65–79

H. Baumgarten, Galen, Über die Stimme. Testimonien der verlorenen Schrift Περὶ φωνῆς, Pseudo-Galen De voce et hanelitu, Kommentar, Diss. Göttingen 1962

A. R. Birley, Marcus Aurelius, London 1966

–, A nickname for Commodus and the date of Fronto's death, Chiron 2, 1972, pp. 463–473

F. Blass and A. Debrunner, A Greek grammar of the New Testament, 10th. ed., trans. R. W. Funk, Chicago 1961

G. W. Bowersock, Greek sophists in the Roman Empire, Oxford 1969

A. Cornelii Celsi quae supersunt, ed. F. Marx, CML I, Leipzig and Berlin 1915

CIL = Corpus Inscriptionum Latinarum

CMG = Corpus Medicorum Graecorum

CML = Corpus Medicorum Latinorum

K. Deichgräber, Die griechische Empirikerschule. Sammlung der Fragmente und Darstellung der Lehre, Berlin 1930 (repr. Berlin/Zürich 1965) (= Emp.)

–, Medicus gratiosus, Akademie d. Wiss. u. d. Lit., Abh. d. geistes- u. sozialwiss. Kl. 1970, 3, Wiesbaden 1970

J. D. Denniston, The Greek particles, Oxford 1934

H. Diels, Die Handschriften der antiken Ärzte, I, Abh. d. Königl. Preuß. Akademie d. Wiss. 1905, phil.-hist. Kl. 3, Berlin 1905

–, Die handschriftliche Überlieferung des Galenschen Kommentars zum Prorrheticum des Hippokrates, Abh. d. Königl. Preuß. Akademie d. Wiss. 1912, phil.-hist. Kl. 1, Berlin 1912

W. L. H. Duckworth, M. C. Lyons and B. Towers, Galen, On anatomical procedures, the later books, A translation, Cambridge 1962 (= Dkw.)

L. Edelstein, Ancient medicine, Baltimore 1967

D. E. Eichholz, Galen and his environment, Greece and Rome 20, 1951, pp. 60–71

Erotiani Vocum Hippocraticarum collectio, ed. E. Nachmanson, Uppsala 1918

Claudii Galeni Opera omnia, ed. C. G. Kühn, 20 Vols., Leipzig 1821–1833 (= K.)

Claudii Galeni Pergameni Scripta minora, ed. J. Marquardt, I. Müller and G. Helmreich, 3 Vols., Leipzig 1884–1893

Claudii Galeni De placitis Hippocratis et Platonis libri novem, ed. I. Müller, I, Leipzig 1874 (= Ml.)

Galeni De usu partium libri XVII, ed. G. Helmreich, 2 Vols., Leipzig 1907/1909

Galeni De uteri dissectione, ed. D. Nickel, CMG V 2,1, Berlin 1971

[1] Works cited once are described in full in the appropriate place; works cited twice only are given first in full and secondly in an easily recognisable form.

Galeni De propriorum animi cuiuslibet affectuum dignotione et curatione, De animi cuiuslibet peccatorum dignotione et curatione, De atra bile, ed. W. De Boer, CMG V 4,1,1, Leipzig and Berlin 1937

Galeni De sanitate tuenda libri, ed. K. Koch; De bonis malisque sucis, ed. G. Helmreich; De victu attenuante, ed. K. Kalbfleisch; De ptisana, ed. O. Hartlich, CMG V 4,2, Leipzig and Berlin 1923

Galeni In Hippocratis De natura hominis comment. III, ed. J. Mewaldt; In Hippocratis De victu acutorum comment. IV, ed. G. Helmreich; De diaeta Hippocratis in morbis acutis, ed. J. Westenberger, CMG V 9,1, Leipzig and Berlin 1914

Galeni In Hippocratis Prorrheticum I comment. III, ed. H. Diels; De comate secundum Hippocratem, ed. J. Mewaldt; In Hippocratis Prognosticum comment. III, ed. J. Heeg, CMG V 9,2, Leipzig and Berlin 1915

Galeni In Hippocratis Epidemiarum libr. I comment. III, ed. E. Wenkebach; In Hippocratis Epidemiarum libr. II comment. V, trans. F. Pfaff, CMG V 10,1, Leipzig and Berlin 1934

– In Hippocratis Epidemiarum libr. III comment. III, ed. E. Wenkebach, CMG V 10,2,1, Leipzig and Berlin 1936

– In Hippocratis Epidemiarum libr. VI comment. I–VI, ed. E. Wenkebach; comment. VI–VIII, trans. F. Pfaff, CMG V 10,2,2, 2nd. ed., Berlin 1956

– In Hippocratis Epidemiarum comment. Indices nominum et verborum Graecorum comp. E. Wenkebach et K. Schubring, CMG V 10,2,3, Berlin 1955

Galens Kommentare zu den Epidemien des Hippokrates, Indizes der aus dem Arabischen übersetzten Namen u. Wörter, ed. F. Pfaff, K. Deichgräber and F. Kudlien, CMG V 10,2,4, Berlin 1960

Galeni Adversus Lycum et Adversus Iulianum libelli, ed. E. Wenkebach, CMG V 10,3, Berlin 1951

Galeni De causis procatarcticis libellus a Nicolao Regino in sermonem Latinum translatus, ed. K. Bardong, CMG Suppl. II, Leipzig and Berlin 1937

Galeni De consuetudinibus cum versione Nicolai, ed. J. M. Schmutte, CMG Suppl. III, Leipzig and Berlin 1941

Galeni De diaeta Hippocratis in morbis acutis, De causis continentibus, De partibus artis medicativae. Versionem Arabicam ed. et in linguam Anglicam vert. M. C. Lyons, CMG Suppl. Or. II, Berlin 1969

Galenos, ΠΕΡΙ ΚΡΙΣΕΩΝ. Überlieferung und Text, ed. B. Alexanderson, Studia Graeca et Latina Gothoburgensia XXIII, Gothenburg 1967 (= Alex.)

Galeno, La dieta dimagrante, ed., with comm. and transl., N. Marinone, Turin 1973 (= Marinone)

Galen, Über die medizinischen Namen, ed. and trans. M. Meyerhof and J. Schacht, Abh. d. Deutschen Akademie d. Wiss. 1931, phil.-hist. Kl. 3, Berlin 1931 (= M.)

Galeni De examinando medico: quotations in: A. Dietrich, Medicinalia Arabica, Abh. d. Akademie d. Wiss. in Göttingen, phil.-hist. Kl. 66, 1966, Göttingen 1966, pp. 190–195; A. Z. Iskandar, Galen and Rhazes on examining physicians, Bulletin of the History of Medicine 36, 1962, pp. 362–365; M. Meyerhof, Autobiographische Bruchstücke Galens aus arabischen Quellen, Archiv für Geschichte der Medizin 22, 1929, pp. 72–86

V. Gardthausen, Katalog der griechischen Handschriften der Universitätsbibliothek zu Leipzig, Leipzig 1898

W. A. Greenhill, Galen, in Smith's Dictionary of Greek and Roman Biography II, London 1854, pp. 207–217

M. Grieve, A modern Herbal, New York 1959

F. Grosso, La lotta politica al tempo di Commodo, Memorie dell'Accademia d. Scienze di Torino, Cl. di Sci. Mor. Stor. e Fil., ser. 4, n. 7, Turin 1964

A. S. Halkin, Classical and Arabic material in Ibn ʿAḳnin's "Hygiene of the soul", Proceedings of the American Academy for Jewish Research 14, 1944, pp. 25–147

J. A. Hall, Lucian's Satire, Diss. Cambridge 1967

C. R. S. Harris, The heart and the vascular system in Ancient Greek medicine from Alcmaeon to Galen, Oxford 1973
W. Herbst, Galeni de Atticissantium studiis testimonia, Leipzig 1911
Œuvres complètes d'Hippocrate, ed. and trans. E. Littré, 10 Vols., Paris 1839–1861 (= L.)
Hippocratis Opera quae feruntur omnia, ed. H. Kühlewein, 2 Vols., Leipzig 1894/1902 (=Kw.)
Ibn abī Uṣaibiʿa, *ʿUyūn al-anbāʾ*, ed. A. Müller, 2 Vols., Cairo 1882
IG = Inscriptiones Graecae
IGR = R. Cagnat, Inscriptiones Graecae ad res Romanas pertinentes, 3 Vols., Paris 1911–1927
J. Ilberg, Aus Galens Praxis, Neue Jahrbücher f. d. klassische Altertum, Geschichte u. Deutsche Literatur 15, 1905, pp. 276–312 (= NJ)
–, Über die Schriftstellerei des Klaudios Galenos, Rheinisches Museum 44, 1889, pp. 207–239; 47, 1892, pp. 489–514; 51, 1896, pp. 165–196; 52, 1897, pp. 591–623 (= Schriftstellerei)
ILS = H. Dessau, Inscriptiones Latinae selectae, 3 Vols., Berlin 1892–1916
L. Jacchinus, Galeni liber de praecognitione, Lyons 1540
S. W. Jackson, Galen – on mental disorders, Journ. Hist. Behavioral Sciences 5, 1969, pp. 365–384
C. P. Jones, Plutarch and Rome, Oxford 1971
O. Kern, Inschriften von Magnesia, Berlin 1900
J. Kollesch, Aus Galens Praxis am römischen Kaiserhof, in E. C. Welskopf, ed., Neue Beiträge zur Geschichte der Alten Welt, II, Berlin 1965, pp. 57–61
M. Levey, The medical formulary or Aqrābādhīn of Al-Kindī, Madison and London 1966
H. Liddell, R. Scott and H. S. Jones, A Greek-English Lexicon, 9th. ed., Oxford 1968 (= L–S–J)
F. Lo Parco, Niccolò da Reggio antesignano del Risorgimento dell'antichità elleniche nel secolo XIV, Atti d. Reale Accademia di archeologia, lett. e belle arti di Napoli, n. s. 2, 1910, Naples 1913
Marcellinus, De pulsibus, ed. H. Schöne, Festschrift zur 49. Versammlung Deutscher Philologen u. Schulmänner, Basle 1907, pp. 448–471
Marinone s. Galen
E. Mayser, Grammatik der griechischen Papyri aus der Ptolemäerzeit, 2 Vols., Leipzig 1906/1934
J. Mesk, Antiochus und Stratonike, Rheinisches Museum 68, 1913, pp. 366–394
J. Mewaldt, Galenos über echte und unechte Hippokratika, Hermes 44, 1909, pp. 111–134
J. I. Miller, The spice trade in the Roman Empire, Oxford 1969
al-Mubaššir, *Muḫtār al-ḥikam*, trans. F. Rosenthal, Das Fortleben der Antike im Islam, Zürich and Stuttgart 1965, pp. 53–57
W. Müri, Der Arzt im Altertum, 3rd. ed., Munich 1962
V. Nutton, Galen and medical autobiography, Proceedings of the Cambridge Philological Society, n. s. 18, 1972, pp. 50–62 (= PCPS)
–, Two notes on immunities: Digest 27, 1, 6, 10 and 11, Journal of Roman Studies 61, 1971, pp. 52–63 (= JRS)
–, The chronology of Galen's early career, Classical Quarterly, n. s. 23, 1973, pp. 158–171 (= CQ)
J. H. Oliver, Marcus Aurelius: aspects of civic and cultural policy, Hesperia Suppl. 13, 1970
Oribasii Synopsis ad Eustathium; Libri ad Eunapium, ed. J. Raeder, CMG VI 3, Leipzig and Berlin 1926
Paulus Aegineta, ed. J. L. Heiberg, Libri I–IV, CMG IX 1, Leipzig and Berlin 1921
J. Pereira, The elements of materia medica, 2 Vols., London 1857

H. G. Pflaum, Les carrières procuratoriennes équestres sous le haut-empire romain, Paris 1960 (=CP)
–, Les sodales Antoniniani de l'époque de Marc Aurèle, Mémoires présentés à l'Académie des Inscriptions 15, 2, Paris 1966 (= Sodales)
PIR² = Prosopographia Imperii Romani saec. I–II–III, 2nd. ed., ed. E. Groag, A. Stein, L. Petersen, 5 Vols., (to L.), Berlin 1933ff.
S. B. Platner and T. Ashby, A topographical dictionary of Ancient Rome, Oxford 1929
Razes (ar-Rāzī), *Kitāb al-ḥāwī fi ṭ-ṭibb* (Liber Continens), Hyderabad (India) 1955ff.
RE = Paulys Real-Encyclopädie der classischen Altertumswissenschaft, ed. G. Wissowa, W. Kroll, K. Mittelhaus and K. Ziegler, Stuttgart 1893ff.
B. P. Reardon, Courants littéraires grecs des II et III siècles après J.-C., Annales littéraires de l'université de Nantes 3, Paris 1971
J. and L. Robert, La Carie, Vol. 2, Paris 1954 (= Carie)
L. Robert, Hellenica, 13 Vols., Limoges and Paris 1944–1965
–, Opera Minora Selecta, 3 Vols., Amsterdam 1969/1970 (= OMS)
E. Rohde, Der griechische Roman und seine Vorläufer, 2nd. ed., Leipzig 1900
ar-Ruhāwī, *Adab aṭ-ṭabīb*, trans. M. Levey, Medical ethics of Medieval Islam. With special reference to al-Ruhāwī's "Practical ethics of the physician", Transactions of the American Philosophical Society N. S. 57, Pt. 3, Philadelphia 1967; rev. by J. Ch. Bürgel, Göttingische Gelehrte Anzeigen 220, 1968, pp. 215–227
W. Schmid, Der Atticismus in seinen Hauptvertretern von Dionysius von Halikarnass bis auf den zweiten Philostratus, 4 Vols., Stuttgart 1887–1896
E. Schwyzer, Griechische Grammatik, Handb. d. Altertumswiss. II 1: I, 2nd. ed., Munich 1953; II, ed. A. Debrunner, Munich 1950
Sorani Vita Hippocratis, ed. J. Ilberg, in: CMG IV, Leipzig and Berlin 1927, pp. 173–178
G. Strohmaier, Galen als Vertreter der Gebildetenreligion seiner Zeit, in E. C. Welskopf, ed., Neue Beiträge z. Gesch. d. Alten Welt, II, Berlin 1965, pp. 375–379
L. Thorndike, Translations of the works of Galen from the Greek by Niccolò da Reggio (c. 1308–1345), Byzantina Metabyzantina 1, 1946, pp. 213–235
M. Ullmann, Die Medizin im Islam, Handb. d. Orientalistik, Ergänzungsband VI 1, Leyden and Cologne 1970
R. Walzer, Galen on Jews and Christians, Oxford 1949 (= JC)
–, Greek into Arabic: essays on Islamic philosophy, Oriental Studies I, Oxford 1962 (= GA)
A. Weisenberg, Handwörterbuch d. gesammten Arzneimittel v. d. ältesten bis auf d. neueste Zeit, Jena 1853
R. Weiss, The translators from the Greek of the Angevin Court of Naples, Rinascimento 1, 1950, pp. 195–226
I. Wille, Überlieferung und Übersetzung. Zur Übersetzungstechnik d. Nicolaus v. Rhegium in Galens Schrift De temporibus morborum, Helikon 3, 1963, pp. 259–277
R. Zazzeri, Sui codici e libri a stampati della Biblioteca Malatestiana di Cesena ricerche ed osservazioni, Cesena 1897

PROLEGOMENA

A. The manuscripts

The reconstruction of the original text of a medical author, even of one as careful in his legacy to posterity as Galen, is beset by many difficulties. Prose is corrupted more easily and with less chance of detection than is poetry, and a technical treatise in which matter was more important than style was always open to alteration in a way in which one whose merit and survival depended upon the beauty and rhythms of its language was not. In a recently published papyrus of the Hippocratic Oath (Oxyrrhyncus Papyrus 2547) difficult and dialect words are replaced by easier ones of an identical meaning, and there is no reason to suppose that the works of Galen were not subject to similar treatment in antiquity. The Galenic papyrus of De comp. med. per genera (Antinoopolis Papyrus 186) reveals words, headings and a general arrangement that differ from the corresponding passages in Kühn's edition, as well as a section, frag. 5a, which is not found elsewhere. Treatises might be combined in order of subject rather than of author, and works and sections not by Galen or extracted from his other writings might be added to another relevant book, as can be seen from the second part of this treatise (below, pp. 51f.). How extensive such revision and reorganisation could be is clear from the Syriac Book of Medicine, whose compiler took long passages from several Galenic treatises and organised them as his own medical vademecum.[1] No matter how careful Galen tried to be in restricting copies of his books to those who were worthy of them and in preventing any loss of meaning through changes in the text by, for example, writing out all numbers in full, the lack of any official text and of any mechanism for ensuring a regular and faithful transmission frustrated his wishes. The Galenic scholars of sixth and seventh century Alexandria who helped to establish an accepted canon of his writings come too late to be able to offer a text in its pristine state, and there is no proof that their comments and recensions, if any there were, stabilised the textual tradition for the Middle Ages. The fragments of the Arabic version, or versions, and the Latin translation, which offer readings

[1] The Syriac Book of Medicine was first edited by E. A. W. Budge, Oxford 1913, and its sources were established by J. Schleifer, Zum Syrischen Medizinbuch, Zeitschrift für Semitistik und verwandte Gebiete 4, 1926, pp. 70–122; 160–195: 5, 1927, pp. 195–237: 6, 1928, pp. 154–177: and Rivista degli Studi Orientali 18, 1940, pp. 341–372: 20, 1942, pp. 1–32; 162–210; 383–398: 21, 1946, pp. 157–182.

that differ from those of the Greek manuscripts and that supplement their deficiencies, demonstrate that considerable changes took place in the text between the ninth century and the period when the five Greek manuscripts of this treatise were written. These, coming at a late stage in the transmission, when corruption and contamination had long occurred and when scribes were capable of collating and correcting the texts they themselves were transcribing, offer us only a 'Byzantine Galen'. It is true that a stemma of the Greek manuscripts can be constructed, but its value is limited: it is a signpost whose reliability diminishes the more trust is placed in it. It enables us to assess the worth of some late manuscripts, not to reconstruct the text as it was taken down from the lips of Galen. Not even the help given by the Arabic and Latin versions permits such a reconstruction in every detail, and it may well be doubted whether the Greek text given here represents more than a variant of the original that would have been in circulation in the ninth century. Some of the changes that had taken place before then can be divined and cured, but, in the absence of any adequate earlier textual quotations, it is impossible to say how far this treatise suffered the mutilations and alterations already noted for other medical writings.

I. The Greek manuscripts

a) Vaticanus gr. 1845

V Vaticanus graecus 1845 (=V) was written in the late twelfth or early thirteenth century on oriental paper, 205 mm. by 145 mm. in size.[1] It has suffered badly from the attacks of worms and the ravages of time, with the result that all that remains of 'On prognosis' is one leaf, fol. 197ᵛ, ending with ὀκνοῦσιν ἐλαχίστῳ (68,19), and even this is badly damaged at the top where the title and many of the opening words have been rubbed or eaten away. A later hand, probably of the fourteenth century, has added in the margin a comment upon Galen's complaints of a decline in medical standards: ὥσπερ (?) κεκλημένον ἀληθῶς. ἄγγελος σαφῶς συ ἐφάνης. Its loss is serious, for its

[1] P. Canart, Bibliothecae Apostolicae Vaticanae codices manu scripti recensiti. Codices Vaticani graeci, Codices 1745–1962, Tomus I, Vatican City 1970, pp. 314–315. It has been widely used and studied by editors of Galen: see especially W. De Boer, Galens Traktat Über die schwarze Galle und seine Überlieferung, Wiener Studien 51, 1933, pp. 56–58; and CMG V 4,1,1, pp. Xf.: and D. Nickel, CMG V 2,1, pp. 13f. H. Diels, in his pioneering catalogue, Die Handschriften I, p. 100, attributed this tract to the sixteenth century, but since elsewhere (pp. 61, 68, 73, 81f., 96 and 101) it is dated to the thirteenth and since there is no change of hand in the text at this point, this discrepancy may be attributed either to a printer's error or to a confusion between the hand of the scribe and the hand of the annotator.

text is by far the best of the Mss. I note only one peculiar error: 68,13 σκεβῶν.

b) Parisinus gr. 2332

Another manuscript can also be dealt with briefly, the collection of fragments preserved in Paris, Bibliothèque Nationale, fonds grec 2332 (formerly Fontebl.-Reg. 3493, =P), written in a poor hand in the P fifteenth century on paper 171 mm. by 112 mm. in size and with 24 lines to the page.[1] It contains 416 leaves, together with a doublet at fol. 9 and two blank preliminary pages. Many of the leaves have been damaged at the top and in the outer margin and have been repaired by pasting paper over the damaged area, with the subsequent loss of the opening lines of each page and of three or four letters in the margin. It consists mainly of extracts from Galen and Hippocrates, including on fols. 198^v–199^v the following passages from 'On prognosis': 76,5–7 ἀπεφηνάμην; 78,13–14 πιεῖν; 78,16 ἐπυνθάνετό – 17; 78,17/18 ἀπεκρινάμην . . . ὡς οὐ – 19; 78,20 ἄπεπτον – 23; 80,2 δεύτερον – 3 δόντες; 80,10–14; 82,10–11 ἰατρῶν; 82,13f. καταγελῶν – ἐκεῖνον; 82,20 ἔφασκεν – 22; 82,25–31; 96,27–98,4; 98,17 καὶ – 22 ἐργάζοιτο. What is preserved confirms the conclusion of Alexanderson (p. 17), that little has been altered during the process of selection, although the only reading of importance to be found here is the omission of οὐ at 98,18.

c) Vindobonensis med. gr. 15

A second Ms. containing the same extracts was overlooked by Diels and his associates, although its existence was known to them.[2] Vienna, Österreichische Nationalbibliothek, med. gr. 15 (= W), W written in the first half of the sixteenth century, is a paper Ms. of 257 pages, 280 mm. by 210/20 mm. with 31 lines to the page. It was acquired by Busbecq at Constantinople, probably among the 240 Mss. he had copied for the Imperial Library in Vienna.[3] P and W are unique among the Greek Mss. in retaining the arrangement of treatises also preserved in the Latin version (below, pp. 51f.), since they are immediately succeeded under the same heading by the following extracts from the short tract 'On prognosis' (XIX, pp. 497–511 K.):

1 H. Omont, Inventaire sommaire des manuscrits grecs de la Bibliothèque Nationale, Pars 2, Paris 1888, p. 242.

2 Handschriften, p. 119. A full description of the Ms. is given by H. Hunger, Katalog d. griechischen Handschriften d. Österreichischen Nationalbibliothek, Vol. 2, Vienna 1969, pp. 55–59. His report of the reading at 76,5 is wrong. 'On prognosis' is found at fol. 137^{r-v}.

3 Cf. E. S. Forster, ed., The Turkish Letters of Ogier Ghislin de Busbecq, Oxford 1927, pp. 242f.

pp. 501,15–502,3 K.; p. 502,8–16 K.; pp. 502,18–503,12 K.; p. 504, 9–11 K.; p. 507,6–10 K.; and p. 508,2–9 K.[1]

d) Ambrosianus gr. 659

We are thus left for most of this treatise with four manuscripts, of which one, Milan, Biblioteca Ambrosiana, cod. graec. 659 (formerly A Q 3 Sup., = A), is itself mutilated. Consisting of 272 leaves, it was written about 1450 on paper, 210 mm. by 139 mm. in size, and contains this treatise on fols. 265^r–272^v. Fol. 265^v has lost its top left hand corner, and the last two leaves have almost a third of the page missing, viz.: 90,6 αὐτίκα – 12 ἐνταῦθα; 92,1 οἱ παρ' ἡμῖν – 12 ψεύδονται; 92,29 ἀπαλλάξομαι – 94,4 νοσή]ματος; 94,21 ἐποιησάμην – 30 αὐ]τὸς; and the codex ends at 96,15 μελλούσῃ γενή-[σεσθαι. Little is known of the history of this manuscript. It was sold in 1466 to Demetrius, the son of a bishop of Media in Thrace, and again in 1611 at Pisa[2]: and if, as I argue below (p. 46), it was used by Scaliger, it may have been at Pavia or Padua around 1575 as "exe(mplum) Papien(se) et cum hoc uno ex s(ancto) Anto(nio)". There are many typical scribal errors:

1. Omissions: 70,20 ὀκνῶν – διαβουλευόμενος; 82,22 τάς τε; 84,17 ὁποίας; 84,18 καὶ θαρρῶν; 86,6 ἀθρόως ἀκηκοότι.

2. Repetitions: 86,9 ὧν ἐπιγενομένων καὶ τῶν ἐπιγινομένων καὶ τῶν ἐπιγενομένων.

3. Single λ for λλ: 86,4 ἀγγέλοιμι.

4. Iotacism: 80,26 ἔτυχεν] ἐπεῖχεν; 84,9 λέγοι] λέγει.

5. Confusion between ο and ω: 70,25 τὸν] τῶν; 94,18 ὁ δ'] ὦ δ'.

6. Orthography: A regularly prefers μικρός to σμικρός, αὑτός to ἑαυτός, while at 78,20–23 it has the variants ἄπεμπτος and πέμψαι for ἄπεπτος and πέψαι.

7. Influence of nearby words and constructions: 70,7 ἀγαπήσειεν] ἀγαπήσειαν, because of the following ἂν; 70,20 ἐρώτημα] εὕρημα; 88,5 θεσπίζειν] θεραπεύειν, from the presence of θεραπεύειν in the following line.

8. Iota subscript is always omitted.

But other readings, which can be categorised only with difficulty, seem to me to reflect the activity of an emending scribe concerned to replace rare words and constructions with easier and more familiar ones. If this contention is accepted, it is probable that readings peculiar to A and simpler than those of L, M and N derive more from the ingenuity of the scribe than from a good manuscript tradition. The following examples adequately demonstrate the problem:

[1] Of the other Mss., V and A end with this treatise and it is possible that, had they survived entire, they would have preserved an arrangement similar to that of P and W.

[2] H. Diels, Die handschriftliche Überlieferung, p. 31.

72,19 μάλιστα μὲν καὶ πρῶτον] πρῶτον μὲν καὶ μάλιστα; 72,23 πρεσβυτέρως] περαιτέρω; 72,30 οὐ θεωροῦσιν] οὐθ' ὁρῶσιν; 74,24 ἐνάτην] ὀγδόην; 80,15 ἐπισκεψάμενοι] ἐπισκεψόμενοι; 82,25 σεμνότητος] σεμνότητι; 86,27 κενώσεως] κινήσεως; 90,17 φύσει πονηρῶν] φιλοπονηρῶν; 94,9 Διομήδους] Δημώδους; 96,4 προτέρως] πρότερος.

e) Laurentianus gr. 74,5

The earliest of the three Mss. offering a full text is Florence, Biblioteca Laurenziana, Plut. 74,5 (=L), a paper Ms. of the twelfth L or early thirteenth century, 290 mm. by 192 mm. in size, in which 'On prognosis' occupies fols. 104r–120v.[1] This part of the codex was written by the (Italian?) colleague of the scribe Ioannikios, who, with a third colleague, shared in the writing of this Ms. K. K. Müller identified this codex with one described in Lascaris' catalogue of the library of Lorenzo dei Medici, and there is thus the possibility that it was already in Italy by 1492.[2]

The following are typical examples of the scribal errors of L:

1. Omissions: 92,8 ὀλιγοχρόνιον] ὀλιχρόνιον.

2. Repetitions: 78,17 οὖν οὖν; 84,9 πυνθανανομένων; 98,3 τμημηθεῖσιν; 128,16 οὐλελέγχθη.

3. Iotacism: ει for οι: 102,33 φοβοῖτο] φοβεῖτο; η for ι: 106,23 μάντιν] μάντην; ι for η: 84,18 σφαλησομένῳ] σφαλισομένῳ.

4. Confusion between ο and ω: 102,17 ὅστις] ὥς τις.

5. Influence of nearby words or constructions: 108,19 μέρος] μέρους, genitive as the supposed subject of σεισθέντος; 126,2 ἔδειξα] ἐδείξατο, making 'prognosis' the subject, not Galen.

6. Smooth for rough accent: 68,12 ἰματίων; 114,2 ἐστάναι.

7. L normally disregards enclitic accents.

8. Iota subscript is always omitted.

9. L regularly keeps ephelkustic nu, especially at the end of a sentence or clause, even when it is not strictly necessary. Many typical scribal errors and confusions of sound are shared between L and N, of οι for ει, οι for η, οι for υ, οι for ι, η for ει, η for υ, ε for αι, and ω for ο.

Many errors of L were corrected either by the scribe himself or by a second emending scribe (Ioannikios?), but the microfilm copy from L²

[1] I am grateful to Mr. N. G. Wilson for this revised dating and information on the scribes, which were given in an unpublished lecture to the University of London: for the previous (fourteenth century) dating, see G. Helmreich, Galeni de elementis ex Hippocratis sententia, Erlangen 1878, pp. VIII f.

[2] K. K. Müller, Neue Mittheilungen über Janos Lascaris und die Mediceische Bibliothek, Zentralblatt für Bibliothekswesen 1, 1894, p. 376. The suggestion of J. L. Heiberg, Beiträge zur Geschichte Georg Valla's und seiner Bibliothek, Beihefte zum Zentralblatt für Bibliothekswesen 16, 1896, p. 38, that this manuscript was used by Valla cannot be accepted because the treatise 'On prognosis' translated by him was the fragment printed in Vol. XIX of Kühn's edition, which is not to be found in this manuscript.

which I worked was not sufficiently clear always to distinguish the two hands with certainty or to suggest a Ms. source for the readings of L².
Examples of such corrections are these:

74,5 λογικῇ L N A: σοφιστικῇ scr. L² super lineam, M; 90,18 πανούργως L: πανουργίας L (e corr.) M N A; 106,5 οἶσθα L N in mg.: ᾖσθα L (e corr.) M N; 130,2 τὸ αὐτὸ super αὐτῶν add. L²; 130,6 ἐπισημαίνθεσθαι L: ἐπισημαίνεσθαι L (e corr.) M N; 130,11 κατὰ add. L super lineam, M N.

f) Marcianus gr. 281

The third major manuscript of this treatise is Venice, Marcianus gr.
M 281 (=M), fols. 81ᵛ–89ʳ, a parchment codex written for Cardinal Bessarion, c. 1468–1472, as part of a set of eight volumes, Marciani gr. 279–286, and, from the absence of any ex-libris, it may not have been completed before Bessarion's departure for France in 1472.[1] It was included in the second inventory of his books, drawn up after his death[2], and was available for borrowing by 1524.[3] Although its script is the clearest and neatest of all the Greek manuscripts, it contains many errors, a selection of which I now give:

1. Omissions: 70,3 ἐσομένην; 78,16 αὐτῶν; 88,9 δέ με; 102,23 παραχρῆμα, omitted through haplography before ταραχθέντα; 102,25 ἰδὼν, also through haplography after πολυειδῶς; 104,20 μακρὸς; 110,7 τέχνης; 114,30 ἰδίᾳ ὧδε; 116,4 ἐδίδουν; 126,25 ἔωθεν; 134,6f. ἐκ τῆς θεωρίας – διαθέσεων, through haplography following διαθέσεων; 134,26 φόβου.

2. Repetitions: 68,19 ἐπαγγελλόμενοι; 70,16 τῷ Ἱπποκράτει; 96,15 γενήσεσθαι; 108,13 ἐπὶ.

3. Single ν for νν: 130,29 Ἄνια.

4. αι for ε: 104,7 ἐξετασθήσεσθαι] ἐξαιτασθήσεσθαι.

5. Iotacism: ι for η: 74,1 κληρονομήσουσι] κληρονομίσουσι; υ for ι: 82,25 ἐπίθετο] ἐπύθετο; 112,8 κεκριμμένον] κεκρυμμένον.

6. Wrong word division: 70,2 τῶν νόμῳ] τῷ νόμῳ.

7. Influence of nearby words or constructions: 70,17 τολμᾶν] τολμᾶ, forgetting that the sentence was in oratio obliqua; 134,18 προσηκόντως] προσηκότες, depending on the preceding nominative ἰατροὶ.

8. Iota subscript is always omitted.

1 A list of its contents is given by H. Hinck, Galeni Scripta minora I, p. IX, note 1: see also H. Diels, Die handschriftliche Überlieferung, p. 25f., G. Helmreich, CMG V 9,1, p. XXXIV, and E. Mioni, Bessarione bibliofilo e filologo, Rivista di Studi Bizantini e Neoellenici n. s. 5, 1968, p. 72 and p. 77.

2 Details of the contents of the inventory are given in the forthcoming book by L. Labowsky, The Library of Cardinal Bessarion, an edition of the oldest inventories.

3 G. Coggiola, Il prestito di manoscritti della Marciana dal 1474 al 1527, Zeitschr. f. Bibliothekswesen 25, 1908, p. 66.

9. Ephelkustic nu is frequently omitted, especially at the end of sentences, 88,3 εἴωθε; 96,26 ἐδήλωσε, even when hiatus results, 116,16 νοσήσειε.

g) Parisinus suppl. gr. 35

The last of the Mss. with a full text, Paris, Bibliothèque Nationale, Supplément grec 35 (=N), which contains 'On prognosis' on fols. 144ʳ–166ʳ, almost escaped the author's notice because of an error in a Paris catalogue. In spite of the fact that the hand-written index to the volume on fol. 1ʳ rightly translates the Greek title as De praecognitione ad Epigenem seu Posthumum, Henri Omont merely described it as 'De praecognitione', which Diels and his collaborators took to refer to the later tract on prognosis, XIX, pp. 497–511 K.[1] They compounded their error by listing it simply as fol. 144, thereby giving the impression that it was only a short fragment. The Ms., written on paper in the late fifteenth / early sixteenth century and consisting of 245 leaves + two preliminary leaves, measures 290 mm. by 200 mm. and has 30 lines to the page. There are many scribal errors: N

1. Omissions: 68,17 ἂν; 72,16. 94,25 νῦν; 72,21 ἀνθρώποις; 76,4f. τῶν σφυγμῶν – μέ; 90,5 οὐ; 108,10 πάντα; 118,23 μεταστάντος.

2. Additions: 68,2 πρὸς Ἐπιγένην.[2]

3. Repetition: 88,18 ἦν ἐκεῖνοι.

4. Confusion of β and μ: 92,15 μαθεῖν] βοηθεῖν; 116,23 μολογέσου; 116,31 μημούρας.

5. Confusion of μ and κ: 76,19. 102,20 μετὰ] κατὰ; 108,8 μετακομίσας] κατακομίσας.

6. Iotacisms: ει for η: 138,10 προμαθὴς] προμαθεὶς; ει for ι: 96,25 φιλονεικίας] φιλονικείας; ι for η: 122,2 πτισάνης] πτησάνης; ι for υ: 76,18. 130,26. 142,12 ἐγγὺς] ἐγγὶς; 98,1. 24 φάρυγγος] φάριγγος.

7. Wrong endings: 70,2 νόμῳ] νόμων; 76,22 συνήθεσιν] συνήθοις; 110,10 συνετοὶ] συνετὸν; 128,32 θαυμαστοτέραν] θαυμαστοτάτην.

8. Confusion of ο and ω: 90,20 φωραθῶσιν] φοραθῶσιν; 94,12 πρωτευόντων] προτευόντων; 124,13. 130,30 αὐτοκράτορι] αὐτοκράτωρι; 128,2 ἀψαμένων] ἀψάμενον.

9. Iota subscript is frequently omitted.

10. Ephelkustic nu as for L (above, p. 17).

Two sets of corrections are found in the text[3]: the first is that of the original scribe, the second that of the writer of the title and of the first letter, who used a much darker ink. N²

[1] H. Omont, Inventaire sommaire des manuscrits du Supplément grec, Paris 1883, p. 6; Diels, Handschriften, p. 112.

[2] Was it through seeing this Ms. that Chartier added the two words in his edition? Possibly, but the Ms. was not then in the Royal Library.

[3] A third hand appears in the margin at fol. 162ᵛ, but it brings no pertinent information.

Most of the corrections of the scribe of N are clearly taken from his original Ms.: 72,27 ἔρουσιν N: αἶρουσιν N (e corr.), or are easy improvements on his text: 106,23 μάντην N: μάντιν N (e corr.), more by his own conjecture than by any second Ms.: 112,27 δεῖν N: δεῖ N (e corr.); 132,14 ἡμεῖς N: ὑμεῖς N (e corr.); 132,28 τὰς N: τῆς N (e corr.). Other changes are not so felicitous: 74,3 ἔχουσαν] ἔχουσιν N: ἔχουσι N (e corr.); 114,6 θλίψας] θλείψας N (e corr.); 138,15f. ἰατρῶν ἰωμένων] ἰατρὸν ἰωμένον N (e corr.).

The impression of the scribe of N is that he is a competent transcriber, careful enough to check his errors against his exemplar and confident to make slight changes in the text where the sense demanded it.

N^2 checked the work of N and made his own corrections and suggestions, probably without the aid of a Ms. or at least with only the exemplar to help him. Most of them are good: 72,24 τετημηκότες N: τετιμηκότες N^2; 80,16 πολὺ N: πολὺν N^2; 80,17 πόλεος N: πόλεως N^2; 82,2 ἔφην N: ἔφη N^2; 82,13 καταγέλων N: καταγελῶν N^2; 94,18 τῶνδε N: τόνδε N^2; 102,5 μοῦ N: μοι N^2; 102,20 ἐχθῶ N: ἐλθῶ N^2; 104,27 νοήσαντος N: νοσήσαντος N^2. But others are mere speculation: 78,21 κακοχυμίαν N: κακοχυμίας N^2; 134,26 φανέντος N: φανέντα N^2. Again the scribe seems to have a competent knowledge of Greek and is not afraid to put forward his own emendations. In both N and N^2 we have the familiar figure of the emending scribe of the Renaissance period, a conclusion that is of some importance for the right understanding of the relationship between the Mss., to which I now turn.

II. The relationship between the Greek manuscripts

Since there is insufficient evidence upon which to base an estimate of the affiliations of V, I begin my enquiry with the two collections of extracts, P and W, which, like V, cannot be brought into a relationship with L, M, N and A.

The first thing to note is that W has no reading superior to that of P and several that are inferior: 76,5 σοῦ om. W; 78,19 ἐργάσεται P: ἐργάσετο W; 80,2 τοῦ φαρμάκου P: τὸ φάρμακον W; 80,10 ἔω P: ἔω W; 80,13f. ἠψάμην – παροξυσμὸν om. W; 82,28 ἠλήθευσα P: ἠλεύθησα W; 98,26 κακωθέντα P: κακοθέντα W. Secondly, the number of tracts excerpted and their order of presentation is identical in both Mss., even to the citation of the excerpts from De simpl. med. temp. et fac., XI, p. 813,12 K. without a heading. The only difference in the order is that in W the anonymous commentary on the Prognosticon follows, not precedes, Aristotle's Problemata and some medical extracts. In none of my sample collations have I found readings in W that are better than P's, and I conclude that W was copied from P or, at best, from a defective twin of P, and I have thus omitted its readings from the apparatus criticus as being a secondary witness when the primary witness is still available for use.

Among the other four Mss., there is no significant error shared by A and M and only one by A and L N: 74,5 λογικῇ L N A: σοφιστικῇ L² M. On the other hand, there are many readings preserved by L, M and N, but not by A, of which I list only a few:

74,24 πέμπτην L M N: ὀγδόην A
76,17f. ἐπισκοπεῖσθαι L M N: ἐπὶ τὸ λοῦτρον ἔχων ἐπισκοπῆσαι A
82,2 πᾶν L M N: πάνυ A
82,21 τριταίους L M N: τεταρταίους A
92,26 ἱκετῶν L M N: οἰκετῶν A
94,30 ὀργάνων L M N: ἔργων A

I conclude from this that A belongs to a branch of the textual tradition that differs from that of L, M and N, and also that neither L, M nor N is closely related to A. How close, then, is the relationship between these three? Since there is no example of words omitted by both L and N being retained by M, we must decide whether M descends from either L or N or a source similar to them solely from the quality of the readings of the Mss. Before 96,15, with the possible exception of 72,2 ἀτολμώτερος L N: ἀτολμηρότερος M A, any difference between L N and M is such that the presence of a good reading in M and not in L N can easily be attributed to scribal correction. After 96,15 the differences are still slight, with M, as I have shown, being more inclined to careless repetition and omission. I give a list of the more significant divergencies so that it will be possible to see upon what evidence the choice rests between an emending scribe who copied L or N and one whose Ms. was closely related to, but not identical with them.[1]

100,2 οὐδεὶς ἐτόλμησεν L N: οὐδὲν ἐτόλμησέ τις M
102,3 πρῶτον L N: πρότερον M
102,5 αὖθις L N: πάλιν M
118,15 Ῥωμαίων L N: Ῥώμην M
120,2 εἰς τὴν Ῥώμην τοῦ βασίλεως L N: τοῦ βασίλεως εἰς τὴν Ῥώμην [M
120,10 καταφανῆ L N: καταφανὴς M
122,11 τὸν πυρετὸν L N: αὐτὸν M
124,18 ὅλης L N: τέχνης M
138,3 ὑπολαβὼν L N: ὑποβαλὼν M

Although this proof is not entirely conclusive, it suggests that although L and N had texts superior to that of M, they were not the source of M but members of the same family descended from a Ms. (y) written in uncial script, as can be seen from the following examples: y

[1] It is just possible on palaeographic grounds that N was the source of M, although it is very unlikely, as will be shown, and I have included N here argumenti causa.

80,11 σῶσαι] ἐᾶσθαι y
108,24 δηλωσάντων] γινωσκόντων y[1]

The relationship between L and N is at first sight very complex. Although they share wrong readings together against M, N lacks the repetitions and fills in the omission in L noted above, p. 17, which should indicate that they both descended from the same source. But we have already noted the activities of an emending scribe (above, p. 20) and none of the improvements of N required great powers of divination. Besides, it several times alone preserves the correct reading against the agreement of L and M, which is impossible if the tradition is closed tightly:

118,3 καμπανιᾳ N : καμπυη L M
118,20 ἐξωρμηκότες N : ἐξορμηκότες L M
136,14 ἴδῃ N in mg. : ἤδη L M N

Besides, there are many examples of the agreement of N and L in errors, and, more significantly, some of N correcting a good reading to correspond to the bad reading of his exemplar:

76,29 ἐπέπειστο N M A : ἐπέποιστο L N (e corr.)
86,20 τέτμηνται N A : τετίμηνται L N (e corr.) : τετίμενται M

Many mistakes in N can also be easily explained as deriving from L, especially when L (or the common exemplar) had a compendium or abbreviation that was wrongly interpreted or completed by the scribe of N: e. g. 112,3 ζητοῦμεν N : ζητοῦ L : ζητοῦσιν M; 128,32 θαυμαστοτάτην M : θαυμαστο^{τρ} L : θαυμαστέραν N.

Even more revealing are the errors in N that come from an exemplar whose script is difficult to decipher. N's confusion of β and μ (above, p. 19) indicates a Ms. akin to L in its cursive script. But two readings above all prove that N can only be a descendant of L since its writing alone provided the invitation to faulty copying. At 70,23 the scribe of L wrote βελτίων with a large, upright beta instead of his usual cursive form (cf. fol. 116^{v},3 for a similar beta), which the scribe of N, mistaking for a theta, turned into θελτίων. Similarly, at 86,23 the scribe of L wrote εἴη with a square, almost majuscule eta (cf. fol. 117^{v},4) whose bar was towards the top of the letter: this was turned into εἴ τι. It is very unlikely that any other Ms. than L preserved these scribal peculiarities, and I therefore conclude that N was copied from

1 This was also the opinion of W. De Boer, CMG V 4,1,1, p. V, who demolished the theory of O. Hennicke, Observationes criticae in Cl. Galeni Pergameni commentarios Περὶ ψυχῆς παθῶν καὶ ἁμαρτημάτων, Diss. Erlangen, Berlin 1902 (also Potsdam 1902), p. 3, that both L and M were copied from Laurentianus, plut. 74,3. E. Heitsch, Überlieferungsgeschichtliche Untersuchungen zu Andromachos, Markellos von Side und zum Carmen de viribus herbarum, Nachrichten d. Akad. d. Wiss. in Göttingen, phil.-hist. Kl. 1963, 2, p. 37, suggests that M was copied directly from L.

L and that where it has superior readings, they have come from scholarly sagacity rather than another and better Ms.[1]

III. The Latin translation and its manuscripts

a) Authorship

Until the publication of the Aldine edition in 1525, the mediaeval Latin versions were the main source of a knowledge of Galen available to the scholars and physicians of Western Europe. A long and distinguished line of translators stretched back to the sixth century, not the least of whom was Niccolò di Deoprepio, a Greek from Reggio **Nic.** di Calabria.[2] Writing under the benevolent rule of Robert of Anjou, he produced a large number of versions designed to preserve the Galenic original by translating "de verbo ad verbum, nihil addens, nihil minuens vel permutans". In a span of over thirty six years, from 1308 until 1345, he developed an accurate method and technical vocabulary whereby to express even the smallest features of the Greek original.[3] R. Weiss argued that he was the major, if not the only, translator of Galen active at that time in South Italy, and endeavoured to show that the absence of any version made after his death proves that there was no school of translators.[4] But the strict rules adopted by Niccolò, once a technical vocabulary is agreed, render the identification of individual translators by their styles

1 My assessment of N, especially in its acceptance of some scribal improvements, amplifies the conclusion of R. Noll, Galeni Περὶ χρείας ἀναπνοῆς libellus, Diss. Marburg 1915, pp. XVIf. (cf. CMG V 4,1,1, p. V) that N was a copy of L.

2 For earlier translations, see A. Beccaria, Il ritorno della scienza classica nel primo medioevo, Rivista Storica Italiana 51, 1937, pp. 17–52; and, Sulle tracce di un antico canone latino di Ippocrate e di Galeno, I, Italia medioevale ed umanistica 3, 1959, pp. 1–56; II, ibid. 4, 1961, pp. 1–75; III, ibid. 15, 1971, pp. 1–23. For the cultural background, see R. Weiss, The Greek culture of South Italy, Proceedings of the British Academy, 37, 1951, pp. 23–50. On Niccolò himself, see F. Lo Parco, Niccolò da Reggio, a major study, but heavily criticised by L. Thorndike, Translations of works of Galen, passim, and by R. Weiss, Translators from the Greek, cf. also R. Weiss, Ancora 'cretico', Rinascimento 4, 1953, pp. 166f., and R. Calvanico, Fonti per la storia della medicina e della chirurgia per il regno di Napoli nel periodo Angioino, Naples 1962, p. 128. I have not seen P. F. Russo, Medici e veterinari calabresi, Naples 1962, which deals with Niccolò on pp. 71–102.

3 The brief notices of K. Deichgräber, Emp., pp. 9–11, have been extended by I. Wille in her edition of De temporibus morborum, Diss. Kiel 1960, and in her article, Überlieferung und Übersetzung, pp. 259–277. Of the published versions by Niccolò, that of De consuetudinibus by J. M. Schmutte, CMG Suppl. III, survived the last war in only a few copies; Wille's dissertation exists in typescript and is not easily obtainable outside West Germany; and Marinone's new edition of De subtiliante dieta has no index (and neglects Paris, Académie Nationale de Médecine, Ms. 53, fols. 263v–273v). I have derived much benefit from discussions on Niccolò's technique with R. J. Durling of the University of Kiel, who has also contributed a few emendations to the text.

4 R. Weiss, Translators, pp. 220–224.

extremely difficult, and the evidence for Niccolò's authorship must be closely examined for each treatise.

Although it has long been assumed that Niccolò was the author of the Latin version of 'On prognosis', the evidence for this assumption is weak, since it comes not from the manuscripts but only from the printed edition of Bonardus of 1490. As I shall show (below, pp. 35–37) that the argument in favour of Bonardus' use of a lost, unrelated manuscript is not strong[1], I believe that Bonardus' ascription is a mere editorial hypothesis which associates other anonymous translations, such as De comate and De introductione medicorum, with a great name. The fact that a, b and d, which together give much information about the authorship of the versions they include, say nothing here about Niccolò lends support to the view that he was not the translator of this treatise. But Thorndike demonstrated that Vatican, Palatinus lat. 1211 (which does not contain 'On prognosis') assigns many versions to Niccolò that are elsewhere anonymous, and it is still possible to believe that Bonardus was using a manuscript now lost which named Niccolò expressly as the translator. Certainly, as the translation of στάσις (92,7) by 'guerra' shows, the translator was an Italian speaker who lived in the fourteenth rather than the thirteenth century, to judge from the style of the version[2], but the treatment of particles in this tract, which differs from that adopted for De temporibus morborum and De consuetudinibus, offers a further argument against identifying him with Niccolò immediately.[3] New manuscript

[1] Marinone, pp. 20–34, argues cogently that for De subtiliante dieta Bonardus had a second translation at his disposal that was independent of Nic., but, if he did use a lost Ms. in his edition of this tract, the indications are that it was a Ms. of Nic. rather than an independent version, of which there is no trace in 'On prognosis'.

[2] Contrast the evidence for earlier translators given by L. Minio-Paluello, Opuscula, Amsterdam 1972, pp. 57–86, and by P. Thillet, Alexandre d'Aphrodise De fato ad imperatores, version de Guillaume de Moerbeke, Paris 1963, pp. 36–59.

[3] The following list of significant words indicates that either there is a second translator (of the school of Niccolò?) or Niccolò changed his technique and vocabulary over a long period (W. = Wille; S. = Schmutte; N. = this edition):

γάρ] enim W. S. passim; enim 39: autem 2: et 1?: igitur 2: itaque 1: namque 1: uero 1: om. 2 N.

γοῦν] denique 4: enim 3: attamen 1: igitur 1: demum 1 W.; sed ... quidem 1 S.; denique 1: enim 1: igitur 1: uero 1 N.

δέ] autem 79: uero 19: sed 5 W.; autem 23: uero 5: enim 1 S.; autem 116: uero 69: sed 15: et 10: cumque 4: igitur 3: itaque 3: etiam 2: om. 6 N.

διό] quoniam 1 W.; quocirca 1: om. 1 S.; quocirca 1 N.

ἕτερος] alius 12: alter 5 W.; alius 4: alter 5 S.; alius 12: alter 6 N.

ἤ] uel 22: aut 3 W.; uel 13: aut 1 S.; uel 18: aut 8: et 1 N.

μὲν γάρ] nam quidem 6: enim 2: nam 1: quidem 1 W.; quidem enim 4: enim 1 S.; namque 1 N.

μὲν οὖν] igitur quidem 13: igitur 2: denique 1: quidem 1: quidem igitur 1 W.; quidem 3: quidem igitur 2: igitur quidem 1: igitur 1 S.; igitur 6: autem 3: quidem 3: itaque 2: sed 1: sed quidem 1 N.

ὅταν] quando W. passim; cum 3 S.; quando 6: cum 3 N.

ὅτι] quoniam 13: quod 3 W.; quoniam 2 S.; quoniam 10: quod 3: quia 1 N.

or archival material or a broader study of mediaeval translation technique may confirm Bonardus' attribution, but until then it is safer to consider the authorship anonymous. This caveat is necessary, if only to prevent an exaggerated estimate of the abilities and activity of Niccolò; it does not diminish the value of this translation for the constitution of the text. Nevertheless, for the sake of convenience, I shall continue to refer to it as if it were by Niccolò, without wishing to imply that I regard the ascription to him as proven.

We must next consider whether this treatise was translated from a Greek original or, as were several of the earlier versions, from an Arabic intermediary. The proof of a Greek origin is simple and conclusive:

68,11 βωμολοχεύεσθαι] bomolochantur Nic.
88,24 γνησίων] gnisiis Nic.
94,25 ἀγῶνα] agonis Nic.
96,23 ἐπιεικῆ] epiykem Nic.
104,21 ἔρωτος] erotis Nic.
110,10 συνετοὶ] sineti Nic.
116,10 σινδόνων] sindones Nic.
130,15 παρισθμίων] parismiorum Nic.
138,2 κῶλα] cola Nic.

These words, with the possible exception of 130,15, are all non-technical and have been retained by the translator for want of an immediately better rendering. In the first three examples, later scribes, uncertain of this mixture of Greek and Latin, altered the Greek transcription to the nearest Latin equivalent or provided a gloss for the Greekless reader. A Greek source is thus certain, and in view of the relative scarcity of Greek Mss. of this treatise surviving to us – and, presumably, a similar scarcity existed in the fourteenth century – it is not an extravagant conjecture that the Greek original of this version was contained in the great collection of Galenic writings presented to Robert of Anjou by Andronicus III.[1] The Latin version offers an opportunity of comparing our existing Greek Mss. with one circulating

οὖν] igitur 18: sed 3 W.; igitur 4: autem 1 S.; igitur 24: autem 16: enim 2: uero 2: ergo 1: etiam 1: itaque 1: tamen 1 N.
οὕτως] ita W. S. N. passim.
πάλιν] rursus 4 W.; rursus 1 S.; rursus 3: iterum 1: om. 1 N.
τοιοῦτος] huiusmodi 11: talis 8 W.; talis 5: huiusmodi 1 S.; talis 18: hic 7: huiusmodi 2 N.
ὥστε] quocirca 5: ut 1 W.; itaque 1 S.; ut 4: itaque 1: unde 1 N.
αὖθις] rursus 5 W.; rursus 3: om. 1 S.; rursus 4: iterum 2 N.
εἶτα] deinde 23: tum 1 W.; deinde 4: iam 1 S.; deinde 14: demum 4 N.
ἐπιεικής] epiykes W. N.

[1] F. Lo Parco, Niccolò, p. 264; R. Weiss, Translators, p. 220, n. 2. A Constantinopolitan source is also suggested by the origin of W, which, together with P, preserves an arrangement of the two treatises on prognosis identical with that of the Latin version.

in Constantinople about 1300, but, before doing so, I shall list the surviving Latin Mss. and discuss their affiliations. A stemma of the Latin codices, unlike that of the Greek, is here very useful, especially since one of them was written less than a generation after the translation was made.

b) The manuscripts

Although Diels' catalogue of manuscripts can claim respectable accuracy when dealing with the Greek tradition, it is much more fallible in its listing of the various versions. There is confusion between works of similar title and subject, a slackness in noting leaf numbers and internal divisions, and a disregard of the anonymous or pseudonymous medical literature in circulation.[1] Reliance upon catalogues, often without personal inspection by a member of the Commission, produced both a commendable speed of execution and the perpetuation of errors to entrap the unwary. A particularly blatant one was the citation of an Oxford manuscript, St. John's College 17, written between 1083 and 1085 with additions of circa 1100, as an early text of Niccolò's version of 'On prognosis'. As I have shown, this is an example of the mediaeval Prognostica Galieni, crude rules of thumb whose only connection with Galen is their title.[2]

1. Parisinus lat. 6865

Probably the oldest Latin manuscript of 'On prognosis' and certainly the most studied of all the manuscripts of the Latin Galen
b is Paris, Bibliothèque Nationale, fonds latin 6865 (=b), a parchment manuscript of 211 leaves, 385 mm. by 302 mm. in size, written in two columns, each 77 mm. wide.[3] The margin is decorated with coloured filigree work; the initial letters of each treatise are multicoloured; the chapter openings are painted in blue and red, the chapter headings in red; internal divisions within paragraphs and, occasionally, within sentences are made in blue or red. The two parts of 'On prognosis' are contained on fols. 179^{v}–186^{r}, with the division between the parts coming at fol. 184^{v}. There are many marginal drawings, ornaments and annotations by at least four hands, of which the most important
b^{2} are the corrections made by the scribe himself, by a second scholar
b^{3} using an Italian hand, and by a third scholar using a French hand, who also contributed the comments and summaries at the foot of the page. Since this codex contains also De disnia, translated in 1345 by

[1] See A. Beccaria, I codici di medicina del periodo presalernitano, Rome 1956, p. 10; R. J. Durling, Corrections and additions to Diel's Galenica, Traditio 23, 1967, pp. 461–476.

[2] V. Nutton, Prognostica Galieni, Medical History 14, 1970, pp. 96–100.

[3] A brief description is given by A. Melot, Catalogus codicum manuscriptorum bibliothecae regiae, pars tertia, tomus quartus, Paris 1744, p. 286.

Niccolò, it must have been written between then and 1353, a date provided by a note on fol. 215^{v}, which reads: J. de S(an)c(t)a Cruce licen(ciatus) in artib(us) et me(dicin)a fuit expectans Uticensis anno primo VIII idus marcii. Undoubtedly this refers to the supplicat made on behalf of Johannis de Sancta Cruce by the University of Avignon on March 8th., 1353, in the first year of Pope Innocent VI[1], and we may conclude from this that the owner of the codex was then at Avignon, attached to the Papal Court, a supposition confirmed by a reference at fol. 215^{r} to the filling of a prebend at Le Mans. An examination of the hand of the first scribe reveals that the codex was written in South Italy, probably in Naples, although the absence of any arms, as on Bibliothèque Nationale, acq. lat. 1365, suggests that it did not form part of the Royal Library of Naples. Its transfer from Italy to Avignon so soon after it was written lends credence to the statement of Guy de Chauliac, often discussed and often rejected[2], that Niccolò delivered some Galenic translations to the Papal Court, and to the hypothesis of Lo Parco that this was the book in question. It was certainly read by several members of the Papal Court who annotated it and ornamented its margin in a manner familiar from other codices circulating in Avignon in the mid-fourteenth century.[3] Little more is known of its later fortunes: in 1650 it was in the possession of Jacobus Mentelius, a nobleman, physician, scholar and bibliophile of Chateau-Thierry[4], from whom it may have passed directly into the library of Colbert and thence into the Royal Library. Orthographically it is the best of the Latin manuscripts, preserving, as far as possible, the spelling of the Greek words left untranslated by Niccolò. It divides 'On prognosis' into seventeen chapters, each with its own heading.

2. Dresdensis Db 92

The beautiful illuminated manuscript of Galen, now in the Sächsische Landesbibliothek in Dresden, Db 92–93 (=d), suffered d
severely in the last war, and the first volume, containing fols. 1–319,

1 This supplicat is printed by M. Fournier, Les statuts et privilèges des universités françaises II, Paris 1891, n. 1247. Schmutte, CMG Suppl. III, pp. VIII f., dated it on palaeographic grounds alone to North Italy in the late fourteenth century. I should like to thank Miss A. C. De la Mare for her help in solving some of the palaeographic problems raised by this Ms.

2 F. Lo Parco, Niccolò, pp. 262 f. and pp. 281 ff.: the story is rejected by L. Thorndike, Translations, pp. 215 f., who gives a full bibliography of earlier discussions. The article of M. S. Ogden, The Galenic works cited in Guy de Chauliac's Chirurgia Magna, Journal Hist. Med. 28, 1973, pp. 24–33, would seem to confirm my thesis.

3 Fol. 211^{r-v} contains 'Dicta philosophorum extracta de t(erti)o libro ystoriali Vincentii' written in a French hand that cannot be securely identified with either that of b^3 or that of the chancery scribe(s) of fol. 215. The extracts come from Vincent of Beauvais, Speculum Historiae II 120; III 24. 25. 33.

4 Biographie Universelle, ed. 2, Paris/Leipzig 1843, vol. 27, p. 658: a letter from him to P. Labbé is printed in the latter's Elogium chronologicum Galeni, Paris 1660.

received irreparable damage from the action of water which has rendered large portions illegible.[1] Its quires have become detached from the binding, the miniatures are a mess of paint, some pages have lost their lettering, others preserve a mere palimpsest of words, and in the absence of any specialised modern equipment an accurate decipherment and a complete collation are impossible. 'On prognosis' is found on fols. 1^{v}–8^{v}, the break between the parts coming at fol. 7^{v}, of which I was able to collate much of fols. 1^{v}–3^{r} and 5^{v}–7^{v} and occasionally parts of fols. 3^{v}–5^{r} (80,21–86,2, 102,22–112,10, 114,12–116,20, 134,30–140,11 are the passages most affected) as well as using the photo-facsimile of fol. 1^{r}. Written on parchment 455 mm. by 343 mm. in two columns each 110 mm. wide and varying in height from 333 to 338 mm., it dates from the second half of the fifteenth century and comes from Northern France or Flanders.[2] It divides 'On prognosis' into sixteen chapters, each with its own heading in red, and begins with a list of contents on fol. 1^{r}.

3. Malatestianus S. V 4

Two other manuscripts are preserved in the Biblioteca Mala-
c testiana at Cesena, the elder of which, S. V 4 (=c), a parchment codex of 264 leaves, with an additional blank leaf at the beginning and end, measuring 405 mm. by 260 mm., in two columns with 56 lines to the page, contains 'On prognosis' on fols. 130^{r}–135^{v}, the division between the parts coming at fol. 134^{v}. The index to the whole volume, fol. 1^{r}, is written over some earlier financial accounts. The script is small and crabbed with many abbreviations and compendia which make it difficult to read. A blank leaf at fol. 158^{v} is followed by a change of hand and then by the remaining treatises: De terapeutica, fols. 159^{r}–198^{r}; De febribus, fols. 198^{r}–209^{v}; De flebothomia, fols. 209^{v}–214^{v}; De sanitatis ingenio, fols. 215^{r}–261^{v}; and by the copiously annotated and corrected Flores thesauri of Petrus Hispanus, fols. 261^{v}–264^{v}. At least three hands can be distinguished among the corrections and marginalia of this treatise; the first that of the scribe, the
c^{2} second that of a later owner, Nicolaus de Leonardis Venetus physicus, a doctor artium et medicinae at Padua between 1424 and 1440, whose

[1] F. Schnorr von Carolsfeld, Katalog der Handschriften der königlichen öffentlichen Bibliothek zu Dresden, Leipzig 1882, pp. 307f., is not always accurate in his listing of the treatises contained in this Ms. A facsimile of the miniatures and of some pages in full was edited by E. C. van Leersum and W. Martin, Miniaturen der lateinischen Galenos-Handschrift der kgl. öffentl. Bibliothek in Dresden, Leyden 1910, who dealt only with artistic problems. I have discussed this manuscript in A forgotten manuscript of Galenus Latinus, Studia Codicologica, Berlin 1977, pp. 332–340.

[2] Brussels and Mechlin are but two of the centres suggested, but none has yet commanded full assent.

signature appears at fol. 264^{v1}, and the third that of Giovanni di Marco da Rimini (ob. 1474).[2] There are no indexes or chapter divisions to any tract: initial letters are ornamented in red and blue, internal divisions are marked in red or blue. The initial letter of this treatise is finely ornamented in a manner not found elsewhere in the codex. Such spellings as paxionis for passionis, inextiuali for inestiuali and ųexicam for vesicam indicate an Italian origin, probably, as Zazzeri thought, in the second half of the fourteenth century. c^3

4. Malatestianus S. XXVI 4

The second Cesena manuscript, S. XXVI 4 (=e), is a parchment codex of 238 leaves and a fly leaf, measuring 312 mm. by 227 mm., which contains the two parts of 'On prognosis' on fols. 67^v–80^r with the division between them coming at fol. 77^v. It is written in two columns with 43 lines to the page in a very clear, well ordered humanist script.[3] Within it there are again two sections, fols. 1–132^v containing the Galenic and Hippocratic treatises described on the fly leaf, then a blank page, fol. 133^r, some medical jottings, fol. 133^v, and then Aristotelis physica cum anonymi commentario, 134^r–238^v. The last treatise, missing from the index, is written in a different and earlier hand, while the medical jottings are in a third hand, probably that of Giovanni di Marco, whose signature appears on the fly leaf and who may have been responsible for combining the two collections into one. I attribute many of the marginalia to him (=e^2), distinguishing them from corrections made by the original scribe. There is no index of chapters and no internal chapter divisions, although on many pages the initial letter of some words protrudes into the margin, clearly awaiting ornamentation, although the words themselves are rarely significant as sentence or paragraph dividers. The initial letter of the first tract, De rigore, fol. 1^r, is beautifully painted in blue and gold, but although it was intended to apply a similar decoration throughout, as can be seen from the opening letter of 'On prognosis', the a of apud, fol. 67^v, which stands alone in a large expanse of blank page, this was never completed. e e^2

1 The date is given by C. Zonta and G. Brotto, Acta graduum academicorum Gymnasii Patavini ab anno 1406 ad annum 1450, Padua 1970, nn. 609, 743, 1430 and 1433: see also below, p. 58.

2 R. Zazzeri, Sui codici e libri a stampati della Biblioteca Malatestiana di Cesena ricerche ed osservazioni, Cesena 1897, pp. 296–300. On Giovanni's activities, see G. Baader, Die Bibliothek des Giovanni Marco da Rimini, Studia Codicologica, Berlin 1977, pp. 43–97: note also Modena Ms. Est. lat. 597, fols. 32^r–39^v, a life of Homer by Pietro Pierleoni of Rimini dedicated to him.

3 The scribe's name is at present unknown, but he may be identified probably with one of the scribes of Malatesta Novello, Ser. Giovanni da Epinal, Jacopo da Pergola, Francesco Bartolomeo da Figlino Valdarno and Bonifacio Paulino de Tradino. Cf. A. Domeniconi, Ser. Giovanni da Epinal, copista di Malatesta Novello, Studi Romagnoli 10, 1959, pp. 261–282.

Zazzeri dated this to the thirteenth century, and was followed blindly by Diels.[1] But this is impossible since it contains, fols. 107^{v}–120^{r}, De disnia, written in 1345, and both A. Minor and J. Schmutte agreed in placing it in the fifteenth century, probably in the second half.[2] Since it can be demonstrated (below, p. 31) that e is copied directly from c, it is an easy supposition that the copying took place at Cesena when Giovanni di Marco was active there, that is, between 1452 and 1474, and, if the illumination was left unfinished because of Giovanni's death, we would be able to date e precisely to 1474. But, as G. Baader points out, Giovanni was interested in obtaining copies of works not in his possession, not in having more beautiful copies made of works he already had, and his signature is more easily explained if he obtained the codex after the death of the intended recipient than if he made notes in it before the illumination was completed. Nevertheless, the costly beauty of the opening initial suggests that it was intended for a wealthy owner or as a gift from one, and it would not be rash to suppose that he was Malatesta Novello and that the codex was in process of illumination at his death in 1465.

5. Parisinus Academicus 51

The apparent finality of the work of Diels and his Commission made the work of editors searching for medical Mss. only too easy and thus several opportunities were lost to utilise later discoveries. In 1909, two years after the publication of Diels' Nachtrag, A. Boinet gave to the world his catalogue of the manuscripts held by the Académie Nationale de Médecine in Paris, among them six codices, 51–56, containing many Latin versions of Galen and Hippocrates.[3] 'On
a prognosis' is found in the first of these, 51 (=a), fols. 180^{r}–201^{v}, with the division between the parts coming at fol. 198^{v}. This paper manuscript, measuring 260 mm. by 205 mm., written in a single column 203 mm. by 125 mm., has never been used in any edition of Galen and thus demands close attention. Two sections can be distinguished within it: the first, fols. 1^{r}–232^{v}, is provided with indexes and chapter headings in red, which are missing from the second, fols. 237^{r}–327^{v}, and the two are separated by four blank pages, 233^{r}–236^{v}, which may mark a deliberate division or indicate that two volumes have been later bound into one. On the evidence of its script, it was written in Northern France or Flanders in the mid-fifteenth century. Two hands can be distinguished among its corrections; the first that of the scribe,
a2 the second a later hand giving alternative readings either in the margin or above the line and explaining difficult words. The scribe made

[1] Sui codici, pp. 480ff.; H. Diels, Die Handschriften, p. 100 and p. 125.

[2] A. Minor, De Galeni libris Περὶ δυσπνοίας, Diss. Marburg 1911, p. 5; J. Schmutte, CMG Suppl. III, pp. XIIIff.; Marinone, p. 14.

[3] A. Boinet, Catalogue général des manuscrits des bibliothèques publiques de France: Paris, Tome 1, Paris 1909, pp. 366–372.

many errors, almost all of which he corrected himself by comparison with his exemplar. The initial letters of sentences and the sixteen chapter headings are rubricated, and the script, although not as regular as that of d and e, is neat and well ordered.

c) The relationship between the Latin manuscripts

There have been few editors of Galen who have devoted great effort to the examination of the Latin manuscript tradition and most have been content merely to note the existence of a Latin version without committing themselves to a further inquiry. Consequently little is known about the relationships between individual manuscripts, and it was thus doubly unfortunate that the conclusions reached by Schmutte in his edition of De consuetudinibus were prevented from gaining wide circulation by the destruction of most of the copies of the work in the last war. For 'On prognosis', the most important of his results was the confirmation of Minor's hypothesis that e was a direct copy of c[1]: many errors in e derive from an incorrect resolution of compendia in c or from the copying of c's errors, and although it would be possible to argue that e was copied from a manuscript with abbreviations and errors similar to those found in c, the length of the list of examples provided by Schmutte is decisive against such a hypothesis. The following selection of readings demonstrates that his conclusion is valid also for 'On prognosis':

74,17 μὲν γὰρ] namque bad: nā ʒ c: naturam e
74,23 ἕνεκεν ἔδοξεν] grā uisum bad: $\hat{g}$ uisum c: gauisum e
76,2 περὶ] de causa ba: de cā c: de ea causam e
90,27 πανουργοῦντας] mala bad: mala mala ce
92,31 γεγόναμεν] generati bad: $\hat{g}$ti c: grati e
94,19 μαντικῆς] diuinatiua ba: d'inata c: d$\overline{ei}$ natiua e
110,26 καθόλου] uniuersalem ba: $\overline{ul}$em c: utilem e
118,30 ἐν ᾧπερ ἂν] ubicumque bad: $\overset{i}{u}$cūque c: licumque e
140,26 αὐτὸς] ipse bad: uxor ce

Nowhere does e supplement a lacuna in c, even when several words are lost: 104,32f. παρακαθημένην ... ἡμέρας] sedentem ... diem ba: *om.* ce. One final example confirms that e is copied from c: 100,7 λοιπὸν ... ἐφεξῆς] reliquum igitur est ut (ut *om.* a) quod promisi deinceps ba: *deest* d: ⌈ reliquum igitur est ut ⌊ promisi deinceps c *in textu*. At almost exactly the same level in the margin c[2] adds the following comment: ⌈ redit ad complendum quod dixit de muliere amante, and next to this c has added the missing ⌊ quod. The scribe of e, mistaking the purpose of the omission sign in the text, incorporates the words of c[2] into his text thus: reliquum igitur est ut redit ad complendum quod de muliere amante di$\overline{x}$it promissi deinceps. We have here not only the

[1] Proved also by Marinone, pp. 16f., without reference to earlier discoveries.

explanation of the error but also the source from which it was taken, for it is extremely unlikely that a lost exemplar of e would have also included in its margin the identical comments of Nicolaus Venetus.

But before rejecting e totally we should note that it occasionally has good readings missing from c, which may derive either from a collation of c with a good manuscript or from the ingenuity of the humanist copyist. Many changes are merely orthographical, especially the substitution of y for i:

78,23 diaforare bac: dyaforare de

86,7 desidero badc: desydero e

116,10 sindones bac: syndones e

Others may be more significant:

68,8 θωπεύειν] adhulari c: adulari bade

84,7 δικαίως] iusste c: iuste bae

88,23 ipsum badc: *om.* e *et codd. graeci*

96,15 παρῆσαν] adherant c: ad~~h~~ erant e: aderant bad

96,24 prebentem ei c: prebentem bae *et codd. graeci*

104,32 αὐτὸν φυλάξαι] obseruare eum badc: eum obseruare e

124,19 Ἀσκληπίου] asclepiadis dac: asclipiadis b: esculapii e

126,23f. ὅλης . . . ἅμα] tota . . . simul *iterat* c: *recte* bade

None of these examples is such as to compel immediate belief in the independence of e: rather they indicate the activity of an emending scribe, who can be seen at work at 96,15. It is as easy to ascribe the omission of ei at 96,24 and the changed order at 104,32 to inadvertence or to an itch for emendation as it is to believe that they come from a lost manuscript, and only at 124,19 is there any real possibility that the good reading comes from a lost source. But even here, the adjacent apollinis may well have suggested the right reading to the scribe.[1] Ms. e can thus be dismissed as a humanist copy of a known manuscript, c.

There can be little doubt also that c was transmitted independently of b, a and d. It agrees in wrong readings only five times with b against a and / or d; once with d against b and a; and three times with a against b, apart from the regular confusion in the Mss. between hoc and hec, and none of these agreements is in any way significant.[2] In

[1] W. John, CMG V 4,2, p. LII, believed that the good readings of e were enough to prove that c and e were derived from a common source, but his argument, based upon one passage only, involves a rigid preconception of what a scribe could or could not do and takes no account of the well known phenomenon of the learned emending scribe. Cf. for further proof, Marinone, p. 17.

[2] c agrees with d: 76,25 πυρέττειν] infebrientem ba: in febriente dc. – c agrees with a: 104,20 ἐρωτικῶς] erotice b: eroice ac: *deest* d; 106,7 κλίνη] lectum b: lectus ac: *deest* d; 114,22 κατὰ τὰς κρήνας] fontanee b: fontane ac: *deest* d. – c agrees with b: 80,4 κατ' αὐτὸν] ei ad: *om.* bc; 94,27 πρότερον] primo ad: prima bc; 96,6 διδα-

its major errors it stands alone with its copy and it can in no way be brought into close relation with b, a or d.

But there is all the difference in the world between a textual stemma composed of two branches and one composed of more than two, and it is essential to determine next whether b, a and d form a group derived from the same ancestor or whether any one of them is a witness to an independent tradition. Again the proof is simple. Thirteen instances where c has an exact translation of the text given by our surviving Greek Mss. and where b, a and d concur in the same wrong reading demonstrate that the three are derived from a common ancestor[1] and thus that their combined reading is equivalent to the testimony of c.

The connection between b and d has long been known and utilised: Kalbfleisch went so far as to say that they were so close "ut in lacunis alter ex altero supplendus, in discrepantiis modo hic modo ille sequendus, interdum etiam utriusque lectio in unum coniungenda sit"[2] and all subsequent editors have concurred. The discovery of a complicates the simple threads of tradition and compels a new investigation of their interrelationship. In an earlier article based partly upon the readings of d in the tracts De causis contentivis and De causis procatarcticis[3] I suggested that a and d were derived from the same source, which itself depended upon the same source as b, and a second inspection of d at Dresden enabled me to offer a similar and cogent proof drawn from the readings of 'On prognosis' alone. It is clear from the agreement between a and d against b both in wrong readings and in right[4] that they cannot derive directly from b, while the presence of good readings in a that are absent from d[5], and vice-versa[6], is enough

σκάλῳ] doctore ad: doctori bc; 116,9 τε] et ad: *om.* bc; 140,2 χρόνον ἅπαντα] tempore toto ad: toto tempore bc.

1 The following are the most important examples: 78,29 πρώτης] prima c: ipsa bad; 80,7 νῦν μέν, ἔφην] nunc dixi c: dixi nunc bad; 90,27 αὐξάνει] auget c: augent bad; 112,18 θύρας] portam c: partem bad; 116,28 ἄφνω] repente c: *om.* bad; 134,23 ἡμεῖς] nos c: mox bad; 142,11 θαυμάζουσιν] mirantur c: opinantur bad. I shall call the common ancestor of bad, w.

2 In his edition of De causis contentivis, Marburg 1904, p. 1.

3 A neglected manuscript, Studia Codicologica, Berlin 1977, pp. 332–340.

4 In right readings, as well as the examples cited in note 2, p. 32 above: 72,19 γνώριμοι δὲ] noti uero adc: uero noti b; 112,29 φροντίζοντί – νύκτωρ] et me sollicito existente per noctem adc: *om.* b; 128,28 fore adc: fere ba[2] *(in mg.)*; in wrong readings: 70,6 τοσοῦτον] in tantum bc: iterum ad; 74,6 πάντων] omnium bc: omnino ad; 80,13 ἐπὶ πλέον] ad plurimum bc: *om.* ad; 96,27 τριχοειδῆ] capilliformem bc: capilli formam habentium ad.

5 ba right against d: 80,11 μεταξὺ] interim bac; iterum d; 86,16 τῷ λόγῳ] uerba tua bac: uerba d; 102,13 βεβαιωθῆναι] confirmari bac: contristari d; 120,24 αὐτῷ γελάσας] ei ridens ba[2] *(in mg.)* c: ei euidens a: euidens d; 122,12sq. ὑποστρέφων ... πυρέττειν] adiuit ... febrire bac: *om.* d; 124,21sq. οἱ ... φιλοσοφίας] qui ... philosophie bac: *om.* d.

6 bd right against a: 118,12 χρόνου] tempore bdc: tempe a; 120,4 ἀναξίοις] indignis bdc: indigno a; 124,9 qui bdc: cui a; 134,25 ἀνεπήδησε] surrexisset bd: surres-

to show that they are independent of each other. The stemma of the Latin manuscripts can be represented thus:

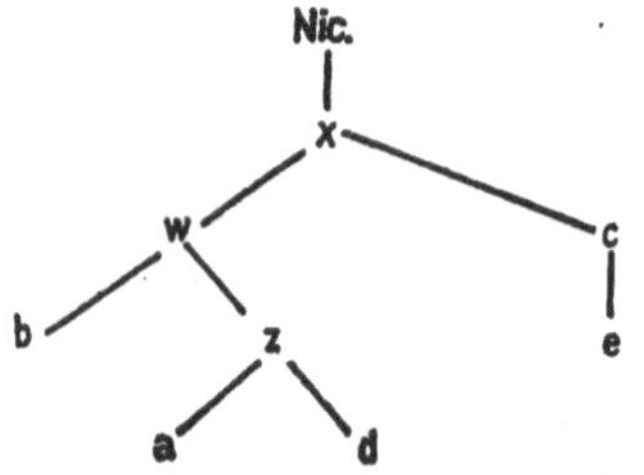

The lost manuscript, z, is likely to have been in Northern Europe in the mid-fifteenth century when the two copies were made from it, and, w from the history of b, it is not rash to conjecture that Ms. w was the copy preserved in the Angevin Library. But the presence of errors common to both w and c which cannot be ascribed simply to Niccolò's method of translation but which are obviously errors of transcription[1] indicates that x was not Niccolò's own manuscript or that, if it was, it was copied from notes that were not always unmistakably clear.

d) The edition of Diomedes Bonardus

The most difficult task of any scholar wishing to define the relationships between manuscripts is to pick up hints of other manuscripts now lost which survived until the Renaissance when they were used by scholars in the compilation of printed editions. The editio princeps of any author might thus be based either on a known manuscript or manuscripts or, on the other hand, on one or more that have since perished. Much still remains obscure concerning the sources of the first edition of the complete works of Galen in Latin, that edited v by Diomedes Bonardus (=v) and printed by Philippus Pincius at Venice in 1490, but now that a stemma of the surviving Latin manuscripts of 'On prognosis' has been established, it becomes possible to isolate those used in the making of the editio princeps and in turn to assess the value of the printed text both within the manuscript tradition and as an example of the art of editing. Not that this is at all easy, for we must take into account both the state of the manuscript tradition, the ingenuity of the editor and the uncertain hazards that attend the transmission of a text from manuscript to printed book. But when the readings of known manuscripts have been isolated, there remains a residue which may be assigned either to an otherwise

sisset c: surrexit a. d right against the others: 78,1 προσταχθὲν] iniunctum d: iniunctum uel inmissum a: inmissum b: inuentum c.

[1] The following serve as examples: 72,17 συρφετοῦ] ceu wc: cetu v; 108,15 μάντις] diuinator v: *om.* wc; 122,21 τρεῖς] tres v: *om.* wc; 128,20 θερμῷ] oleo wc: calido v; 138,27 περὶ τῶν ἀμυδρῶν ... διάγνωσιν] indebilium ... dignotionem wc: in debilium ... dignotione Durling.

unknown source or to the editor himself. In attempting to distinguish the readings of individual manuscripts, good readings, that is, readings that correspond to a translation of the Greek text, are rarely as informative as bad, since an error shared between the printed edition and one known manuscript is more likely to come from that manuscript than from elsewhere.

There has been little dispute that b was used by Bonardus in the preparation of his edition. Mewaldt stated that the printed text of De comate came "e codice Parisino 6865 mea quidem sententia . . .; nam ubicumque editio Latina a codice discrepat, aut correctum est lene codicis mendum aut e contrario neglegenter lecta vel aliter depravata integra et perlucida codicis memoria."[1] The evidence for the use of b in 'On prognosis' is clear: 70,5 predixit bv: predixerit adce; 70,26 asclipiadum bv: asclepiadum ad: asclepiadis ce; 88,24 gnisiis bv: grafiis certis ad: ueris ce; 90,20 eos ignorant bv: ignorant eos a: eos ignorauerunt c: ignorauerunt eos e; 104,32 iuxta eum bv: iuxta a: *om.* ce; 124,8 amoueo bv: admoueo adce; 124,19 asclipiadis bv: asclepiadis adc: esculapii e; 124,31 ego adce: eꝯũ so b: econuerso v; 134,29 emoragiare bv: emorogiare ce: emorrogiare ad; 138,30 quos bv: quod ace.

Two examples out of many are enough to show that b was not the sole source: 114,2 et plorabant acev: *om.* b; 116,11 deinde . . . durissimas acev: *om.* b; and we must thus examine each manuscript in turn for evidence of its employment. Significant indications of the use of c are few: 74,9 respiciunt solum ba: aspiciunt solum c: solum aspiciunt e: aspiciunt necessariam solum v; 102,33 requirere acv: inquirere e: requisitionem b; and by no means conclusive, especially when compared with the evidence in favour of the use of e[2]: 68,15 allicientes badc: alicientes ev; 84,21 saltim adc: saltiim b: saltem ev; 90,27 cotidie adc: coctidie b: quottidie ev; 98,8 pyronios c: pironios ev: pironeos b: piroynos ad; 106,13 uxorem bac: uxorem suam ev; 118,2 quod bac: quidem ev; 130,12 uero badc: *om.* ev; 138,9 cataforas c: catoforas ev: cathaforas ba. In addition ev always read mihi, while a and d have michi, b and c either $\overset{i}{\mathrm{m}}$ or michi.

The loss of much of d greatly hampers any investigation into the use of a Ms. belonging to the same family as a and d or identical with one of them, and complete certainty cannot be attained. However, a list of selected readings will show what possible solutions can be considered. First, instances where v agrees with a and d: 76,3 esse me bce: me esse adv; 76,6 quo sine bce: sine quo adv; 78,7 quartam adv: q^{am} c: quartanam be; 82,28 uerificatus adv: iurificatus b: iustificatus ce; 112,12 euenire bce: aduenire adv; 112,22 afferre adv: offerre be: affere c; 114,15 inclinamus bce: inclinauimus adv; 122,4 xvii^{o} die

[1] J. Mewaldt, CMG V 9,2, p. XV, n. 1; confirmed also by K. Bardong, CMG Suppl. II, p. VII. Only W. John, CMG V 4,2, p. LII, and J. Schmutte, CMG Suppl. III, pp. XXf., discounted the use of b in the treatises they edited.

[2] W. John and J. Schmutte, loc. cit. (see above, n. 1) both confirm the use of e for their treatises.

hora tertia adv: xiii° die hora tertia b: xvii° die c: *om.* e; or with a in the absence of d: 110,17 monet bce: mouet av; 116,9 et av: *om.* bce; 118,7 egressum bce: regressum av; 138,2 cola bce: colla av. But since there is no clear instance of the use of a when d survives and two possible examples of the use of d: 76,19 Eudimus dv: Eudinus bce: Endinus a; 78,1 iniunctum dv: iniunctum uel inmissum a: inmissum b: inuentum ce: inuinctum e *(e corr.)*, it may be legitimate to conclude that either d or a lost relative of d was used. If the latter solution is adopted, it is essential to remember that the place of this lost manuscript in the stemma makes it extremely unlikely that many of the good readings found only in v could come from this source without leaving any trace elsewhere in the tradition.[1]

One possible source of v's good readings, as W. John and J. Schmutte rightly saw, is a Greek manuscript or a Latin manuscript annotated or corrected from the Greek.[2] The following readings support that conclusion: 72,17 συρφετοῦ] ceu badce: cetu v; 78,20 ἔτ' εἶναι] esse adhuc badce: adhuc esse v; 96,2 προπηλακιζόμενος] cum iniuriaretur bace: cum iniuriarer v; 100,10 σφυγμοὺς] pulsu bace: pulsibus v (and wrongly, for Niccolò's version was 'pulsu pulsantibus hiis'); 102,17 δηλοῖ] significabat bac: significabar e: significat v; 108,1 μάντεως] diuinatoris v: diuinationis bac: *om.* e; 108,15 μάντις] diuinator v: *om.* bace; 108,24 ἐμήνυσα] sic coniecturaui bace: sic *om.* v; 120,25 ἐξωτέρω] extra v: circa badce; 122,19 ὑποστροφῆς νοσήματος] redita (reddita ad) egritudine badce: reditu egritudinis a²v; 132,31 ἀρρώστους] egritudines badce: egros v; 140,15 ἄνθρωπον] hominem v: *om.* bace. Other readings may be attributed with less certainty to a Greek manuscript source, since they could equally well be derived from a lost Latin source or by editorial conjecture: 72,31 κατασκευὴν] constitutionem badce: constructionem v; 80,27 ὡς] quod v: que bace; 82,4 Βάρβαρος] Barbarus v: Barbatus badce, but cf. 98,13 where all Mss. read Barbarus; 96,19 Φαβωρίνου] Fauorni b: Fauorii ace: Favorini v; 128,20 θερμῷ] oleo badce: calido v, but cf. 128,22 calidum adcv: oleo b: *om.* e. Only in

[1] My collations of De causis contentiuis and De causis procatarcticis seem to exclude the use of a: if that is so, support for a third Ms. of the ad group may come from the ascription to Niccolò of a version of De sequela found only in d, a (PAM 53, fols. 324ᵛ–339ᵛ) and in v. No translator is named in d (cf. Thorndike, p. 229); a, fol. 339ᵛ, has: translatus a nicolao de calabria; v, I, p. 120ᵛ, has: translatus a magistro Nicolao de Regio Calabria. v calls the tract De sequela operationum anime...; a De sequela potenciarum anime ...; and the differences between the two exclude the use of a. Did Bonardus invent the ascription himself? or did he have a lost Ms.?

[2] I am not convinced by Marinone's objections to Bonardus' use of a Greek text, p. 22, especially if some corrections were made to his copy by a friend glancing at a Greek Ms., which would account for the sporadic readings that can only come from the Greek and would explain why Bonardus said nothing about his borrowings in his preface. If John Clement could correct the Greek of the Aldine with the help of the Latin (below, p. 41), it is not impossible that Bonardus used a Ms. either Greek or corrected from the Greek. Nor do I think it necessary to posit a complete series of pre-Niccolò translations for all Galen's works.

two places is there a reading that must come either from a lost Latin manuscript or from an editorial conjecture. The first is the strongest evidence for the use of a lost manuscript: 68,2 *titulus*] translatus a Nicolao de Regio de Calabria v: *om.* badce. But it is difficult to understand why, if this superscription stood in w, it should have been omitted by the scribes of b, a and d, who are meticulous in distinguishing between translators, unless this manuscript derived independently of the surviving manuscripts. But I regard such a hypothesis as unlikely and prefer to assign this ascription to the ingenuity of Bonardus. A similar conjecture, but a correct one, may be found at the second passage, 132,28, τὰς y: tres v: *om.* badc: quattuor e: τρεῖς Cornarius. Cornarius' emendation, which is probably correct, was without doubt owed to his knowledge of v, and all the manuscripts of Niccolò's version have a reading equivalent to that of the Greek manuscripts, with the significant exception of the emended manuscript e. Here the humanist scribe, shrewdly noting the absence of a necessary numeral, conjectured the wrong number, which was in turn corrected by Bonardus.

When Diomedes Bonardus was editing the Latin Galen, knowledge of the Greek Galen was already reaching Western scholars, especially in Venice, with its many Greek refugees, and it would have been easy for a humanist editor to check the accuracy of the versions he was printing by an occasional glance at the Greek original. The result of this cross-check is that the printed text improves upon the translation it purports to represent: it is occasionally more faithful to the words of Galen than to the rendering of Niccolò. The use of a Greek manuscript removes the possibility of collating the editio princeps as a manuscript[1], especially as its sources can be isolated and identified with tolerable certainty. Its basis is the two manuscripts b and e, supplemented by a third manuscript of the ad group, which I am inclined to identify with d itself. To posit a fourth manuscript preserving some good readings and a title ascribing the translation to Niccolò is excessive if room is to be left for Bonardus' conjectural powers and for his borrowings from the Greek. Thus v is not cited as a manuscript in the apparatus criticus, but only for readings peculiar to it.

IV. The Latin translation and the Greek manuscripts

Before full use can be made of the Latin translation as evidence for a Greek manuscript it is essential first to make some general comment upon the translator's ability and technique, if only in order to prevent conclusions about his Greek manuscript or manuscripts

[1] This conclusion was also forcefully argued by J. Schmutte, CMG Suppl. III, p. XXII.

being drawn from what are merely idiosyncrasies of his style.[1] There can be no doubt that he was a very faithful translator, usually keeping close to the word order of the Greek without much concern for Latin elegance, but recognition of this virtue should not blind us to the fact that he could make mistakes or lead us to assume that all the novelties in his translation imply a corresponding reading in his Greek text; many of them are imposed on him by the differences between the two languages in which he worked.

There are times when he omits words in his translation which are either irrelevant to his purpose or untranslatable into Latin, e. g. 94,5f. μὲν – ἀττικίζοντες and 96,18f. δημοσίᾳ – λέξεως, both of which are incomprehensible to a mediaeval reader: at others, especially when re-organising the Greek clause structure to fit into Latin, he omits connecting words and pronouns that are superfluous in Latin, e.g. 124,5 με and 130,2 αὐτῶν. J. N. Mattock's comments upon the Arabic translators of Galen also apply well to the Latin.[2] "Most translators were at home in an easy passage: when they came across something they did not understand they translated word for word, in the hope that some sense might emerge or they paraphrased what they hoped might be the sense." A good example is found at 142,2f. αὐτὸς – αὐτό, where 'secundum ineptitudines discentium anni multiplicantur' gives meaning to the corrupt Greek of the manuscripts, even if it is wrong itself. It is much more difficult to decide, in passages where the Latin has an expanded version, between good readings preserved only in Latin, additions necessary in Latin to give sense to what is understandable only in Greek, and amplifications introduced by the translator himself.[3] Some additions can be immediately discounted, e. g. 126,14 Commodi, filii Pitholai, but others are much more problematic and their aptness often deceived the Basle editors into accepting them into the Greek text (below, p. 43). I may possibly have gone too far in reaction to this by relegating a few readings preserved only in Latin from the text of Kühn to the apparatus criticus, e. g. 130,18 locis. But minor alterations, positive adjectives for comparative, the bringing forward of a noun or participle to give clarity and emphasis[4], rarely demand a corresponding change in the Greek or the attention given to, e. g., the transposition of the sentences at 124,26–31. One final point should be made about the translator's technique as a warning to those who rely blindly upon him. Compound words in Greek are often split up in the Latin (and vice-versa) and prepositional phrases, adverbs and even nouns can replace the prefix of the verb, e.g. 68,18 παρανομεῖν is rendered by 'enormia satagere'; 72,23 πρεσβυτέρως τετιμηκότες by 'preferentes'. Wille's cautious conclusion

[1] Cf. F. Kudlien, CMG V 10,2,4, p. 108, n. 3.

[2] In a review printed in Bulletin of the School of Oriental and African Studies 34, 1971, p. 147.

[3] I. Wille, Überlieferung, pp. 270–273; D. Nickel, CMG V 2,1, pp. 25f.

[4] I. Wille, Überlieferung, pp. 273–275.

must be noted.[1] "Man darf sich also in all den Fällen, wo keine offenkundigen paläographisch erklärbaren Abweichungen von N festzustellen sind, nicht einfach auf die wörtliche Übersetzungstechnik des Nicolaus verlassen, sondern muß sorgfältig prüfen, ob nicht eine freiere Wiedergabe des Textes vorliegt."

When these qualifications have been made, the Latin version can be used to indicate a Greek text, current in the first half of the fourteenth century, and possibly earlier, that is an older, if not in parts a better, witness than some of the surviving manuscripts. As is clear from the later chapters of 'On prognosis', it preserves a tradition that is independent of that of L and M:

122,13 ἐπορεύϑη πρὸς αὐτὸν] adiuit ipsum Nic.: *om.* y

132,5 καὶ – μὴ] et aridum – nequaquam Nic.: *om.* y

136,32 ἠξίωσα – ἐνερείδοντα] nosti – pruritum Nic.: *om.* y

There are also several instances in which it appears to have readings akin to those preserved by A:

72,6 ἀδικημάτων A: nequiciarum Nic.: ἀδοκιμωτάτους y

80,4 ἐχωρίσϑησαν A: recesserunt Nic.: ἐχωρίσϑη y

82,2 πάνυ A: ualde Nic.: πᾶν y

86,5 ἀγαϑά A: omnia bona Nic.: ἀγαϑόν y

86,12f οὖσαν ἔν σοι μοχϑηρίαν A: existentem in te prauitatem Nic.: νόσον ἔν σοι μοχϑηρὰν y

Only once does Nic. follow A in a bad reading; 82,6 ὥσπερ καὶ A: sicut et Nic.: ὥσπερ y, but this cannot be termed a significant error. Similarly, Nic.'s agreement with y at 80,14 cannot be considered important: τρίτον A: tercie Nic.: τρίτου y. Thus, although it is possible that the Greek source of Nic. was a member of the same family as A, a safer conclusion is that it belongs to a different one from L and M. A stemma of manuscripts, excluding V, P and W, although the latter pair have links with Nic. because all three contain the second part of this treatise, can be represented thus:

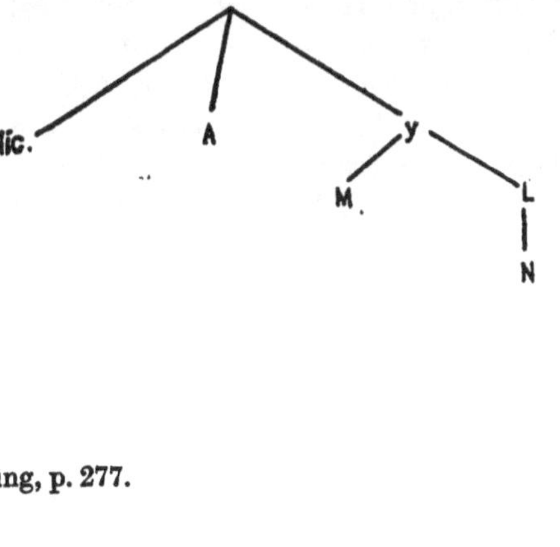

[1] I. Wille, Überlieferung, p. 277.

B. Editions and annotations

The great Aldine edition of Galen, edited by Opizzoni and Asolano and printed at Venice in 1525, which contains 'On prognosis' in Volume III, pp. 135–142, has been the foundation of previous editions of this treatise.[1] To assess its quality and reliability it is essential first to know upon what manuscript sources it is based and whether any manuscripts were used in its composition that have since been lost. Wenkebach's demonstration[2] that some manuscripts once in the possession of the English humanist, John Clement, and now in the Bibliothèque Nationale in Paris, fonds grec 2164, 2165, 2167 and 2173, were used is here of little value since none of them includes this treatise. We must therefore turn to the extant manuscripts, A, L, N and M, to see whether any of them lies at the base of this edition.

It is at once clear that LN was never used: many readings that are rightly preserved there were omitted in favour of poorer ones, to be restored occasionally by conjecture or from the Latin tradition. There is no reading peculiar to LN given in the Aldine before 96,15, and after that, only a handful of readings, all simple corrections of M: 96,15 γενήσεσθαι LNAld.: γενήσεσθαι iter. M; 108,13 ἐπὶ LNAld.: ἐπὶ iter. M. There are also over sixty instances of the readings of M being preferred to better ones in LN, including 102,25 παραχρῆμα LN: confestim Nic.: om. MAld.; 102,25 ἰδὼν LN: uidens Nic.: om. MAld.; 104,20 μακρὸς LN: longa Nic.: om. MAld.; 110,7 τέχνης LN: arte Nic.: om. MAld.; 116,4 ἐδίδουν LN: dabam Nic.: om. MAld. From this we may conclude that LN was not used in the preparation of the Aldine and that M was a basic manuscript.[3] As further proof of the latter assertion, against the hypothesis that the second half of 'On prognosis' was taken from a lost manuscript akin to M, it is enough to note 88,18, where LNA and M all read κινήσεως but the Aldine καὶ νήσεως. The error derives from a hurried reading of M, which apparently shows a space after the iota and the remains of a link between kappa and iota which resembles the contraction for καί. Greater familiarity with the hand of M (cf. fol. 83^r,47, and fol. 83^v,2) reveals that this is M's normal way of writing κινήσεως.

There is also evidence for the use of A: 74,24 ὀγδόην AAld.: πέμπτην LMN: nonam Nic.; 76,5 τῷ δὲ AAld.: in eo quod Nic.: οὕτω LMN; 76,17 ἐπὶ τὸ λουτρὸν ἔχων AAld.: om. LMN Nic.; 82,21 τεταρταίους APWAld.: quartanas Nic.: τριταίους LMN; 92,25 ἀναιρεθῆναι AAld.: ἀναιρεθέντα LMN: interfectum Nic.; 94,30 ἔργων

[1] N. Mani, Die griechische Editio princeps des Galenos, ihre Entstehung und ihre Wertung, Gesnerus 13, 1956, pp. 29–52.

[2] E. Wenkebach, CMG V 10,3, pp. XIIIff., with the references there cited.

[3] Cf. CMG V 9,1, p. XXVII with p. XXXVII, 20.

AAld.: opera Nic.: ὀργάνων LMN. While it is possible to argue that some of these readings could derive from editorial conjecture or from the Latin, those at 74,24 and 76,17 can only come from a Greek manuscript, presumably A.[1] There is also the possibility that the Aldine editors used the Latin version, especially since Nickel has collected strong evidence for its use in other treatises[2], but there is no sure proof of its employment here. The best examples are: 112,10 ἐπεπιστεύκειμεν Ald.: confidebamus Nic.: ἐπεπιστεύκει μὲν LMN; and 126,23 βραχύ Ald.: modicum Nic.: τραχύ LN: τράων M. I thus conclude that the text of the Aldine edition was based primarily on M and A, supplemented by editorial conjecture and an occasional glance at the printed Latin version.

But, even when it is recognised that the editors relied largely upon the poor manuscript M, how well did they perform their task of producing a sound text? I have accepted only ten of their emendations into the text, none being of outstanding merit[3], and the small number of improvements made by the Aldine editors is surpassed by the number of errors and misprints they introduced.[4] While it cannot be denied that the publication of the Aldine gave a great boost to Galenic studies, its text of this treatise confirms the opinions of Erasmus and Guinther that an opportunity had been thrown away. Erasmus' criticism is justified: "Discrucior tantum autorem tantis impendiis tam mendose proditum".[5]

The effect of this edition is immediately apparent in the Latin versions of this treatise.[6] Niccolò's version, which was printed in the Juntine edition of 1528, was superseded by translations made directly from the Aldine, the first of which, that of Guinther of Andernach, published at Paris in 1536, survived to be reprinted as the Latin version appended to 'On prognosis' in Kühn's edition of 1827.[7] I credit him with the correct solutions to the difficulties of the Aldine text at 68,17f. οὐ – ὑπειλήφασιν] quum vera bona non sint, ipsi falso opinantur; 100,12 where he followed Nic. in omitting καὶ – παλλακῆς;

1 Further evidence for the use of A was assembled by C. Gabler, Galeni libellus de captionibus quae per dictionem fiunt, Diss. Rostock 1903, pp. VII ff.

2 D. Nickel, CMG V 2,1, p. 26.

3 Examples of them are: 130,26 ὧν LM: ὂν NAld.; and 138,25 bis μέγα LMN: μέγαν Ald.

4 Examples are: 68,18 ψευδῶς] ψευδεῖ Ald.; 96,26 ante Ἀλέξανδρος add. καὶ Ald.; 128,9 παρὰ] περὶ Ald.; 136,10 ἀπὸ] ὑπὸ Ald.

5 Erasmus, Ep. 2049, cf. Epp. 1707, 1713; and Guinther's preface to his edition of De semine (Claudii Galeni Pergameni Libri duo de Semine Ioanne Guinterio Andernaco interprete, Paris 1533, fol. a iii^{v}).

6 R. J. Durling, A chronological census of Renaissance editions and translations of Galen, Journal of the Warburg and Courtauld Institutes 24, 1961, p. 289.

7 In his preface Guinther says, "Exemplar graecum quod unicum in his laboribus, plurimum mihi uti alias facessit negotii ... in sequenti commentario, nempe de praenoscendo, plura castigavi quam hic repeti debeant." Although Chartier and Kühn made some improvements in Guinther's text, they did not include his own corrections or bring his version into line with their own text.

134,11 δεδειγμένον] monstratum Guinther: δεδειγμένων LMNAld.; 140,5–8, where he followed Nic. in rejecting αἰσθανομένους – πολλῆς; and 140,21 χρόνον] tempore Nic. Guinther: λόγον LMNAld. The years 1540/41 saw three new versions produced in different parts of Europe; by A. Ludovicus at Lisbon[1]; by L. Jacchinus at Lyons, with a useful commentary[2]; and by J. M. Rota, whose version became standard in the later Juntine editions. The harvest to be gleaned from them is exceptionally meagre: all translate ἐαθῆναι, 80,11, by some form of servare, and Rota produces satisfactory versions of 68,17f. and 140,5–8, almost certainly copying Guinther. The two later productions of J. Cornarius in 1549 and J. B. Rasarius in 1562 are of no value in the reconstruction of the Greek text since they rely heavily upon the Aldine, occasionally supplemented by the Basle edition.[3]

This is by far the most important edition of 'On prognosis' and was made by H. Gemusaeus and published at Basle in 1538 by A. Cratander as part of Volume III of the Omnia Opera Galeni, pp. 451–462. As well as removing some typographical errors, the editor also used the Latin tradition[4], probably through a printed book rather than a manuscript, from which he took readings which he placed either in the text or in the margin. The corrections made without the aid of the Latin version are small: e. g., 70,21 μέλλειν Bas.: μέλειν LMNAld.: μέλλον A; 118,28 κακοηθείας Bas.: κακοηθίας LMNAld.; and see also 96,11 and 108,14. Those derived from Niccolò are numerous and, for the most part, good: e. g., 80,4 ἐχωρίσθη LMNAld.: recesserunt Nic.: ἐχωρίσθησαν ABas.; 86,20 τέτμηνται AAld.: τετίμενται M: τετίμηνται LN²: ordinatae Nic.: τετάχαται Bas.; and 114,32 ἡμέραις ὡς add. Bas.: diebus ut Nic.: om. LMNAld.; and see the apparatus, passim.[5] But because the technique of the Latin translator was but little understood, several errors were introduced that were not removed by later editors. Sometimes, when the translator broke up a long Greek sentence by making two connected main verbs out of a main verb and participle, the Basle editor followed him and altered

[1] A Ms. of Ludovicus' translations is preserved in the Biblioteca da Ajuda in Lisbon, see Machado Santos, Manuscritos de filosofia do seculo XV existentes em Lisboa, Catalogo, Coimbra 1951, pp. 143ff., but this treatise does not appear to be among them.

[2] This was reprinted in A. Ricci and V. Trincavelli's edition of the Omnia Opera Galeni, Sectio Tertia, pp. 847–888, which appeared at Venice in 1544, by which time Ricci, the shrewd annotator of the first volume, was dead; and formed the basis of Andres a Laguna's Epitome Galeni, Basle 1551, pp. 645–652 and 860.

[3] One example is 74,24 ἐννάτην Bas. in mg.: nonam Nic. Cornarius.

[4] As E. Wenkebach observed, CMG V 10,3, p. XLI: cf. also D. Nickel, CMG V 2,1, p. 27.

[5] Twice Bas. restored a good reading from Latin, but in the wrong place: 102,25 ἰδὼν om. MAld.: uidens eum Nic.: ὁρῶντα inepte post αὐτὸν restituit Bas.; 134,26 φόβου om. MAld.: nullo timoroso presente Nic.: μηδενὸς φοβεροῦ πάροντος rest. Bas.

the Greek [1], at others he excluded words not translated into Latin [2], or added words that were unnecessary in Greek [3]. Some of the changes introduced are owed to a credulous faith in the accuracy of Nic.[4], without regard either for differences among the constituent Latin manuscripts [5] or for the possibility that the Latin translation was an adequate version of the Greek of the Aldine.[6] But on balance the improvements brought by Gemusaeus to the Greek text far outweigh the occasional zealous failing, and although many cruces were left unsolved and many corrupt readings left uncorrected, the editor could justly claim to have forwarded the cause of Galenic scholarship. His edition was as superior to the Aldine as that had in its turn been to any of its constituent manuscripts.

In 1550 a small edition was edited anonymously and printed in Paris by Guillaume Morel, who was just embarking upon a career as a scholar-printer that was to carry him to the office of Royal Printer.[7] The only pocket edition of 'On prognosis', it was one of a series of single treatises printed by Morel, presumably for students unable to afford the complete works of Galen. Although largely dependent on the Basle edition, it contains a few emendations, of soundness rather than brilliance, e. g.: 94,29 ἤδη LNM: ἴδιοι Bas.: ἴδοι

1 92,14 δυνάμενοι LMNAld.: possunt Nic.: δύνανται Bas.; 122,17 καὶ κελεύσας LMN: iussit Nic.: ἐκέλευσε Bas.; 128,14 εἰπὼν LMN: dixit Nic.: εἶπεν . . . καὶ Bas. The reverse correction, participle for main verb, was made at 76,16, rightly, if asyndeton is not allowed: ἔφην LMNAAld.: dicens Nic.: φήσας Bas.

2 90,19 τό τε] τότε LMNAAld.: om. Nic. Bas.; 104,22 δήποτε LN: μηδέποτε MAld.: om. Nic. Bas.

3 At 90,12, 110,25 and 126,23 Bas. inserted καὶ, following Nic.'s 'et', although Nic. had broken down the sentence structure into two main verbs connected by 'et'; at 120,11 Bas. added ἔσται, following 'erit' in Nic.; others are: 130,18 τόπων sec. Nic. (locis) add. Bas.; 136,22 ὀλίγον sec. Nic. (modicum) add. Bas.; at 112,9 the correct text τοῦ γυναικείου ῥοῦ was preserved in LN: τοῦ ῥοῦ τοῦ γυναικείου MAld., and Bas. addition ὄντα, following Nic.'s 'existentia', was a fair attempt to solve the difficulty. The addition of σοῦ (te Nic.) at 134,9 may well be correct.

4 80,3 ἡμέρας sec. Nic. (die) add. Bas., wrongly for the supplement should refer to 'hour', not 'day'; 120,9 Κοιντιαλίων LN: Κυιντιαλίων M: Κυιντιαλίου Ald.: Κυιντιλιάνου sec. Nic. (Quintiliani) scr. Bas.; 120,16 'Αντωνίνου υἱὸς sec. Nic. (Antonii filius) add. Bas.; in three places: 126,14 ἐπιδημίαν LNMAld.: ἀποδημίαν sec. Nic. (in peregrinatione) scr. Bas.; 128,2 δυοῖν sec. Nic. (duobus) add. Bas.; and 128,5 τότε δὶς LNMAld.: ὅτι δύο sec. Nic. (quoniam hii duo) scr. Bas., the Latin version appears to have a different Greek text, as opposed to a fuller text, than that of y. In the first example the Latin may be right, in the others it is not.

5 78,25 αἰδεσθέντι LNMAAld.: uerecundante eo Nic.[bad]: uerecundante Nic.[v]: uerecundanti Nic.[ce]: αἰδεσθέντος scr. Bas.; 122,4 tercia hora Nic.[badv]: om. Nic.[ce]: τρίτῃ ὥρᾳ post ἡμέραν add. Bas.

6 94,14 πολλὴ δόξα παρὰ πᾶσιν ἦν LNMAAld.: in magna gloria ut nosti eram Nic.: ἐν πολλῇ δόξῃ παρὰ πᾶσιν ἦν Bas., sed cf. 84,4 δόξα μεγάλη . . . ἦν LNMAedd.: in gloria magna erat Nic.; 98,4 and 106,23 ὑποτυχὼν LNM: interloquens Nic.: ὑπολαβὼν Bas.; 108,8 στορεσθῆναι LNMAld.: transuerti Nic.: ἀναστορεθῆναι scr. Bas., sed cf. 108,14 στρώννυσθαι; 122,16 μὲν . . . τε LNMAld.: quidem . . . autem Nic.: μὲν . . . δὲ scr. Bas.

7 M. Maittaire, Historia typographorum aliquot Parisiensium, I, London 1717, pp. 33–46; P. Renouard, Répertoire des imprimeurs parisiens, Paris 1965, pp. 314f.

Mor.; 102,5 μοῦ LNMBas.: μοί Mor.; 106,16 πρότερον LNMBas.: πότερον Mor.; 140,25 τινι om. Ald.Bas., add. Mor., sed post ῥήτορα.[1] But neither its text nor its handiness preserved it from an unjustified neglect by subsequent editors, and it became a bibliographer's rarity, not a student's delight.

Certainly René Chartier, who edited this tract in Volume VIII of the collected works of Galen and Hippocrates, Paris 1679, pp. 829–852[2], made little use of it, although he accepted or, more likely, made himself the same emendations at 106,16, 118,20, 126,7, 136,12, and 140,17, which typify the sort of conjecture of which he was capable. He wrote out in full many abbreviated numerals, e. g. 116,12, 120,17, and made minor improvements in the spelling of proper names and technical terms, 98,8, 118,9, but when these changes are set aside, the worth of his emendations becomes clearer. I give the following examples of his ability: 74,7 τὸ LNMABas.: τῷ Chart.; 108,24 γινωσκόντων LNMBas.: δηλωσάντων Chart.; 112,25 τῷ add. Chart.; 120,23 ἀδύνατον LNMBas.: ἀδυνάτων Chart. They can be characterised as the correction of trivial errors such as any competent editor can make in a long text or series of texts, and possibly Chartier should not be blamed for failing to do more than that.

But few have been found to speak a word in favour of C. G. Kühn, an editor whose zeal outran his abilities and whose edition unfortunately remains the most accessible even today.[3] W. Herbst curtly dismissed his work thus[4]: "constat editionem Kuehnianam scatere erroribus et mendis", and there is no need of a lengthy indictment. With a few exceptions[5], wherever he emended the text or permitted the printers' Greek to stand he introduced chaos and error into what was once clear and true.

If the editions of 'On prognosis' are disappointing in their quality and if an examination of their contents imparts into the reader a sense of human weakness and scholarly frailty, three collections of manuscript notes lighten his mind and encourage his spirit, for here at last he is in the company of scholars whose philological acumen would have been worthy of Galen himself. The earliest and by far

[1] See also the apparatus at 126,7, and 140,17. I cannot accept 124,25 ἀγγελοῦντας for ἀγγέλλοντας, also conjectured by Cobet, for reasons I give at p. 215.

[2] J. Kollesch, René Chartier, Herausgeber und Fälscher der Werke Galens, Klio 48, 1967, pp. 183–198; René Chartier als Herausgeber der Werke Galens, Antiquitas Graeco-Romana, Prague 1968, pp. 525–530.

[3] A biography of him is given by K. Schubring in the reprint of Galeni Omnia Opera, Hildesheim 1965, XX, pp. IX–XV. 'On prognosis' is contained in Vol. XIV, pp. 599–673, originally published at Leipzig in 1827. There was a second impression of the first edition which removed a few minor imperfections.

[4] W. Herbst, Galeni Pergameni de atticissantium studiis testimonia, Leipzig 1911, p. 157.

[5] 86,9 τ' for τε; 88,3 εἴωθεν for εἴωθε; 114,30 διελέχθην for διειλέχθην; 124,29 ᾔδεσαν for εἴδεσαν; 130,3 ἂν added; 130,9 ὅτε for οὗ; 130,30 εἶδε for οἶδε; 138,11 προσεπελογισάμην for προσεπιλογισάμην.

the most important of these collections of annotations was written by Janus Cornarius of Zwickau in the margin of his copy of the Aldine, now in the University Library at Jena. Although he had purchased his copy in September 1532, he did not set down his conjectures and emendations to this treatise until March 1544, from the ninth until the twelfth. He knew the Basle edition, for he cites its readings either by name or simply as 'alii', but he makes no reference to any other commentator. Since elsewhere he carefully lists the sources of some emendations in his introductory title to each tract, e. g. Fuchs, Leonicenus and Guinther, I conclude that the editions of 1540–1542 were unknown to him.[1] Nevertheless, despite the speed with which his annotations were inscribed, their quality reveals his high ability and confirms the eulogies of later scholars. He uses Niccolò's version well: e. g. 68,16 οὗτοι LNMAAld.: ipsi Nic.: αὐτοὶ Corn.; 114,11 τυροῦ LMAld.: om. Nic. Corn., and his own emendations are impressive: e. g. 92,3 ποιοῦντες LNMAld.: ποιοῦνται Corn.; 96,24 τὸ om. LNMAld.: add. Corn., and are often confirmed by the evidence of manuscripts unknown to him: e. g. 98,3 βλαπτόμενον PCorn.: βλαπτομένου yAld.; 98,20 κατεσχισμένα PCorn.: κατεχημένα M: κατισχημένα L: κατεσχημένα Ald.; 140,25 τῶν ἑταίρων τινὶ LNMCorn.: τινὶ om. Ald. His diagnosis of the difficulties of the text is often as important as his solution, for he was the first Greek scholar to attack seriously the corruptions of the later sections of this treatise, e. g. 142,2 ἐμοι τοῦ LNM: μὴ διὰ τὴν τοῦ Corn. The violence of some of his conjectures should not obscure the merits of his work, which in its fecundity is a reproach to successive editors, who slavishly reproduced the Basle edition, and an encouragement to modern scholars. His death robbed the world of the edition of Galen he had long projected, and postponed for three centuries or more the production of even competent texts of Galen.

A different problem is raised by the series of marginalia written by Joseph Justus Scaliger into his copy of the Aldine, now preserved at Wolfenbüttel.[2] Since few of the Renaissance editors of Galen have

[1] Since I was able to see Cornarius' notes at Jena, I have made no use of the fallible production of C. G. Gruner, Iani Cornarii coniecturae et emendationes Galenicae, Jena 1789, or of the transcript of them referred to by V. Gardthausen, Katalog der griechischen Handschriften der Universitätsbibliothek zu Leipzig, Leipzig 1898, Ms. gr. 58. On Cornarius, see Biographie Universelle IX, Paris 1813, pp. 597ff.; J. Mewaldt, CMG V 9,1, pp. XXIff.; O. Clemen, Janus Cornarius, Neues Archiv f. Sächsische Geschichte 33, 1912, pp. 36–76; T. O. Achelis, Zu Janus Cornarius, ibid. 34, 1913, pp. 163f.; E. Wenkebach, Pseudogalenische Kommentare zu den Epidemien des Hippokrates, Abh. d. Preuß. Akad. d. Wiss. 1917, phil.-hist. Kl. 1, 1917, pp. 8–12, 53f.; and P. Uhlig, Auf der Suche nach Stadtärzten, Sudhoffs Archiv f. Gesch. d. Med. u. d. Naturwiss. 31, 1938, p. 335.

[2] Now Cod. Gud. 8 lat.: for some of the history of this volume see F. Koehler and G. Milchsack, Die Gudischen Handschriften (Marquard Gude), Wolfenbüttel 1913 (repr. Frankfurt a. M. 1966), p. 81. A copy of these notes was transcribed in the late eighteenth or early nineteenth century in four volumes and is still preserved at Leipzig, V. Gardthausen, Katalog, ms. gr. 57.

any claim to be recognised as philologists of the first rank, the annotations of a man who was the greatest scholar of his age have demanded pious citation and approval. Not all have concurred. Wenkebach dismissed them thus[1]: "quo impensius illius coniectaneis studium impertiendum putavi, eo segnius huius mihi videbantur tractari posse emendationes in Aldinae Guelferbytanae marginibus adscriptae, ut quae nobis per haec quidem commentaria nulli fere essent usui; . . . omnia divinationem meram viri docti litterarum renatarum aetatis redolere sentiebam." My estimate of their value is the same as Wenkebach's, but for a totally different reason. Far from displaying the learning of a Renaissance scholar and emendations divined by the "smoky fire of Scaliger's genius", they reveal another side of the abilities of that great critic. "Um Handschriften hat er sich eifrig bemüht." Thus Wilamowitz praised him[2], and, indeed, his Galeniana are, as far as concerns this treatise, little more than the variant readings offered by A. The proof is simple: almost every variant given by A, with the exception of 78,20 and 21 ἄπεμπτον and 88,5 θεραπεύειν, is recorded by Scaliger, even when they are clearly wrong: 78,23 πέψαι] πέμψαι A Scal.; 88,19 ἀκριβῶς om. A Scal., and his last annotation, at 96,5, ἔσχον Ald.: ἔσχεν LNMA Scal., occurs shortly before A breaks off at 96,15.[3] There can thus be no doubt that he had seen and used A, possibly during one of his Italian visits around 1565, and great care must be taken to distinguish manuscript variants, which may or may not have been accepted by the critic, from the emendations which rest upon the authority of their maker. The latter number only seven: 70,11 οὖν] γοῦν Scal.; 70,22 πρώτη LNMAAld.: πρῶτον Scal.; 72,19 μάλιστα μὲν καὶ πρῶτον LNMAld.: πρῶτον μὲν καὶ μάλιστα A: μάλιστα πρῶτον μὲν καὶ Scal.; 76,24 ante μετὰ add. τὴν A, τῇ Scal.; 80,13 ἀπεφηνάμην] ἀποκρινάμενος Scal.; 82,17 γνώσεσθαι] γνώσοντες Scal.; 84,19 ἀφικέσθαι] ἀφικεῖσθαι Scal., of which only those at 72,19 and 76,24 merit serious consideration. If any praise is to be given to Scaliger for his suggestions, it is not for his conjectural ability, which falls far below that of Gemusaeus and Cornarius, but for his discovery and use, albeit uncritical, of another manuscript to set against the Aldine: among the early Galenists, he alone returned to the manuscripts.

I have also used the marginalia of H. Schöne, which are preserved in the CMG Archive in Berlin and which include suggestions for com-

[1] CMG V 10,2,1, p. XXVI.

[2] U. von Wilamowitz-Moellendorff, Geschichte der Philologie. Einleitung in die Altertumswissenschaft I, 1, Leipzig/Berlin 1921, p. 24.

[3] It must be stressed that my observations apply only to this treatise and that I have not compared the annotations in other treatises with A. But note the view of K. Koch, Berliner Philologische Wochenschrift 32, 1912, p. 1217, referring to De usu partium: "Diese Bemerkungen . . . sind zwar z. T. Korrekturen oder nur Inhaltsangaben, z. T. aber Kollationen guter Hss. . . . jedenfalls stimmen die Lesarten vielfach mit Helmreichs cod. A überein . . ." (A = Paris, Bibliothèque Nationale, fonds gr. 2253).

ment as well as for the improvement of the text. He produced conjectures for over seventy places, often where Cornarius had gone before, of which I choose two examples: 88,16 φίλος LNMAedd.: φιλόσοφος Schöne; 142,2 ἐμοὶ τοῦ κατὰ γνώμην LNMedd.: ἐμαυτοῦ καταγνοίην Schöne. I have noted his suggestions in the apparatus, even when I have discounted them in the text, for his long familiarity with Galen and his fine intelligence rarely led him to conjectures that were entirely frivolous.

Four other scholars must be mentioned briefly for their work on 'On prognosis'. The Dutchman C. G. Cobet amassed and published a large number of conjectures on Galen, although his successes here were few, basing them, not upon manuscripts, but upon his great familiarity with Attic prose authors, which in consequence led him to over-estimate the Atticism of Galen's style.[1] More recently, W. Müri edited two sections, 90,6–92,32 and 126,16–130,10, together with a German translation and notes in his anthology of Greek medical writings, but, apart from improving the punctuation, he brought little benefit to the text.[2] The last scholar to have dealt in any detail with any portion of this treatise, H. Baumgarten, in his commentary on the fragments of the lost Galenic tract 'On the voice', made five changes in the small amount of text he edited, of which one, at 98,24, ἡ add. Baumgarten, was a correction of a misprint in Kühn, and two, at 98,1 and 98,19, almost certainly correct.[3] Finally, no English translator of Galen can fail to acknowledge the merits as a translator of A. J. Brock[4]: how much I owe to his witty and lucid version is only too apparent.[5]

1 Ad Galenum, Mnemosyne, n. s. 13, 1885, pp. 12f.: his emendations are at 76,29; 94,5; 118,4 (ἀναγομένην, like N); 124,25 (ἀγγελοῦντας, wrongly); 126,12 (ἔδοξεν for ἔταξεν, a correction of Kühn's error); and a change in the punctuation at 68,8.

2 W. Müri, Der Arzt im Altertum, ed. 3, Munich 1962, pp. 50–59; 128,27 is his only sure emendation, although those at 90,29 and 92,12 are possible if Galen always wrote good Attic Greek.

3 H. Baumgarten, Galen, Über die Stimme, Diss. Göttingen 1962, pp. 102f. His other two changes, at 96,27 and 98,24, indicate the problems there without providing a certain solution.

4 A. J. Brock, Greek Medicine, London 1929, pp. 200–220 being a version of 68,3–82,2; 82,17–92,32; 100,15–104,15; 120,16–126,7; 126,16–128,30; and 134,9–138,4. Through the kindness of Prof. K. Deichgräber I have been able to use the unpublished German translation of J. Ilberg, which has occasionally been helpful in locating difficulties.

5 The annotations inscribed by N. Moranghelli of Viadana, flor. 1569, in his copy of Jacchinus' edition, now in the University Library, Cambridge, although of interest for the medical and social conditions of the time, are of little value in the reconstruction of the text. The same applies to the comments of A. Lopez de Corella, In omnia opera Galeni annotationes, Saragossa 1565, pp. 106ff. Although Leo Allatius scribbled annotations prolifically throughout his copy of the Basle edition, now in the Sudhoff Institut in Leipzig, he made no comment upon or emendation to 'On prognosis'.

C. The treatise

I. Authenticity

Galen refers four times directly and possibly once indirectly to a treatise he composed upon prognosis and to incidents described therein. At In Hipp. Progn. comm. I 8 (CMG V 9,2, p. 219,4), after mentioning briefly the celebrated tale of Erasistratus and the love-sick prince, he refers to his own discovery of a man's infatuation by taking his pulse and to his fuller exposition of the case in 'On prognosis'. The same incident, which concerned a woman, not a man, is also noted at In Hipp. Epid. libr. II comm. II (CMG V 10,1, p. 208, 28) and In Hipp. Epid. libr. VI comm. VIII (CMG V 10,2,2, p. 495,2), where there is a brief discussion of the physical symptoms produced by certain mental states. At In Hipp. Progn. comm. III 42 (CMG V 9,2, p. 369,23) he talks about the various signs which either indicate the future course of a disease or are present naturally in the body and are therefore harmless, among which he includes an intermittent pulse, about which he has said more in 'On prognosis'. Finally, in Über die medizinischen Namen (p. 21,20 M.), after describing how he has come to be regarded as a magician and wonder-worker as a result of his prognostic cures, he attacks the ignorance of many of his opponents: "zu anderen Zeiten leugnen sie, daß (überhaupt) einer der Ärzte in einem Buche etwas über die Prognose der zukünftigen Entwicklung des Falles eines Kranken geschrieben habe." But, although there are several close verbal parallels between 'On prognosis' and Über die medizinischen Namen[1], the doctor referred to here is only possibly Galen, and the argument in favour of authenticity must rest upon the other four citations. All the incidents and problems there mentioned occur also in this treatise: the story of Galen's cure of the love-sick wife comes furnished with appropriate Erasistratean trimmings at 100,7–102,28, and his treatment of the man with the naturally intermittent pulse is the concluding case in the book, 138,13–142,14.

Only one objection can be brought against the identification of this treatise with that mentioned by Galen with a similar title; the absence of any reference to it in the lists of his writings, under the heading either of prognostic or of therapeutic works (Scr. min. II,

[1] Compare Über die medizinischen Namen, p. 20,21 M. with 68,3–21, 90,10–92,5, and 110,16. That the doctor in question was not Galen is suggested by a reference at De diff. puls. II 10 (VIII, p. 635,4f. K.) to Über die medizinischen Namen as already completed, since undoubtedly De diff. puls. preceded 'On prognosis' (cf. 132,28; 140,4). But it is very likely that the reference in De diff. puls. is a later addition, coming, as it does, right at the end of Book II, and thus it is still possible to believe that Über die medizinischen Namen followed, or at least was written at the same time as, 'On prognosis'.

pp. 109,4–111,8 Müller = XIX, pp. 30,17–33,13 K.), but there is a simple reason for its exclusion (discussed below, p. 50) and the argument for authenticity remains compelling. Ḥunain, who was better acquainted than we with the corpus of Galen's writings, did not hesitate to include 'On prognosis' among the genuine works of Galen which were omitted from the 'Pinakes', and there is no cogent reason to dispute his opinion.[1]

II. Date of composition

At 100,2–6, after describing his anatomical demonstrations, Galen boasts that no one has dared to contradict his conclusions even though fifteen years have intervened. Since these exhibitions occurred during the spring and summer of 163, Ilberg concluded that 'On prognosis' was composed in the year 178.[2] This date was challenged by Bardong in his subtle re-dating of many Galenic writings, who argued for a date of composition early in 177[3]: "Aber im Jahr 177 befand sich Galen immerhin im 15. Jahr, und nichts ist natürlicher, als daß er nach oben auf volle 15 Jahre abrundet, zumal er stets das Bestreben hat, möglichst viel zu seinen Gunsten herauszuholen."[4] A choice between the two dates is not easy. By placing 'On prognosis' early in 177 Bardong was able to spread the dates of other Galenic treatises over a slightly longer period, but to suggest that it was written early in the year, before even fourteen years had elapsed, stretches the evidence unduly. Ilberg's interpretation fits the Greek better, and 'On prognosis' may thus be dated to 178 or, with less likelihood, to late 177 or even early 179.[5]

Bardong's essay was written too early to profit greatly from the information given in the Arabic version of In Hipp. Epid. libr. VI comm. VIII (CMG V 10,2,2, p. 495,2–12), which has consequently remained unknown. In Pfaff's translation it reads: "Da schrieb ich über diese Prognose unter diesem Titel ein Buch. Leider verbrannte dieses Buch kurz nach seiner Vollendung bei dem großen Brand, bei dem der sogenannte Friedenstempel abbrannte, zusammen mit vielen anderen Büchern, welche auch verbrannt sind. Ich hoffe noch immer, eine Abschrift von der einen oder der anderen Schrift wieder zu finden,

[1] G. Bergsträßer, Neue Materialien zu Ḥunain Ibn Isḥāq's Galen-Bibliographie, Abhandlungen für die Kunde des Morgenlandes 19,2, 1932, p. 94: "Was die Wissenschaft der Prognostik anlangt, so haben wir (darüber) von ihm ein einziges Buch gefunden, nämlich (n. 147) Über prognostische Merkwürdigkeiten" *(nawādir taqdimat al-ma'rifa)*.

[2] J. Ilberg, Schriftstellerei, II, Rheinisches Museum 47, pp. 493, 497: on the date of the exhibitions, see the commentary on p. 187.

[3] K. Bardong, Beiträge, pp. 609f.

[4] Ibid., p. 610, n. 1.

[5] D. W. Peterson, Observations on the chronology of the Galenic Corpus, Bull. Hist. Med. 51, 1977, p. 488, argues for 178 or early 179.

welche sich in den Händen von Schülern befindet, die sie abgeschrieben haben. Deshalb habe ich eine neue Abfassung dieses Buches immer noch zurückgestellt. Ich schiebe also die Neuabfassung dieser verbrannten Bücher noch auf."[1] We know from Cassius Dio (LXXIII, 24,1) and Herodian (I,14,2) that the great fire which destroyed the Templum Pacis occurred just before the assassination of Commodus, that is about 192, but can such a date be said to be "kurz nach seiner Vollendung", if on other evidence 'On prognosis' appears to have been completed some fourteen years earlier? Ancient authors are notoriously vague about chronology and, although events may be narrated in sequence, the distances between them are often distorted. Galen is no exception: at De libr. propr. 2 (Scr. min. II, p. 98,13 Müller = XIX, p. 17,16 K.) a period of at least a year, and possibly two, is telescoped into the adverb, εὐθέως, and thus one of fourteen years could easily be denoted by "shortly afterwards". Much more serious is Galen's assertion that he could find no surviving copy of this treatise on which to base a second edition. Two questions immediately arise: to what date does this statement belong; and have we in this text of 'On prognosis' a later re-writing of an earlier treatise? No definite answer can be given to the first question, except to recall that, by accepting Suidas' date of death for Galen, 199, Bardong was compelled to bunch several works into the period 192–199 which, on the Arabic date of Galen's death, c. 215, could be spread out over some fifteen more years. But, if we assume with Bardong that, shortly after 192, Galen could not find a copy of this treatise in existence, we must decide how the present treatise came to be preserved. Is it a new edition or the fortunate survival of the original? Galen, we know, was always adding cross-references and tinkering with the text of tracts already in public circulation. 'Anatomical Procedures', of which the first eleven books were already published when the Templum Pacis was burnt, contains several indications that additions were made to the text after it had been distributed to his friends.[2] It is therefore strange that in 'On prognosis' there are no hints of similar additions: we are not told of Alexander's philosophical chair at Athens (Anat. admin. I 1: II, p. 218,6–8 K.), and the prosopographical references and the style of the polemic are consistent with a date of composition in the seventies rather than with one some twenty years or more later. I conclude that 'On prognosis', as we have it, was written in 178 and that a copy of it still existed after the fire of 192, although unknown to Galen, who, because he found no trace of it, made no mention of it in the catalogue of his own writings. As he tells us in his preface (De libr. propr. prooem.: Scr. min. II, p. 92,4–24 Müller = XIX, pp. 9,13–10,14 K.), he wrote De libris propriis to authenticate the treatises circu-

[1] Pfaff thought that the references here and at In Hipp. Epid. libr. II comm. II (CMG V 10,1, p. 208,28) were to the fragment preserved at XIX, pp. 497–511 K., but, as I have shown above, they are to this treatise.

[2] K. Bardong, Beiträge, pp. 615f.

lating under his name, and there was thus little point in including a tract which, as far as he knew, had disappeared completely.

III. The second part of 'On prognosis'

All the surviving Latin manuscripts are divided into two parts, the first being 'On prognosis', the second bearing the title at a fol. 179ᵛ and d fol. 1ʳ of 'De cautelis ad recte pronosticandum obseruandis et recto regimine uerutrorum (neutrorum d) tam decidentis (decidentie a) quam conualescentis (conualescentie a)'; and at b fol. 184ᵛ of 'Secunda pars de pronosticatione'; and being marked off by a space at c fol. 134ᵛ and e fol. 77ᵛ. Its incipit is: De pronosticatione igitur consequenter dicimus quoniam utilis nobis; and its explicit is: et adhuc (adhanc e) passionum inuentionem similiter. fecit et eos qui secundum singulam earum modos sanationis (singula eorum ce: singulam eorum b). No trace of it is found in the Greek manuscripts L and M, which continue with De temp. morb., or in the defective A and V, but the collection of extracts in P and W retains an identical arrangement, which proves that the juxtaposition of these two parts was not due to the Latin translator but already existed in a Greek source. The excerpts in P and W can be identified as coming from the smaller treatise 'On prognosis', first edited by Chartier from Paris, Bibliothèque Nationale, fonds grec 2269, and printed by Kühn, XIX, pp. 497–511, they are respectively: pp. 501,15–502,3; p. 502,8–16; pp. 502,18–503,12; p. 504,9–11; p. 507,6–10; and p. 508,2–9. But, as K. Kalbfleisch showed[1], this is not an independent treatise but an excerpt from the larger De constitutione artis medicae (I, pp. 289,1–304,3 K.) which was separated from the main body of the treatise, possibly as early as the time of Oribasius, and thenceforth enjoyed an existence in its own right. At a later date it was attracted in some manuscripts to the larger treatise of the same name and subject, to which it served as a second part or as an appendix.[2] Since the translator presumably found it already united with 'On prognosis' in his Greek source, he made no separate translation of it, and thus there is no Latin version recorded in Diels' Katalog, p. 112. The conjunction of the two tracts was not universal, as we have seen, and Ḥunain, who describes 'On prognosis' as a single book (above, p. 49, n. 1) was using a manuscript which contained only the first part.

The list of chapter headings in bad is as follows:

Cap. primum in quo premittit quedam necessario attendenda in pronosticatione (attendenda . . . quedam ad; necessaria ad, fol. 7ᵛ).

[1] K. Kalbfleisch, Zu Galenos, Berliner Philologische Wochenschrift 16, 1896, pp. 59f.; see also G. Helmreich, Zu Galenos, ibid., pp. 317f.

[2] On the ease with which this could happen to technical treatises, see above, p. 13.

Cap. ii in quo presupponendo possibilitatem pronosticationis ponit considerationes attendendas circa eius certificationem (rectificationem ad).

Cap. iii in quo remouens quandam opinionem falsam et dans rectum modum circa pronosticationem declarat intentiones quibus debet medicus attendere ut recte pronosticet (ut sit pronosticus ba, fol. 198^{v}).

Cap. iv in quo ponit considerationes que ad intentiones predictas perducunt (dictas in precedenti capitulo b).

Cap. v de intentione preseruatiue (perseuerantie d) et noticia eorum que accidunt hiis qui subserpunt ad egritudines (et – egritudines *om.* b).

Cap. vi de correctione quarundam dispositionum et sinthomatum pertinente ad preseruatiuam (preseruatiua d; symptomatum. que curatio pertinet ad preseruatiuam b).

Cap. vii de intentione resumptiue (resumptione d) cum methodo totius (tocius d) opere sanatiue (cum – sanatiue *om.* b).

Cap. viii in quo quia medicina est ars comparat eam ad alias artes ostendendo in quibus cōicat (communicat?) et in quibus differt ab eis quantum ad eius constōnem (constructionem? *vel* constitutionem?) b: in quo comparat medicatiuam cum sit ars ad artes ostendendo in quibus conuenit et differt ab eis quantum ad eius constructionem (constrictionem d: constructionem eius a, fol. 201^{v}) ad.

IV. Transmission and influence

It is impossible to specify at what point and by what means this treatise, which Galen himself believed lost, survived and was incorporated in the Corpus Galenicum, although in view of the spread of Galenic writings in his lifetime (cf. De loc. affect. IV 2: VIII, p. 224,9 K.) it is not difficult to conjecture that a copy survived in the provinces and was re-integrated in the mass of his writings during the third century [1], or possibly not until the time of Oribasius.[2] The evidence of Oribasius is equivocal. In his discussion of the feminine flux in his Synopsis ad Eunapium (IV 111: CMG VI 3, p. 487,1–25) he makes no mention of the cure of Boethus' wife, yet in that in the Synopsis ad Eustathium (IX 46: CMG VI 3, p. 306,1–12), although depending largely in lines 1–7 on De sympt. caus. III 11 (VII, p. 265,10–17 K.), he quotes at lines 8–12 from 114,20–23 and 116,3–5, without acknowledging his source. It is possible that in the course of his search for rare or missing Galenic works (cf. RE Suppl. VII, 1940, cols. 805–807, s. v. Oreibasios) he discovered a copy of this

[1] On the formation of the Galenic corpus, see F. Kudlien, The third century A. D., in L. G. Stevenson and R. P. Multhauf, Medicine, science and culture, Baltimore 1968, pp. 25–34.

[2] The similarity between 108,22–24 and Marcellinus, De pulsib. 20ff. Schöne, is not enough to prove dependence either way.

tract, from which he excerpted an important therapeutic prescription into his latest synthesis. Of the later encyclopaedists, Aëtius (Tetrabibl. XVI 67) has only the section from the Synopsis ad Eunapium, but Paulus (III 62: CMG IX 1, pp. 278,24–279,25) conflates both sections almost verbatim. At what date the second part was added to 'On prognosis' remains uncertain, but its absence from L and M may indicate that it was at a late stage in the tradition.

It is interesting also to speculate on the origin of the gloss at 142,5–8, for ἀπὸ στόματός μου suggests either a didactic commentary or at least advice given to a mediaeval copyist.[1] The fact that the gloss is itself wrong – for the work in question is 'On prognosis' – leads me to favour the first interpretation and suggests that, at some point, this passage was discussed and interpreted by a teacher of medicine.[2]

It is a relief to turn from shadowy possibilities to the accuracy of the Arabic scholars. In his list of the treatises of Galen and their translations Ḥunain ibn Isḥāq records this tract under the title 'On remarkable cases of prognosis', *Nawādir taqdimat al-maʿrifa,* with these comments[3]: "This treatise consists of a single book, in which he encourages the practice of prognosis and teaches sophisticated techniques leading to it, and also describes the wondrous things that he foresaw and predicted from the patients' states of health and for which he gained public admiration. Ayyūb translated it into Syriac. I had a Greek manuscript with me but I had no time to translate it. Then I turned it into Syriac. ʿĪsā ibn Yaḥyā made a version of it for Abū l-Ḥasan which satisfied me." A later writer adds, "He (Ḥunain) collated it (ʿĪsā's version) with the original (Greek) almost entirely, and this collation was afterwards completed by his son, Isḥāq." Ibn an-Nadīm and Ibn al-Qifṭī preserve similar notices, almost certainly deriving from Ḥunain, except that both entitle this tract 'On prognosis'.[4] These ninth century versions, first into Syriac and then from Syriac into Arabic, have not survived entire, although traces of the Arabic can be discerned that bear Ḥunain's title.

The first Arab author who quotes from 'On prognosis', as opposed to merely referring to its existence, is Isḥāq ibn ʿAlī ar-Ruhāwī, a fellow townsman of the translator Ayyūb ar-Ruhāwī, who composed

[1] M. Richard, Ἀπὸ φωνῆς, Byzantion 20, 1950, pp. 191–222, esp. pp. 204–212.

[2] C. D. Pritchet, Johannis Alexandrini Commentaria in Sextum Librum Hippocratis Epidemiarum, Leyden 1975, was wrong to see an allusion to this tract at p. 116 = 128 A, 46f.

[3] G. Bergsträßer, Ḥunain ibn Isḥāq, Über die syrischen und arabischen Galen-Übersetzungen, Abhandlungen für die Kunde des Morgenlandes 17,2, 1925, p. 27. The translation was made for me by Dr. Strohmaier after collating this edition with Ms. Aya Sofya 3631.

[4] Ibn an-Nadīm, *Fihrist,* p. 289 Flügel = p. 684 Dodge; Ibn al-Qifṭī, *Ta'rīḫ al-ḥukamā',* p. 130 Lippert; cf. L. Leclerc, Histoire de la médecine arabe, Paris 1876, p. 246, and M. Steinschneider, Virchows Archiv 124, 1891, p. 288 (repr. in: Die arabischen Übersetzungen aus dem Griechischen, Graz 1960, p. [340]).

his *Adab aṭ-ṭabīb* towards the close of the ninth century.[1] Unlike his successors, who were content to paraphrase and abbreviate, he includes large sections, keeping close to the original Greek as far as can be seen, and citing the case of the wife of Iustus (p. 71a Levey = fol. 79b = 100,15–104,23), the envy of the physicians at Galen's cures of Eudemus and Charilampes (p. 72a Levey = fol. 81a = 94,4f.) and the case of the frightened steward (p. 90a Levey = fol. 105b = 102,27–104,8). The most interesting quotation by far is that of the prologue, 68,3–14, which is given at length (pp. 88f. = fol. 103b) and which makes no further appearance in later authors.[2] It is unfortunately impossible to tell whether he is using the Arabic version of ʿĪsā ibn Yaḥyā or translating himself from the Syriac either of Ayyūb or of Ḥunain and his son, whom he mentions twice (pp. 23a and 84a Levey = fols. 10a and 98a), simply because not enough comparative material is available.[3] Ar-Ruhāwī's interests in this work are in medical ethics; those of later authors more in practical medicine, and thus the passages cited do not overlap. It is important to see just how much of 'On prognosis' he quotes, far more than any other author, and how, in dealing with medical ethics, he uses the authority of this Galenic treatise to buttress his own solutions.

At the same time as ar-Ruhāwī was preaching about ethics, ar-Rāzī was compiling his great medical encyclopaedia, *Kitābu l-ḥāwī*, which in the Latin version of Faraghius, Liber continens, transmitted much Arabic learning to the West. 'On prognosis' is cited twenty-two times within it[4], mostly in a compressed or abbreviated form which reduces the value of the citations for the establishment of the true Galenic text. Many of them can be swiftly identified: two refer to the case of Sextus (XVII, 96,9; XVIII, 218,10), two to that of the man relieved by an involuntary nose-bleed (III, 76,20; XVIII, 46,11), four to that of Boethus' wife (VII, 185,1; IX, 3,1; 53,5; XVI, 217,3),

1 Translated with an introduction by M. Levey, Medical ethics of mediaeval Islam with special reference to Al-Ruhawi's 'Practical ethics of the physician', Transactions of the American Philosophical Society, n. s. 57,3, 1967; but note the justly severe review by J. C. Bürgel, Gött. Gelehrte Anzeig. 220, 1968, pp. 215–227, cf. idem, Die Bildung des Arztes, Sudhoffs Archiv f. Gesch. d. Med. u. d. Naturwiss. 50, 1966, pp. 337–360.

2 It is impossible from Levey's translation to be sure either of where the quotation ends or of the exact Greek text represented by the Arabic version. A better translation was made for me by Dr. Bürgel.

3 Dr. Bürgel informs me that he thinks it likely that ar-Ruhāwī, as elsewhere, made his own translation, but the proof is not conclusive.

4 The references are given, to varying degrees of accuracy, by M. Ullmann, p. 69, and by F. Sezgin, Geschichte des arabischen Schrifttums, III, Leyden 1970, pp. 114f. Dr. Strohmaier provided me with the reference to VII, 185,1, and with a German translation of it and Dr. Iskandar kindly translated for me the references at III, 76,20; V, 80,9; XVIII, 46,11; and XXIII B, 214,7. I have as yet been unable to verify the brief reference to 'On prognosis' given by an Istanbul Ms., Nuruosmaniye 3553, fol. 15b, in a collection of prognoses from Hippocrates and Galen, cf. A. Dietrich, Medicinalia Arabica, Göttingen 1966, p. 29.

five to that of Eudemus (XVI, 101,5; 113,6; 123,16; XVII, 219,12; XIX, 138, paen.) and five to that of Marcus Aurelius (V, 80,9; 111,6; XIV, 14,8; XVII, 39,10; 42,13). Four others present greater difficulties. XIV, 47, ult. reports Galen as saying, "If a man is attacked by fever, one should try to discover what type it is (?), and, if not, he should keep a light diet until the fourth day is past, refrain from bathing and heavy work, and eat nothing on the day of the next attack until the hour of the attack is past." As it stands, this passage cannot be found in 'On prognosis', unless it is taken as a paraphrase of some of the instructions given to Eudemus by Galen and others, 74,20–24, which ar-Rāzī has forced into his own pattern for his own purposes.

The references at XVI, 198,5 (repeated in his 'Clinical Observations', ed. M. Meyerhof, Thirty-three clinical observations by Rhazes, Isis 23, 1935, p. 340 and p. 354), to a collyrium and at XXIII B, 214,7, to the red hair of fishermen could not be identified, but the fourth citation at XIX, 175,4–183,6, comes in fact from Galen's 'Commentary on the Prognosticum', CMG V 9,2, pp. 279,19–289,14.

Only two extracts offer readings significantly different from those of the Greek Mss. At XIX, 138, paen. (= 80,11), ar-Rāzī's *ḥabasa* (= σωθῆναι) confirms the suggestion of the Renaissance translators, seruari, for the Mss. ἐαθῆναι but the second extract, VII, 185, 1–17, demands fuller quotation and discussion. It reads as follows:

"From 'Remarkable cases of prognosis': A woman had an issue of watery blood. She was cured by the following treatment, which can be applied also to sufferers from dropsy although it is particularly for an issue of blood. I gave her a hydragogic potion and then a decoction of celery and asarabacca for three days, then the hydragogic potion again, then the decoction for three days, and then the hydragogic potion again. I began to rub her with cloths and to anoint her body with honey that had first been heated and then cooled to an appropriate degree. She recovered in fifteen days. Anointing with honey removes moisture, especially if it is well heated until it becomes thick; then it is cooled and applied. As a substitute one may use walks and burial in hot sand, a hot dry bath, etcetera. However, repeated purges, the removal of urine and a dry diet is the best treatment, when possible, for sufferers from dropsy. It is possible that the patient can be purged and his urine removed without any heat, but a presupposition of this treatment, should it ever be repeated, is the increasing of physical strength through potable drugs and the like, so that purgation does not diminish the patient's strength, and the dressing of the liver, for two hours a day after digestion, with whatever strengthens it, and of the stomach with a styptic drug. This treatment is always successful. However, it is true that dropsy results from a hard swelling in the liver: so, even though the water is dried up, the cause of the dropsy is not removed unless this hard tumour goes away. Nonetheless, it is necessary for the tumour to be treated first by drying up the water, then it drains itself away."

This passage can be divided into two parts, each with its particular problem. Down to 'etcetera', much can be traced to Galen: 1–2 = 112,14; 4–7 = 116,3–10; 7–11 = 114,21f.; 11 = 114,15, and the rest, with one exception, can be attributed to ar-Rāzī's method of commenting upon a Galenic extract. The exception is line 6. At 116,3–10, the Greek mentions only two draughts of the potion and only one application of the decoction over a period of three days, not three and two respectively, as the Arabic has. Does ar-Rāzī here preserve a passage missing from the Greek or have we a doublet that occurred either in the Greek or the Arabic transmission? Since there is no trace of the longer version in either Oribasius or Paulus, I conclude that we have a scribal doublet, not a new line of Galen. From line 12 onwards, there is nothing corresponding in the Greek tradition, and it is possible that we have a new fragment of Galen. But this possibility seems to me to be remote, partly because I find no immediately suitable place for it to fit into and partly because it reads like a commentator's addition to and correction of his chosen text, cf. XVII, 219,12–220,2, although ar-Rāzī's comments are usually briefer. Besides, in contrast to Galen's leisurely exposition of his methods in 'On prognosis', this excerpt resembles more the compilations of the later encyclopaedists, who brought together in one place treatments of similar diseases.

Even if, as I believe, the second half of this extract belongs to ar-Rāzī rather than to Galen, it is not without value, for it illustrates the lengths to which the Arab would go in emulating and supplementing his Greek predecessor. Even the literary form influenced him, as can be seen in his 'Clinical observations' or, in the mediaeval Latin version, 'De mirabilibus que ei acciderunt in medicina', where thirty three cases are selected and described.[1] It is true that the tradition of case histories goes back to Hippocrates, but the model here is more likely to have been Galen, since the methods of treatment and the insistence on the merits of the author, described at length in 'On prognosis', are given greater emphasis than in the Hippocratic Epidemics, which concentrate more on the disease. Besides, the title recalls one of the Arabic names for 'On prognosis' (above, p. 53) and since ar-Rāzī elsewhere uses as his stylistic models other Galenic tracts, some of which are lost to us[2], there can be little doubt that he is adapting the formal arrangement of 'On prognosis' to his own use. In this he had no successor, for I know of no author whose case-histo-

[1] M. Meyerhof, Thirty-three clinical observations by Rhazes, Isis 23, 1935, pp. 321–372; O. Temkin, A medieval translation of Rhazes' clinical observations, Bull. Hist. Med. 12, 1942, pp. 102–117.

[2] In his 'Spiritual physick', he relies upon the lost works 'On the avoidance of grief', pp. 68–74 tr. Arberry, and 'Good men profit from their enemies', p. 37 tr. Arberry. Cf. Walzer, GA, pp. 15ff.

ries go back so clearly to the Galenic rather than the Hippocratic model.[1]

The celebrated biographer, Ibn abī Uṣaibiʿa, also knew this work, for he twice refers to Galen's cure of Boethus' wife (I, p. 85,14–18; p. 97,23–25 Müller), and quotes in a somewhat garbled form from Galen's account of his cure of the lovesick wife of Iustus (II, p. 128,15–22 Müller). It is clear from the manner in which he comments on 'On prognosis' that he had read it for himself and had not obtained his information at second hand.

It would be pleasant to associate this treatise with another great oriental physician, Maimonides, whose Aphorisms, in the Basle Latin edition of 1579, XVI 28, pp. 356–358, give an extended quotation summarising in two parts the cure of the wife of Boethus, 110,13–116, 19. But this edition, which in its preface claimed to do no more than polish and emend the Latin of earlier versions, is an "arbitrary forgery"[2], and there is no reference to 'On prognosis' in the earlier Hebrew version[3]. If Maimonides knew this tract, he made no use of it in any extant writing. This is scarcely surprising, for its influence was minimal, even on the Arabic biographers, who prefer the notices given by Galen in Anat. admin. and in the Pinakes, and it was only used by a physician such as ar-Ruhāwī, whose interests were not only in medicine, and by scholars such as ar-Rāzī and Ibn abī Uṣaibiʿa, whose knowledge of Galen was far broader than normal. Not being one of the major technical treatises, 'On prognosis' was left in obscurity to be studied only by an expert or an eccentric.

There is even less evidence for its use in the West and in Byzantium. It was not included in the early Western canon of Galen's writings, and the whole tradition of Prognostica Galieni, both in Latin and in the vernacular, derives from Hippocrates, not from Galen.[4] The scholar-physician, Bernard Gordon, who wrote his Compendium pronosticorum de crisi et criticis diebus in 1295, is well acquainted

[1] The cases cited by ar-Ruhāwī in the closing sections of his *Adab aṭ-ṭabīb* also reflect the influence of Galen. Dr. Iskandar reminds me of the *Kitāb an-Nawādir aṭ-ṭibbīya* of Ibn Māsawaih; cf. M. Ullmann, p. 113. Cf. also the literary reminiscences of other Galenic treatises collected by F. Rosenthal, Die arabische Autobiographie, Studia Arabica I, Rome 1937, pp. 5ff., 15f.

[2] M. Steinschneider, Die Hebräischen Übersetzungen des Mittelalters und die Juden als Dolmetscher, Berlin 1893, p. 766. See also J. O. Leibowitz, The Latin translations of Maimonides' Aphorisms, Koroth 21, 1973, pp. 273–281 and XCIII–XCIX.

[3] Edited by S. Muntner, Jerusalem 1959. Muntner provided a list of quotations contained in the Aphorisms in: Galenus' books listed by Maimonides in his Aphorismes (sic), Homenaje a Millas-Vallicrosa, Barcelona 1956, pp. 118–130.

[4] See Medical History 14, 1970, pp. 96–100. Later examples of the Prognostica Galieni in their first form are given in: Vatican, Palatinus lat. 1098, saec. 14, fol. 61^{v}; Cambridge, Gonville and Caius College, Ms. 97 (49), saec. 15, fol. 138^{v}; Berlin, Staatsbibliothek, Ms. Lat. 908 (fol. lat. 88), circa 1440, fol. 242vb; and possibly Erlangen, Universitätsbibliothek, Ms. Lat. 674, saec. 15, fol. 141^{v}; and in a vernacular translation, J. Follan, Festschrift für G. Eis, Stuttgart 1968, p. 35, citing Edinburgh, Ms. 329, fols. 203^{r}–204^{v}.

with such Galenic works as De crisibus, De diebus decretoriis and De praesagio ex pulsibus, but makes no reference to 'On prognosis'.[1] Even a text which at first sight appears to make great use of 'On prognosis', the Questio circa commentum Galieni per pronostica ubi dicit, ille medicus plures sanat de quo plures confidunt, Vatican, Palatinus latinus 1246, late fifteenth century, fols. 97^{v}–112^{v}, derives its discussion of 'species sensibilis' and the effects on the body of passions and outside stimuli, not from that treatise, but from Galen's commentary on the Prognosticum.[2] This is hardly surprising, for this commentary was among the earliest works of Galen to be translated into Latin and it retained a much greater popularity than did 'On prognosis', as its manuscripts show.[3] The author of this Questio may have known both treatises, but this is impossible to prove from the internal evidence of the commentary.

The last reference to be noted fittingly unites both the Arabic and the Western traditions. Nicolaus de Leonardis of Venice, doctor of arts and medicine at the University of Padua and the annotator of Ms. c, adds in the margin at fol. 130rb that the title of the treatise in Latin is wrong: ego uero dico hunc librum intitulari debere liber de proverbiis pronosticorum. sic illum nominat Rasis 16 Continentis post principium per duas cartas. Nicolaus knew his Continens for the references in it to 'On prognosis' are to De proverbiis pronosticorum, and it is fitting that a Western physician with some claims to scholarship should use the work of an Arab to comment upon the translation of a Calabrian. At the same time the triviality of his comments does not speak highly of his intellectual abilities or of his sympathy with Galen.[4]

The paucity of references in both East and West, although they are scattered over five centuries, demonstrate a lack of interest in 'On prognosis', a treatise which, however important it might be for Galen's biography, could not impart much medical information to its readers and was for that reason neglected.

[1] K. Sudhoff, Zur Schriftstellerei Bernhards von Gordon und deren Zeitalter, Sudhoffs Archiv f. Gesch. d. Med. 10, 1917, pp. 168–171; L. Thorndike and P. Kibre, A catalogue of incipits of mediaeval scientific writings in Latin, ed. 2, Cambridge, Mass. 1963, col. 1428, to which add Oxford, Bodleian, Ms. Digby 46, saec. 14, fols. 64^{v}–99^{v}.

[2] The words medicus – confidunt belong to the 'antiqua versio' of the Commentary and are printed by Scipio Ferrarius in the margin of the Latin translation of Galen's Commentary in the Omnia Opera Galeni, Pavia 1516, III f.CXVI. The author is unknown, although it is possible that it was Taddeo (? Taddeo de Parma, fl. c. 1400; or even Taddeo Alderotti), the writer of a tract which precedes this commentary without a break. The fact that a plague tractate of 1467 opens the manuscript, fols. 1^{r}–70^{v}, is no indication of the age of the commentary.

[3] J. Heeg, CMG V 9,2, p. XXVIII.

[4] Two examples suffice: at fol. 132va (=108,11), construxisset tibi, Galiene, modica tela amplum mataratium; and at fol. 133rb (= 120,24), risus abundat in ore stultorum, dicerem, nec timerem ut mihi indignum videaretur medicina, ut supra dixi.

V. Form, style and language

Of all the writings of Galen 'On prognosis' offers the greatest links with other productions of the Second Sophistic Movement and an opportunity to study his ability and technique as a writer as opposed to a lecturer on medicine. Here, although clarity is one of his aims, literary reminiscences and the flowers of rhetoric often obscure much of the background to the cases he describes and reveal almost everything except the truth. Even when, as in the prologue, the exasperation of Galen appears to be genuine and his complaints to be justified, the commonplaces of popular philosophy and the phrases culled from Plato hint at the artifice that has gone into the passion and vividness of the writing. More than anywhere else in the corpus of his works Galen displays the value of his expensive education, the power of his rhetoric, and a talent for sophistic oratory that would rival any of his contemporaries. Brought up in a tradition of extempore displays of speaking by passing philosophers and rhetoricians and himself lecturing regularly in public on medicine and logic, he comes close at times to the style and language of a popular preacher. Aelius Aristeides' Hieroi logoi show a sophist's knowledge of medicine: 'On prognosis' shows a doctor's knowledge of sophistry.

It is not easy to fit this treatise into the traditional genres of literary criticism; its varied subjects, the combination of an autobiographic and a didactic purpose, the mixture of styles, all contribute to an impression of originality rare in an age when rhetorical creation on the basis of known models was the fashion.[1] Certain aspects can be isolated and identified, but the resultant whole remains an unusual and individual production.

Certainly Galen never thought of it as his autobiography; that was the tract 'On slander' (De libr. propr. 12: Scr. min. II, p. 122,2 Müller = XIX, p. 46,5 K.), even though there are many personal reminiscences recorded here, and even though their inclusion goes beyond the normal practice of doctors in referring to their own cases. They cited them sporadically; here the tract is based almost entirely upon such incidents. There can be little doubt of the formal model for such an exposition, the renowned Epidemics of Hippocrates, but there are great differences between the two. In the Epidemics the patient and his illness are always in the forefront: the doctor stands back to permit others to use his descriptions and to analyse the symptoms he describes. In 'On prognosis', where Galen's personality obtrudes strongly, such discussion upon the cases he gives is impossible and a general guide to medical prognosis is hard to find. The incidents described show that prognosis is possible; they rarely spell out how it is

[1] B. P. Reardon, p. 8. The following argument is pursued further by me in: Galen and medical autobiography, Proceedings of the Cambridge Philological Soc., n. s. 18, 1972, pp. 50–62.

to be attained. Nor are the cases themselves of medical interest or value – with the exception of that of the wife of Boethus – but they are selected and arranged to illustrate Galen's own merits rather than the disease, and their purpose is the furtherance of polemic, not of medicine. In this respect 'On prognosis' is akin to the justificatory commentarii of politicians and public men; it is designed to set the record straight, to offer a true version of events against the onslaughts of doubting opponents, and besides, every physician worth his salt, from Ctesias to Callimorphus[1], thought it right to give to the world his own unprejudiced view of the great deeds he was privileged to witness or perform.

But these literary precedents go only part of the way to explain the peculiar liveliness of this treatise, especially in the prologue, 68,3–74,11, and in the excursus put into the mouth of Eudemus, 90,8–92,20. Here we are in the realm of popular philosophy, the diatribe of the travelling orator or moralist, the extempore sermon denouncing the evils of society. Galen was only too well aware of such performances, having been educated and brought up at two of the great centres of the Sophistic movement, and the list of his writings shows that he did not shrink from indulging in moral homilies when the need arose.[2] His own emphasis on the moral qualities necessary for a doctor in his training and practice, on the need for a doctor to be a philosopher as well as a physician, led him naturally to discuss such topics in his medical writings and to condemn his opponents bitterly on moral grounds when they propounded theories that contradicted his own.[3] Ilberg, in his unpublished translation, also noted the heavy Platonizing tone of much of the treatise and connected it with the dialogue form. As Galen tells us himself, he not only summarised some of the Platonic dialogues but also, like many of his contemporaries, wrote dialogues himself.[4] The conversation between Galen and Eudemus, between Galen and Martianus, the lively scenes over Commodus demonstrate his fluency in this genre and a command over Platonic style that extended to details.[5]

The literary form of this treatise is thus an unusual mixture of genres; the Epidemic case-history, possibly the Pinax, the diatribe, the apologetic commentarius and the dialogue, all brought together

1 F. Gr. Hist. III, C, 1, n. 688 Jacoby: Lucian, Quomodo historia 16,24f.

2 De libr. propr. 12–16: Scr. min. II, pp. 121,5–124,5 Müller = XIX, pp. 43,8–48,7 K.

3 E. Wenkebach, Der hippokratische Arzt als das Ideal Galens, Quellen u. Studien z. Gesch. d. Naturwiss. u. d. Med. III, 4, 1935, pp. 155–175, is a re-edition, not always satisfactory, of Quod optimus medicus, Scr. min. II, pp. 1–8 = I, pp. 53–63 K. The Arabic version has been edited by P. Bachmann, Nachrichten d. Götting. Akad. d. Wiss. 1965, pp. 1–67. See also K. Deichgräber, Medicus Gratiosus.

4 De libr. propr. 13 and 11: Scr. min. II, pp. 122,13 and 120,14 Müller = XIX, pp. 46,15 and 44,16 K.: cf. also R. Hirzel, Der Dialog: ein literarhistorischer Versuch II, Leipzig 1895, pp. 1–365, esp. 364.

5 Note the idiomatic use of ὅς at 90,1 and 124,9.

to illustrate the growth of Galen's reputation.[1] The choice of this form cannot have been fortuitous, for the contrasts of stylistic organisation and subject, and the allusions scattered throughout give it a coherence and a finish that is often missing from his writings. As A. D. Momigliano has stressed[2], the Hellenistic and Roman periods saw a great development in the forms of autobiography – it cannot be forgotten that to the lifetime of Galen belong the Hieroi logoi of Aristeides, the Nigrinus, Somnium and Bis accusatus of Lucian and the Apology of Apuleius – and 'On prognosis', which is largely autobiographical in content, is another variation on the basic theme.

The style of an ancient work depended to a large extent upon the subject: a history need not be written in the same manner as a philosophical dialogue, and thus we should not be surprised at the differences between 'On prognosis', a non-medical text, and Galen's medical writings on similar topics, such as 'On crises'. There may be stylistic divisions even within the treatise, for each chapter has its own character and this juxtaposition of diverse styles and genres gives both a pleasing *variatio* and a distinct rhythm to the episodes. The heavy moralising prologue, with its long complicated sentences and its Platonic phraseology, is succeeded by the more colloquial cure of Eudemus, which is itself broken up by subsidiary encounters with Antigenes and Martianus and by the sermon preached by Eudemus on the wickedness of contemporary physicians. The humorous highlight of the treatise, the cure of Boethus' son, is preceded by the romantic tale of the wife of Iustus and followed by the more strictly medical cure of Boethus' wife, all of which employ a vocabulary and a style appropriate to the subject.[3] What might thus be a mere literary pastiche or a dull collection of anecdotes is held together by the contrasts of organisation, by the personality of the author and, to a certain degree, by the variety of the dialogue, which is far greater in extent than in any other of Galen's writings.

All this makes stylistic comparison with other treatises dangerous, if not impossible, and the colloquial tone in general and the thin line of transmission, which suggests that 'On prognosis', as we have it, was not subjected to Galen's final scrutiny before being put in circulation (above, pp. 49f.), help to explain the presence of many non-Attic words and constructions rarely found elsewhere in his writings. However much he might claim to write a clear Greek prose, uncontaminated by solecisms of the market place or by hyper-Attic refinements (De diff. puls. II 2–4: VIII, pp. 567,1–583,4 K.), he could not but be influenced by the contemporary Koine and fall occasionally into errors of grammar and syntax himself. Although it would be pos-

1 For the possible chronology of the cases, see the commentary on pp. 217 f.

2 A. D. Momigliano, Quarto contributo alla storia degli studi classici, Rome 1969, pp. 78–89.

3 See especially the details of domestic furniture (106,6–108,18), which are entirely suited to a comic situation.

sible to remove many of them by emendation and to assert that they are the products of the mistakes of the scribe, not of Galen, comparative studies of other contemporary prose authors indicate that even the best writers nodded in their imitations of Attic prose and that, for the most part, there was never a uniform Koine to be used as a touchstone of acceptable Greek.[1]

Some of the unusual features of this treatise can be listed briefly:
1. Hyper-Atticisms: 70,12 σφέτερος; 72,17 συρφετός; 72,23 πρεσβυτέρως; 74,3 κῦρος; 90,1, 124,9 καὶ ὅς; 96,16 ἀτὰρ οὖν καί and possibly 136,22 χρόνον.
2. Attic constructions: 116,20 ἕτοιμος τό + infinitive; and the complicated sentence structures at 70,19–72,12 and 106,13–20.
3. Ionicisms: 70,4, 116,25, 118,5, ἐς for εἰς.
4. Rare words: 72,2 ἀτολμηρότερος; 100,21, 108,18 ταραντινίδιον; 106,12 βάθρα; 108,4 γλωττόκομον.
5. Colloquialisms: 82,16 οὐκ οἶδ' ὅτι δόξαν αὐτῷ; 84,1 κατὰ γῆς ἐδύετο; 84,2, 94,9 ὅς ... αὐτός; 86,16 τούτων τῶν ἰαλέμων ἰατρῶν.
6. Simple word for compound: 98,28 σχεῖν; 108,8 στορεσθῆναι; and 108,14 στρώννυσθαι, both in *variatio* with ἀναστ-; 110,4 ἴσχειν; 118,3 γενόμενος.
7. κελεύω + dative: 106,28, 128,23, 130,17.
8. 124,3, 128,14 εἶπες; 124,12 εἶπας.
9. Confusion between μήτε and μηδέ: 88,21.
10. Overuse of τε: 122,8.
11. εἰ + subjunctive: 92,12 (?).
ὅταν + indicative: 90,28.
12. Accusativus pendens: 74,1, 94,24 (?), 120,8f.
13. Genitive absolute, followed by accusative: 78,4, 94,22; by dative: 76,29; by nominative: 78,16.
14. Present or aorist for future (i) participle: 80,15, 102,19, 124,1[2], 136,25, 138,22; (ii) infinitive: 78,31, 82,26, 120,26, 124,10, 136,7.
15. Accusative of the point of time: 78,34.
16. Constructio ad sensum: 82,24f.

The impression given by the style and language of this treatise is that its author was a man of considerable linguistic learning, with a rich vocabulary to suit every occasion, whose zeal occasionally

[1] As well as F. Blass, A. Debrunner and R. W. Funk, A Greek grammar of the New Testament and other early Christian literature, Cambridge/Chicago 1961, see also: W. Schmid, Der Atticismus in seinen Hauptvertretern, Stuttgart 1887–1896; the editions by G. Dalmeyda of Xenophon of Ephesus, Paris 1926, and of Longus, Paris 1934; and L. Radermacher, Koine, SB d. Akademie d. Wiss. in Wien, phil.-hist. Kl. 224, 5, Vienna 1947, esp. his warning on p. 70. The remarks of E. Nachmanson, Galenos' Epidemikommentar, Festschrift V. Lundström, Gothenburg 1936, pp. 108–148, require further substantiation from other treatises before his view of the non-Attic nature of Galenic prose can be totally accepted.

[2] Cf. the combination of aorist and future participles given by the Mss. of Quod animi mores 11: Scr. min. II, p. 78,14 Müller = IV, p. 820,11 K. Editors since Chartier have chosen to emend this to two future participles.

prevented him from writing the purest Attic. His Greek is, for the most part, clear and precise: it is only in the manipulation of long periodic sentences that obscurity and error intervene. A frequent use of variation, both in vocabulary and in syntax, avoids dullness, even in repetitive passages, and asyndeton, especially at 108,7–14, gives speed and vigour to the narrative. Galen's rhetorical training made him a master of all the techniques of literary composition. Although in power 'On prognosis' is inferior to the Epode that closes De usu partium (XVII: II, pp. 437–452 Helmreich = IV, pp. 346–366 K.), by its greater variety of tone and style, by its wit and sarcasm and by its use of many rhetorical devices it can justly be ranked with the most attractive productions of the Second Sophistic and among the finest of Galen's literary works.

D. Principles adopted in this edition

In the apparatus criticus to this treatise I have included the readings of the Latin version only when it appeared to present a text largely different from that of the Greek manuscripts, and I have excluded such minor differences as word order or the replacement of a participial phrase in Greek by a temporal clause in Latin. Where no reference is made to it in the apparatus, it may be assumed that the reading of the Latin version agrees with that in the text or is not incompatible with it. As for the Greek Mss., I have not included the errors of W and N, the copies of P and L respectively, and their absence from the apparatus does not mean that they have the reading given in the text. Where N, N^2 has the right reading and L and M have not, that has been noted in the apparatus.

I have not indicated changes of punctuation, except where a new interpretation is thereby produced, nor have I indicated elisions and crases, on which I have attempted to employ a greater, though not a complete, consistency. I have also endeavoured to standardise spelling throughout, although this may be more consistent than Galen himself wrote. In noting the source of emendations I have given the name of only the proposer (or proposers) and it may be assumed that subsequent editions all include that emendation. I have normally excluded those cases where the correct manuscript reading, either wrongly reported or omitted by the Aldine or later editions, has been correctly emended by a later scholar, even though, by so doing, I have done less than justice to the Basle editors and to Cornarius. I have likewise excluded erroneous conjectures and misprints: a comparison between this edition and that of Kühn will soon reveal the improvements I have made, without stigmatising further the profundities of human error.

Many friends have aided me in the making of this edition. Dr. J. Diggle and Dr. G. Giangrande criticised early drafts of the text; Mr. B. T. Rothwell and my wife helped me to revise my translation; and Miss J. M. Reynolds discussed with me many points of interpretation in the commentary. Whatever expertise I have shown in the collation, description and history of the manuscripts is owed to the teaching and example of Dr. A. H. McDonald, at whose suggestion I began this edition. I should also like to thank Prof. K. Deichgräber for many kindnesses; and the editorial staff of the Corpus Medicorum Graecorum, especially Dr. J. Kollesch for her helpful advice and Dr. G. Strohmaier for translating the Arabic testimonia for me. My thanks go also to the Zentralinstitut für Alte Geschichte und Archäologie of the Akademie der Wissenschaften der DDR for the decision to include my edition in the series of the Corpus Medicorum Graecorum. My visits abroad to inspect manuscripts were supported by grants from the Wellcome Foundation and the Faculty Board of Classics at Cambridge. My greatest debt is to my own College, where, first as a Research Fellow and later as a Lecturer, I was able to pursue my work in congenial and stimulating company and whose Governing Body generously gave me leave of absence to complete this book.

Selwyn College, Cambridge
May 1975

Vivian Nutton

ΓΑΛΗΝΟΥ

ΠΕΡΙ ΤΟΥ ΠΡΟΓΙΝΩΣΚΕΙΝ ΒΙΒΛΙΟΝ

GALEN

ON PROGNOSIS

CONSPECTVS SIGLORVM ET COMPENDIORVM

V	= Vaticanus 1845; s. XII/XIII
L	= Laurentianus 74,5; s. XII/XIII
L^{2}	= eiusdem codicis correctiones manu altera factae
M	= Marcianus 281; s. XV
A	= Ambrosianus Q 3 Sup.; s. XV
P	= Parisinus 2332; s. XV
N	= Parisinus suppl. graec. 35; s. XV/XVI
y	= consensus codicum LM
Nic.	= Nicolai versio Latina; s. XIV
Nic.^{b}	= Nicolai versio codice Parisino 6865; s. XIV tradita
Nic.^{a}	= Nicolai versio codice Parisino Academico 51; s. XV tradita
Nic.^{d}	= Nicolai versio codice Dresdensi Db 92; s. XV tradita
Nic.^{c}	= Nicolai versio codice Malatestiano S. V 4; s. XIV tradita
Nic.^{c3}	= eiusdem codicis correctiones ab Iohanne de Arimino factae
Nic.^{e}	= Nicolai versio codice Malatestiano S. XXVI 4; s. XV tradita
Nic.^{e2}	= eiusdem codicis correctiones ab Iohanne de Arimino factae
Nic.^{v}	= Nicolai versio editione Latina Venetiis a. 1490 typis exscripta
Nic.^{z}	= consensus codicum Nic.^{ad}
Nic.^{w}	= consensus codicum Nic.^{bad}
Nic.^{x}	= consensus codicum Nic.^{badce}
Ald.	= editio Aldina, Venetiis a. 1525
Bas.	= editio Basileensis, a. 1538
Morel	= editio Morelii, Lutetiae Parisiorum a. 1550
Chart.	= editio Charterii, Lutetiae Parisiorum a. 1679
Kühn	= editio Kühnii, Lipsiae a. 1827
Corn.	= Cornarius in Aldinae exemplari suo nunc bibliothecae universitatis Ienensis proprio
Scaliger	= Scaliger in Aldinae exemplari suo nunc bibliothecae Guelferbytanae proprio
Schöne	= Schöne in editionis Kühnii exemplari suo nunc in archivo Corporis Medicorum Graecorum Berolinensi conservato
Cobet	= Cobet in commentariis Ad Galenum, Mnemosyne, n. s. 13, 1885, p. 12sq.
Guinther	= Guinterii versio Latina, Lutetiae Parisiorum a. 1536
Ludovicus	= Ludovici versio Latina, Olisipone a. 1540
Iacchinus	= Iacchini versio Latina, Lugduni a. 1540
Rota	= Rotae versio Latina, Venetiis a. 1541

ΓΑΛΗΝΟΥ

ΠΕΡΙ ΤΟΥ ΠΡΟΓΙΝΩΣΚΕΙΝ ΒΙΒΛΙΟΝ

XIV 599 K. 1. Ὅσον μὲν ἐπὶ τοῖς πολλοῖς τῶν ἰατρῶν, ὦ Ἐπίγενες, ἀδύνατόν
ἐστι προγινώσκειν τὰ τοῖς κάμνουσιν ἐσόμενα καθ' ἑκάστην νόσον. ἀφ' οὗ
γὰρ οἱ τὸ δοκεῖν μᾶλλον ἢ εἶναι σπουδάσαντες οὐ κατὰ τὴν ἰατρικὴν
μόνον ἀλλὰ καὶ κατὰ τὰς ἄλλας τέχνας ἐπλεόνασαν, ἠμέληται μὲν τὰ
600 κάλλιστα τῶν τεχνῶν, ἤσκηται δ' ἐξ ὧν | ἄν τις εὐδοκιμήσειε παρὰ τοῖς
πολλοῖς, εἰπεῖν τε καὶ πρᾶξαι πρὸς ἡδονήν, κολακεῦσαι, θωπευτικῶς
προσαγορεύειν ἑκάστης ἡμέρας τοὺς πλουτοῦντάς τε καὶ δυναμένους
ἐν ταῖς πόλεσι, συμπροέρχεσθαι, παραπέμπειν, προερχομένους οἴκαδε
2 δορυφορεῖν, ἐν τοῖς δείπνοις βωμολοχεύεσθαι. τινὲς δ' αὐτῶν οὐ ταῦτα
μόνον ἀλλὰ καὶ τῇ τῶν ἱματίων καὶ δακτυλίων πολυτελείᾳ καὶ τῷ
πλήθει τῶν ἀκολουθούντων καὶ σκευῶν ἀργυρῶν παρασκευῇ τοὺς
3 ἰδιώτας ἀναπείθουσιν ὡς ἀξιοζήλωτοί τινες ὄντες. ἐκ τούτων οὖν
ἁπάντων τὰ μὲν ᾄδοντες, τὰ δ' ἐκπλήττοντες ἀνθρώπους ἀπείρους
ἀληθινῆς κρίσεως πραγμάτων, ὡς μὲν αὐτοὶ νομίζουσιν, ἀγαθῶν πολλῶν
τυγχάνουσιν, ὡς δ' ἐγὼ φαίην ἄν, οὐ τῶν ὄντως ἀγαθῶν ἀλλ' ὧν
4 αὐτοὶ ψευδῶς ὑπειλήφασιν. ἅτε δ' ὄντες τοιοῦτοι, τἆλλα παρανομεῖν
οὐκ ὀκνοῦσιν ἐλαχίστῳ τε χρόνῳ τὰς τέχνας ἐπαγγελλόμενοι διδάσκειν
ἀθροίζουσι πλῆθος μαθητῶν ἐξ ὧν καὶ αὐτοὶ προσλαμβάνουσι τὸ
δύνασθαι κατὰ τὰς πόλεις ἐν αἷς διατρίβουσιν.

5 Αὕτη μὲν οὖν κοινὴ τῶν τεχνῶν ἁπασῶν δυστυχία κατείληφε τὸν
601 νῦν βίον, ἡ δὲ τῆς | ἰατρικῆς ἐστι μὲν πολυειδής, ἀλλ' ἕν τι τῶν κατ'

3–14] *exc.* ar-Ruhāwī *Adab aṭ-ṭabīb* fol. 103b: p. 88b,43–89a,12 Levey 4–8 πολλοῖς] *cf.* Gal. De dign. puls. I 1: VIII p. 773,8–15 K. De comp. med. sec. loc. II 1: XII p. 534,10–14 K. 8 εἰπεῖν – 11] *cf.* Gal. Meth. med. I 1: X p. 2,15–19 K.; I 9: X p. 76,11–17 K.; II 5: X p. 114,14sq. K.; IX 4: X p. 609,11–14 K. De aff. dign. III 4: CMG V 4,1,1 p. 7,10–13 De exam. medico: Meyerhof, p. 75,14–18 = Iskandar, p. 364,31–36 19sq. ἐλαχίστῳ – μαθητῶν] *cf.* Gal. De dign. puls. I 1: VIII p. 770,13–15 K. De crisib. II 1: p. 127,12–15 Alex. = IX p. 642,8–12 K. Meth. med. I 4: X p. 30,12 K. 20sq. ἐξ ὧν – πόλεις] *cf.* Gal. De ord. libr. suor. 4: Scr. min. II p. 89,1–4 Müller = XIX p. 60,1sq. K. Meth. med. II 5: X p. 115, 2 K.; III 2: X p. 172,12f. K.

2 *ante* ΒΙΒΛΙΟΝ *add.* ΠΡΟΣ ΕΠΙΓΕΝΗΝ N² *Chart.*: ad Epigenem *Nic.*adc3 6 ἠμέλληται y 8 τε] τι Vy: quidem *Nic.*adc: quid *Nic.*b κολακεύεσθαι y: κολακεύειν *coni. Cobet* 9 τούς] τοῦ L 10 συμπροέρχεσθαι *secl. Schöne* προερχομένους *del.* L²: ἐκπροερχομένους *Schöne* 13 σκεβῶν V 16 αὐτοὶ] οὗτοι VyA: *sec. Nic.* (ipsi) *corr. Corn. Schöne* 17 οὕτως ὄντων y ἀλλ' ὧν] ἄλλων y 18sq. παρανομεῖν *(spatio 14 litt. relicto)* τῷ τέλει χρόνου A 19 *post* διδάσκειν *add.* ἐπαγγελλόμενοι M

GALEN

A TREATISE ON PROGNOSIS

1. How impossible it is, Epigenes, for the majority of doctors
to foretell what is going to happen to their patients in each illness.
For since those who are eager for the semblance of ability rather than
the reality have come to predominate in medicine as well as in the
other arts, the finest aspects of these arts are now neglected and atten-
tion is lavished upon what may bring them a high reputation with the
general public – a gratifying word or act, a bit of flattery, a toadying
salutation each day of the rich and powerful men in the cities, ac-
companying them when they go out, staying at their side, escorting
them on their homeward journey, amusing them at dinner. Some of 2
them not only do this but persuade the unsophisticated that they are
men of importance by their expensive clothes and rings, their abundant
retinue and their flashy silver equipment. By all this, by humouring or 3
impressing men who lack any real discrimination in these matters,
they gain great rewards – or so they believe: rather, I should say, they
fail to win a true reward but only what they themselves wrongly
assume to be so. And being such men as that, they do not shrink from 4
further enormities. They announce that they can teach their arts in a
very short time and so assemble a host of pupils through whom they
themselves acquire influence in the cities where they live.

This malaise, common to all the arts, afflicts our modern civili- 5
sation, and its manifestation in medicine has many aspects: but there

6 αὐτὴν ἔγνωκα προχειρίσασθαι τῶν ἐμοὶ μάλιστα διαφερόντων. ὅταν
γάρ τις ἰατρὸς τῶν νόμῳ μεμαθηκότων αὐτὴν ἢ παραφροσύνην
ἐσομένην ἐπὶ νοσοῦντος ἢ ῥῖγος ἢ καταφορὰν ἢ αἱμορραγίας ἢ παρωτί-
δας ἢ ἀπόστασιν ἄλλην ἐς ὁτιοῦν μέρος ἢ ἔμετον ἢ ἱδρῶτας ἢ κοιλίαν
ἐκταραχθησομένην ἢ συγκοπὴν ἤ τι τῶν τοιούτων προείπῃ ἄλλο,
ξένον τε καὶ τέρας τοῖς ἰδιώταις ὑπ' ἀηθείας φαίνεται καὶ τοσοῦτον
ἀποδεῖ τοῦ θαυμάζεσθαι παρ' αὐτοῖς ὁ προειπὼν ὥστ' ἀγαπήσειεν ἂν
7 εἰ μὴ καὶ γόης τις εἶναι δόξειεν. ὀλίγοι δέ τινες αὐτῶν οὐκ ἀπογινώσκουσι
μὲν ὡς ἀδυνάτου τῆς τοιαύτης θεωρίας, ἐρωτῶσι δ' εὐθέως καὶ αὐτὸν τὸν
προειπόντα καὶ τοὺς ἄλλους ἰατροὺς εἰ καὶ τοῖς ἔμπροσθεν εὕρηταί τι
8 τοιοῦτον ἢ μόνον αὐτοῦ τοῦ προειπόντος ἐστὶν εὕρημα. τοὐντεῦθεν οὖν
ἀναγκαῖον γίγνεται τοὺς μὲν ἰατροὺς ἀποκρυπτομένους σφετέραν
ἀμαθίαν, ἴσως δέ τινας καὶ ὄντως ἀγνοοῦντας, οὐδενὶ φάναι τῶν
602 ἔμπροσθεν οὐδὲν | τοιοῦτο γεγράφθαι, γόητα δ' εἶναι τὸν ἐπιδεικνύμενον
τοιαύτην πρόρρησιν· αὐτὸν δὲ τὸν προειπόντα μήθ' ὅτι γέγραπται
πολλοῖς τῶν ἔμπροσθεν καὶ μάλιστα τῷ Ἱπποκράτει, τῷ πάντων
ἡμῖν τῶν καλῶν ἡγεμόνι, τολμᾶν εἰπεῖν αἰδοῖ θ' ἅμα τῶν παρόντων
ἰατρῶν καὶ μίσους ὑποψίᾳ μήθ' ὡς αὐτὸς εὑρηκὼς εἴη· ψεύδεσθαι γὰρ
9 οὕτως καὶ μᾶλλον μισηθήσεσθαι πρὸς αὐτῶν. ἄπορον δὴ πανταχόθεν
ἐρώτημά τις ὑποσχόμενος, ὀκνῶν, οἶμαι, καὶ διαβουλευόμενος, αὐξάνει
μὲν τὴν τῆς γοητείας ὑποψίαν αὐτῷ τῷ μέλλειν ἀεί, τελευταῖον δὲ
φθόνον ἐφ' ἑαυτὸν ἤγειρεν ὥστ' ἐπιβουλεύεσθαι πρὸς αὐτῶν, πρῶτον
μὲν τῇ τῆς φαρμακείας ἐνέδρᾳ, δεύτερον δ' ᾗ Κόιντος ἥλω, βελτίων μὲν
ὢν ἰατρὸς τῶν καθ' ἑαυτόν, ἐκβληθεὶς δὲ τῆς πόλεως ὡς ἀναιρῶν
τοὺς νοσοῦντας, ὥστε δυοῖν θάτερον ἀναγκαῖον γίνεται παθεῖν τὸν
φιλοσόφως τὴν τέχνην μετιόντα καὶ τῶν Ἀσκληπιαδῶν ἀξίως ἢ

2 ἢ – 5 τοιούτων] *cf.* Gal. De crisib. II 14: p. 109,15–17 Alex. = IX p. 614,10–12 K.; III 11: p. 211,17sq. Alex. = IX p. 767,11sq. K. 6 ξένον – 11] *cf.* Gal. Quod opt. med. sit etiam phil. 1: Scr. min. II p. 2,9–11 Müller = I p. 54,16–55,2 K. 15–18] *cf.* Gal. De usu part. X 14: II p. 109,7–9; 110,10–14 Helmr. = III p. 835,16–836,1; 837,7–11 K. 16sq. τῷ[I] – ἡγεμόνι] *cf.* Gal. De crisib. III 11: p. 200,1 Alex. = IX p. 752,14 K. In Hipp. Epid. III comm. I 12: CMG V 10,2,1 p. 41,1sq. 21sq. τελευταῖον – αὐτῶν] *cf.* Gal. De pecc. dign. 3,10sq.: CMG V 4,1,1 p. 48,14sq. De nominib. medic. p. 20sq.

1 διαφερόντων *ex* συμφερόντων *corr.* M 2 τῶν] τῷ M 3 ἐσομένην *om.* M νοσοῦντα L ἢ[III] *om.* y 4 ἢ ἔμετον *om.* *Nic.* 5 ταραχθησομένην M 7 ἀγαπήσειαν A 8 *ante* αὐτῶν *add.* ἐξ A οὐ καταγινώσκουσι *Schöne*: non desperant *Nic.* 10 εἴρηταί A 11 μόνον αὐτοῦ] ipsius solius (-lis *Nic.*[d]) *Nic.* οὖν] μὲν A: γοῦν *Scaliger* 12 ἀποκρυπτομένους – 13 ἀμαθίαν] fingentes se ignorare *Nic.* *ante* σφετέραν *add.* τὴν *Schöne* 13 τινος A 15 μήδ' A 16 τῷ Ἱπποκράτει *iter.* M 17 τολμᾷ M: τολμᾷς L 18 εὑρηκὼς] uidit *Nic.* 18sq. ψεύδεσθαι – μισηθήσεσθαι] mentietur itaque aut odio (hodio *Nic.*[c]) habebitur *Nic.* 19sq. ἄπορον – ὑποσχόμενος *om.* *Nic.* 20 εὕρημά τι ὑπεσχόμενος A ὀκνῶν – διαβουλευόμενος *om.* A: hesitans autem undique sed ueritati tandem adherens *Nic.* 21 τῆς γοητείας *om.* *Nic.* αὐτῷ τῷ μέλειν y: αὐτὸ τὸ μέλλον A: et in futuro *Nic.*: *corr.* *Bas.* δὲ *om.* y 22 πρώτη yA: primo *Nic.*: *corr.* *Scaliger* 23 μὲν τῇ] μέντοι y τῆς *om.* A δευτέρῳ A: δευτέρα y: secundo *Nic.*: *correxi*: ἡ δευτέρα *Schöne* ἥλω yN (ἥλω N[2]) 24 *ante* ἀναιρῶν *addiderit* ἂν *Durling*, *fort. recte* 25 γίγνεται A τὸν] τῶν A

is one that I wish to examine since it has particular relevance to me. Whenever a doctor who has been properly trained predicts the occurrence in a patient of delirium, rigor, depression, haemorrhages, abscessions to the ears or elsewhere, vomiting, sweating, a stomach upset, a fainting fit, or anything of the kind, he appears a strange monstrosity to the laity because of his rarity. The predicter is so far from gaining their respect that he would think himself lucky if he did not seem to be a sorcerer. There are, of course, a few who do not reject 7
such a theory as impossible, yet they immediately ask the man who made the prognosis and his medical colleagues whether this sort of thing was also known to earlier authorities or whether it is the personal discovery of the forecaster. As a result, to conceal their sketchy 8
learning, or possibly because some in fact know nothing, the doctors say that nothing like this was written earlier and that the man who has advanced such a prediction is a sorcerer. The forecaster himself dare not say that this subject was expounded by many of his predecessors and especially by Hippocrates, our guide to all that is good, both through respect for the other doctors present and from suspicion of their hatred. Nor dare he say that it is his own discovery: for then he would be lying – as well as incurring even greater enmity. Thus, as he is subjected to this difficult questioning on all sides, while, 9
I suppose, he delays and debates with himself, he increases their suspicion of sorcery by his everlasting hesitation. Finally he stirs up such envy against himself that they conspire against him, first by plotting poisoning, secondly by the trap in which they caught Quintus, the best physician of his generation, who was expelled from Rome on a charge of murdering his patients. Thus, whoever wants to pursue the art of medicine in a philosophic manner worthy of the sons of Asclepius must suffer one of two things: either he can go into

παραπλησίως Κοΐντῳ φυγαδευθέντα λαμπρὰ τῆς αἰσθήσεως τἀπίχειρα
603 κομίσασθαι ἢ διαβαλλόμενόν γε φα|νερῶς, εἰ μὲν ἀτολμηρότερος εἴη, τὰ
μὲν ἀπολογούμενον, τὰ δ' ὑποπτήσσοντα λαγῶ βίον ζῆν, ἀεὶ τρέμοντα
καί τι πείσεσθαι προσδοκῶντα πρὸς τῷ καὶ τὴν τῆς γοητείας ὑποψίαν
10 αὐξάνειν· εἰ δ' εὐτονώτερος ὢν ὁμόσε χωρεῖ καὶ διαμάχεται μόνος πολλοῖς πανούργοις ἀνθρώποις καὶ πολλοὺς ἀδικημάτων τρόπους ἠσκηκόσιν αὐτὸς ἐκ παιδείας καὶ μαθημάτων ὁρμώμενος καὶ τῶν τοιούτων ἄπειρος κακῶν, ἤτοι κατὰ κράτος ἁλόντα γενέσθαι τὸ λοιπὸν ἐπ' ἐκείνοις, ὅτι ἂν αὐτῷ χρῆσθαι βουληθῶσιν· ἢ εἴπερ ἐπὶ πλέον ἀντέχοι καὶ διαγωνίζοιτο τύχῃ τινὶ χρησάμενος θαυμαστῇ, τὸ μὲν οὖν ἀεὶ πολεμεῖν τε καὶ πολεμεῖσθαι τὸν χείριστον τῶν πολέμων, ὃν ὀνομάζουσιν ἐμφύλιον, ἐκφεύγειν μὴ δύνασθαι.

11 Συμβαίνειν οὖν ἀναγκαῖον [ἐν] πολλοῖς τῶν οὕτως παρεσκευασμένων καὶ τῶν ἄλλων ὅσοι τετιμήκασιν ἀλήθειαν εἰλικρινῶς, οὐ διά τι τῶν ἔξωθεν ἀλλ' αὐτὴν δι' ἑαυτῆς, ὅταν ἅπαξ πειραθῶσι τῆς κατεχούσης τὸν νῦν βίον ἀδικίας καὶ γνῶσι σαφῶς ὡς οὐδὲν ἔσονται τοῖς ἀνθρώποις ὄφελος, ἐξαναχωρεῖν τοῦ τῶν πολλῶν συρφετοῦ [καὶ] ὥσπερ ἐν χειμῶνι
604 12 μεγάλῳ | καὶ ζάλῃ πνευμάτων ἑαυτοὺς γοῦν σῶσαι σπεύδοντας. οὗτοι δὴ τοῖς πολλοῖς μὲν ἄγνωστοι, γνώριμοι δὲ καὶ φίλοι μάλιστα μὲν καὶ πρῶτον θεοῖς, εἶτα τῶν ἀνθρώπων τοῖς ἀρίστοις ἐν ἡσυχίᾳ βιοῦσιν, ἐπιτρέψαντες τοῖς πανούργοις εὐδοκιμεῖν παρὰ τοῖς πολλοῖς ἀνθρώποις.
13 ἁπάντων δὲ τούτων τὰ αἴτια τοῖς ἀνθρώποις ἐστὶ τῶν πλουτούντων ἐν ταῖς πόλεσι καὶ δυναμένων ἡ τρυφή, οἳ πρεσβυτέρως ἡδονὴν ἀρετῆς τετιμηκότες ἐν οὐδενὶ λόγῳ τίθενται τούς τι καλὸν ἐγνωκότας τοῖς τ' ἄλλοις ὑφηγήσασθαι δυναμένους, ὅλοι δ' ἐπὶ τοῖς τὰς ἡδονὰς ἐκπορίζουσίν εἰσι καὶ τούτους πλουτίζουσι καὶ θαυμάζουσι καὶ ὑψηλοὺς αἴρουσιν ὥστε τῶν μὲν ὀρχηστῶν καὶ τῶν ἡνιόχων εἰκόνας ποιοῦνται τοῖς τῶν θεῶν ἀγάλμασι συνέδρους, τοὺς δ' ἀπὸ τῶν μαθημάτων το-
14 σαῦτα τιμῶσιν ὅσα τῆς χρείας αὐτῶν δέονται. τὸ γὰρ ἐν ἑκάστῳ καλὸν οὐ θεωροῦσιν οὔτε τῶν δεινῶν αὐτῶν ἀνέχονται, ἀλλὰ γεωμετρίας μὲν καὶ ἀριθμητικῆς ὅσον εἰς ἀναλωμάτων λογισμοὺς καὶ οἰκίας κατασκευήν,

1sq. λαμπρὰ – κομίσασθαι] *cf.* Plat. Resp. 608 C 3sq. λαγῶ – προσδοκῶντα] *cf.* Demosth. De corona 263: p.163,6 Sandys 17sq. ἐξαναχωρεῖν – σπεύδοντας] *cf.* Plat. Resp. 496 D 27sq. εἰκόνας – συνέδρους] *cf.* Gal. De caus. procat. 11,142: CMG Suppl. II p. 36,15sq. Meth. med. I 1: X p. 3,4 K. 28 τοὺς – 74,2 μουσικῆς] *cf.* Plut. De divinatione, fr. 147 Sandbach

1 φυγαδευθέντων A λαμπρὰ – 2 κομίσασθαι *om. Nic.* τὰ ἐπείχειρα L 2 γε] τε A: τε καὶ y: *corr. Bas.* ἀτολμώτερος L 3 ὑποπτήσσοντα *in* -ήσοντα *mut.* L 4 τι] τινα A τῆς γοητείας *om. Nic.* 6 ἀδικημάτων] ἀδοκιμωτάτους y: nequitiarum *Nic.* 8 ἀλλόντα L 9 εἴ πω y 10 μὲν *om.* L οὖν *om.* A 13 ἐν *secl. Bas.* 13sq. τῶν οὕτως – ἄλλων *om. Nic.* 14 ἄλλως A 15 αὐτῆς A πειρασθῶσιν L 16 γνῶσιν L *(ante corr.)* N 17 καὶ *om. Nic.*, *secl. Schöne* 17sq. ἐκ χειμῶνος ... ζάλης A: ab igne et ualida tempestate *Nic.*[w]: ab hyeme ualida et tempestate *Nic.*[v] 18 οὕτω y 19 *post* δὴ *add.* οἱ A 19sq. πρῶτον μὲν καὶ μάλιστα A 20 ἄριστα y 21 πανούργως y 22 αἰτία *Schöne*: causa *Nic.* τοῖς ἀνθρώποις *om. Nic.* 23 πρεσβυτέρως] περαιτέρω A 24sq. ἄλλοις τε τοῖς L: ἀλλ' οἵ τε τοις M: ἄλλοις τέ τισι τῶν A: *corr. Bas.*: τοῖς τε ἄλλοις *Schöne* 25 δυναμένοις y ὅλοι] ἄλλοι A 27 μὲν *om.* A ἡνιόχων] adulatorum *Nic.* 30 οὐθ' ὁρῶσιν A

exile like Quintus and keep the rewards of his perception untarnished, or, leaving himself wide open to calumny, he can, if he lacks spirit, put forward a justification and then cower back, living like a hare, trembling in constant expectation of disaster – and still increase their suspicions of sorcery. If he has greater courage and joins battle, 10
fighting alone against many wicked men well practised in many ways of crime, himself relying upon his education and learning and innocent of such evils, he will be taken by force, and from then on he will be in their power, however they should wish to use him. Even if he holds out longer and continues the struggle by some remarkable luck, he cannot escape being caught up in that most dreaded of wars, internecine strife, both as attacker and attacked.

Consider, then, what inevitably happens to many who come thus 11
prepared or with a pure regard for truth, not for its externals but for itself alone. As soon as they experience the injustice which has taken hold of modern life and realise clearly that they are going to be of no use to mankind, they desert the popular rabble and seek to save at least themselves 'as if in a great storm and raging tempest'. They will 12
pass their lives in peace, unnoticed by the crowd, and in the knowledge and friendship, first and foremost of the gods, and secondly of the best of men, leaving it to scoundrels to gain a popular reputation. The 13
causes of all this in the world lie in the materialism of the rich and powerful in the cities, who, honouring pleasure above virtue, consider of no account those who possess some finer knowledge and can impart it to others. They are entirely in the hands of the purveyors of pleasure; they enrich them; they admire them greatly; they exalt them so much that they place statues of dancers and jockeys alongside the images of the gods. But the respect they give to men of learning corresponds only to their practical need of them. They do not see the particular 14
beauty of each study and they cannot stand intellectuals. Geometry and arithmetic they need only in calculating expenses and in improv-

605 ἀστρονομίας δὲ καὶ μαντικῆς ὅσον εἰς τὸ προγνῶναι τίνων κλη|ρονο-
15 μήσουσι χρῄζουσιν, ὥσπερ γε καὶ μουσικῆς ὅσον εἰς ἡδονὴν ἀκοῆς. τὴν
δὲ τούτων συμπάντων τὸ κῦρος ἔχουσαν φιλοσοφίαν, ἀποδεικτικῆς
θεωρίας οὐδὲν αὐτοῖς μέλει πλὴν ὅσον ἡ χρεία προσάγει τινὰς τῶν
ῥητορικῶν ἀνδρῶν ὀργάνῳ πανούργῳ, τῇ σοφιστικῇ καλουμένῃ
θεωρίᾳ, χρῆσθαι. φιλοσοφίας γὰρ αὐτῆς οὐδὲν ἐπαΐουσιν ἀλλὰ πάντων
μαθημάτων ἀχρηστότατον τοῦτο νενομίκασιν ὁμοίως τῷ κέγχρον
16 τρυπᾶν. οὗτοι τοίνυν εἰσὶν οἳ καὶ τῆς ἰατρικῆς τὴν ἀναγκαίαν χρείαν
ὁρῶσι μόνην, οὐδὲ ταύτην ὀρθῶς· ἀλλ' ὡς ὁ Πλάτων πού φησιν, εἰ
δέοι κρίνεσθαι παρὰ παισὶν ἢ ἀνθρώποις ἄφροσιν ἰατρὸν καὶ μάγειρον,
[ὡς] ὁ μάγειρος ἂν οὐκ ὀλίγῳ δή τινι πλέον ἐνέγκαιτο.

2. Ταῦτ' οὖν ἀγνοῶν ἐγὼ κατὰ τὴν προτέραν ἐπιδημίαν ἐν Ῥώμῃ
μοι γενομένην οὐδὲν ὑφορώμενος ἐπεδεικνύμην οὐ διὰ λόγων ψιλῶν
ἀλλὰ τοῖς ἔργοις τάς τε τῶν ἐσομένων προγνώσεις καὶ θεραπείας ἄχρι
τοῦ γενέσθαι τι τοιοῦτον, ὡς ἐπίστασαι σὺ ὁ μάλιστα παρὼν τῇ νόσῳ
606 πάσῃ μέχρι τέλους ἀπ' ἀρχῆς Εὐδήμου τοῦ Περιπα|τητικοῦ φιλο-
2 σόφου. ἤρξατο μὲν γὰρ ἡμέρᾳ τινὶ μετὰ λουτρὸν ἀνωμαλία τις αὐτῷ,
φρίκη δ' ἀφ' ὥρας ὀγδόης δι' ἧς ἀναγκασθεὶς ἀσιτῆσαι, κατὰ τὴν
ὑστεραίαν ἀμέμπτως διάγων ὑπέλαβεν ἀσφαλέστερον εἶναι τὴν ὀγδόην
3 ὥραν ὑπερβάλλειν. ὡς δ' οὐ κατ' αὐτὴν ἀπήντησέ τι δυσχερὲς ἀσιτήσαντί
γε μέχρι τῆς ἐνάτης καὶ πρόσω οὐδεμία παραλλαγή τις ἐφαίνετο, λουσά-
μενός τε καὶ βραχέα προσενεγκάμενος ἐπὶ τῇ τρίτῃ ἡμέρᾳ συνεγένετο μὲν
ὡς ἔθος ἡμῖν, ἀσφαλείας δ' ἕνεκεν ἔδοξεν αὐτῷ καὶ κατ' ἐκείνην ὑπερβάλ-
4 λειν τὰς ὑπόπτους ὥρας. ἐλούσατ' οὖν μετὰ τὴν ἐνάτην καὶ τραφεὶς
εὐφόρως ἐπέπειστο μηδὲν αὐτῷ γενήσεσθαι δυσχερές. ἐν τῇ τετάρτῃ δὲ
τῶν ἡμερῶν ἐν ᾗ συγγενόμενος ἡμῖν ἐπὶ τὸ βαλανεῖον ἐστέλλετο, μει-
διάσας θ' ἅμα καὶ ἀποβλέψας πρός σε, «πότερον», ἔφη, «καὶ κατὰ τήνδε
τὴν ἡμέραν τετάρτην οὖσαν ἀσφαλέστερόν ἐστιν ὑπερβάλλειν τὴν
5 ὀγδόην ὥραν ἢ τῷ λουτρῷ χρηστέον ἤδη;» σὺ μὲν οὖν ὡς οὐδενὸς

1sq. ἀστρονομίας – χρῄζουσιν] *cf.* Iuv. Sat. XII 93–130 Lucian. De merced. conduct. 27: I p. 311,10–18 Jacobitz 9 ὁ Πλάτων – φησιν] Plat. Gorgias 464 D–E Politicus 289 A 16 Εὐδήμου] *eandem curam multo brevius narrat Galenus:* In Hipp. Epid. I comm. III 17: CMG V 10,1 p. 125,19–26 *cf.* Gal. De temperam. 6: p. 76, 23–77,19 Helmr. = I p. 631,6–632,12 K. In Hipp. De victu acut. comm. II 29: CMG V 9,1 p. 187,16–188,19 20–24] *exc.* Razes *Kitāb al-ḥāwī* XIV 47 ult.

1 ἀστρονομίαν y δὲ] τε M μαντικὴν y κληρονομίσουσι M: κληρονομίζουσι L 2 χρήζουσιν *ex* χρήσουσιν *corr.* M, *in* χρήσουσιν *mut.* L 3 φιλοσοφίαν *om. Nic.* 4 αὐτῆς A μέλλει LA 5 ὀργάνῳ – 6 χρῆσθαι] ut ea *(om. Nic.*[cv]*)* uelut organo in eorum astutia utantur *Nic.* πανούργως L σοφιστικῇ *scr.* L[2] *super lineam*: λογικῇ LAN 6 ἐπαίσουσιν y 7 μαθημάτων *om. Nic.*: μαθήματα A τῷ] τὸ yA: *corr. Chart.* 8 οἱ A 9 ταύτης y ὁ *om.* y πού *om. Nic.* 11 ὡς y: οἷς A: *secl. Ald.* ἐνέγκατο y 12 ἐγὼ ἀγνοῶν y: ego ignorans *Nic., fort. recte si hiatum probaueris* 14 ἀλλὰ τοῖς ἔργοις *om. Nic.* τάς] τῆς yA: *corr. Chart.* προγνώσεις *om.* y *ante* θεραπείας *add.* τῆς A, τὰς *Chart.* curam *Nic.* 15 παρὼν] παρὰ M 16 πάσα L 17 μὲν *om.* A 19 ὑστερέαν y 20 ὑπήντησε A 22 μὲν *om.* A 23 ὡς ἔθος *post* ἡμῖν *trsp.* A 24 πέμπτην y: ὀγδόην A: *sec. Nic.* (nonam) *in mg. corr. Bas.* 25 εὐφόρως] *sec. Nic.* (copiose) εὐπόρως *fort. praeferendum* 26 ἐτέλλετο L 27 πότερα y: πρότερον A: *correxi* 29 τὸ λουτρὸν y

ing their mansions, astronomy and divination only in forecasting
whose money they are going to inherit, and music simply for auditory
titillation. As for philosophy, which holds the key to all these, their 15
only concern with demonstrative theory comes when need compels
some of the rhetorical gentlemen to use that disreputable instrument,
the so-called sophistic theory. They have no time for philosophy itself,
but consider it to be the most useless of all studies, like boring holes
in millet seed. These, then, are the people who see even in medicine 16
only its necessary utilitarian aspect, and not even that properly. At
any rate, as Plato says somewhere, in a contest between a doctor and
a cook before a jury of children or fools, the cook would win by a
substantial margin.

2. I was completely ignorant of this when I first stayed in Rome.
All unsuspecting, I made not only verbal but also practical prognoses
of the future and cures until the following event took place, as you
well know, since you were present from beginning to end throughout
the whole illness of Eudemus the Peripatetic philosopher. One day 2
he began to feel a little indisposed after his bath, and at the eighth
hour he had a shivering fit which prevented him from taking food.
Although he passed the next day without incident, he thought it best
to let the eighth hour go by. When nothing unpleasant occurred then, 3
although he fasted until the ninth hour, and there was no appa-
rent change later, he took his bath and then a light meal. On the third
day he came to visit me, as was his custom, but for safety's sake he
thought it best on that day also to let the suspected hours go by. He 4
waited until after the ninth hour to take his bath, had a comfortable
meal and was then convinced that nothing untoward would happen
to him. On the fourth day, when he was with us on his way to the bath,
turning to you with a smile, he said, "Will it be safer to let the eighth
hour go past on this particular day, the fourth, or should I take my
bath now?" Expecting no trouble, you told him to go and take his 5

ἐσομένου δυσχεροῦς ἐκέλευσας ἀπιέναι λουσόμενον οἵ τ' ἄλλοι πάντες οἱ
607 παρόντες, ἐγὼ δ' ἐσιώπων μόνος. ἐρομένῳ | δ' αὐτῷ περὶ τῆς σιωπῆς
ἀπεκρινάμην οὐκ εἶναί μοι τελέως ἀνύποπτον ἀρχὴν γεγονέναι τεταρ-
ταίας περιόδου κατὰ τὴν πρώτην ἡμέραν ἡνίκα με τῶν σφυγμῶν ἐκέλευσας
6 ἅψασθαι. τῷ δὲ μὴ προεγνωκέναι μέ ποτε τὸν κατὰ φύσιν σου σφυγμὸν
ὁποῖός τις ἦν, οὐ χωρὶς οὐχ οἷόν τε τὰς βραχείας αὐτοῦ μεταβολὰς εἰς τὸ
παρὰ φύσιν ἐπιγνῶναι σαφῶς, οὐδὲν ἀπεφηνάμην, ὥσπερ οὐδὲ νῦν
7 πλέον ἔχω τι τῆς τότε μοι γενομένης ὑποψίας εἰπεῖν. ἐλούσατό τ' οὖν
εὐφόρως καὶ ἐτράφη μετρίως, εἶτα περὶ τὴν ἑσπέραν μετακαλεσάμενός με
καὶ πάλιν τῶν σφυγμῶν αὐτοῦ κελεύσας ἅψασθαι τὴν αὐτὴν ἀπόφασιν
8 ἤκουσεν ἣν πρὸ τοῦ λουτροῦ καὶ μᾶλλον ἔτι θαρραλεωτέραν ἢ τότε. διὰ
τοῦτ' οὖν ἔδοξε τὴν ἑξῆς ἡμέραν ἑβδόμην μὲν ἀπὸ τῆς ἀρχῆς τετάρτην δ'
ἀπ' ἐκείνης ἀκριβέστερον παραφυλάξαι καὶ διατρίψας ἐπὶ τῆς οἰκίας
ἐλούσατό τε καὶ σιτίων προσηνέγκατο, πλειόνων ὡς οἶσθα τελέως
9 ἀπύρετον αὐτὸν εἶναι φάντων. ἐγὼ μὲν οὖν ἐρομένῳ σοι – μέμνησαι γὰρ
πάντως καὶ τοῦτο – τὴν ὑποψίαν μου νῦν ἔφην ὡς σμικροτάτης τινὸς
608 αὐτῷ τε|ταρταίας περιόδου προοίμιον εἴη συμβαῖνον, ἐχωρίσθην ἔχων
ἐπισκοπεῖσθαί τινα περὶ τὴν ἑσπέραν ἄρρωστον οὐκ ἐγγὺς οἰκοῦντα.
10 λουσάμενος δ' Εὔδημος ἐτράφη μὲν εὐθέως, οὐ μετὰ πολὺ δὲ θερμασίας
ᾔσθετο δι' ὅλου τοῦ σώματος ἣν ἐπὶ τῷ ποθέντι πόματι γεγονέναι
νομίσας – οἴνου γὰρ παλαιοῦ προσενήνεκτο – κατὰ τὴν ὑστεραίαν αὐτὸ
τοῦτο διηγήσατο τοῖς συνήθεσιν ἰατροῖς, αἰτιασαμένων τε κἀκείνων
ἑτοίμως τὸν οἶνον, οὐδὲν ἔτι νομίσας ἔσεσθαι δυσχερὲς ἐν τῇ τετάρτῃ
μετὰ τὴν γενομένην θερμασίαν ἐλούσατό τε καὶ διῃτήθη τῷ συνήθει
11 τρόπῳ. σαφῶς δὲ πυρέττειν ἀρξάμενος ἐπείσθη τεταρταίου μὲν εἶναι τὴν
περίοδον, ἐπῄνει δὲ τοὐντεῦθεν ἐμὲ μόνον ὡς ἀκριβῶς ἁπτόμενον σφυγμοῦ
κατὰ τὸν ἔμπροσθεν χρόνον, ἐν φιλοσόφῳ θεωρίᾳ μόνῃ πεπεισμένος
ἀξιόλογον ἕξιν εἶναί μοι, τῶν δὲ κατὰ τὴν ἰατρικὴν ἐν παρέργῳ πεφρον-
12 τικέναι. καὶ γὰρ ἐπέπυστο τοῦ πατρὸς ἐπὶ φιλοσοφίαν ἄγοντός με

3–17 συμβαῖνον] *exc.* Razes *Kitāb al-ḥāwī* XVI 101,5   29–78,2] *cf.* Gal. Meth. med. IX 4: X p. 609,6–11 K. De ord. libr. suor. 4: Scr. min. II p. 88, 10sq. Müller = XIX p. 59,4–7 K.

1 ἐπιέναι A   1sq. οἱ παρόντες *om. Nic.*   2 ἐρωμένῳ y   3 τελείως y   4 ἡνίκα] ἐν ᾗ A: in quo *Nic.*   τὸν σφυγμὸν y: pulsum *Nic.*   5 τῷ δὲ] οὕτω y   9 εὐφόρως] *sec. Nic.* (copiose) εὐπόρως *fort. praeferendum*   10 καὶ *om.* A   πάλιν *om.* y *Nic.*   τὸν σφυγμὸν y: pulsum *Nic.*   αὐτοῦ *ex* αὐτῷ *corr.* L   11 θαρραλεώτερον yA: audacter *Nic.*: *correxi*   12 τὴν ἑξῆς *om. Nic.*   14 σιτίων – οἶσθα] et confestim obtulit cibaria, sicut nosti *Nic.*   πλεόνων A   15 φάντων] φάσκων *sec. Nic.* (dicens) *Bas.*   ἐρωμένῳ L   γὰρ *post* πάντως *(lin. 16) trsp.* y   16 πάντως *om. Nic.*   μοι yA: *correxi*   μικροτάτης A: μακροτάτης *Corn., fort. recte*   17 τετάρτης LA   *ante* ἔχων *add.* ἐπὶ τὸ λουτρὸν A   ἔχων *om.* y, *fort. recte*: uisitaturus *Nic.*   18 ἐπισκοπῆσαι A   20 ἐπὶ] ἐν y   21 προσηνένεγκτο L: προσηνέγκατο M   22 τοῖς συνηθεσι L: τῶν συνηθῶν M   αἰτησαμένων y   23 ἐν τῇ τετάρτῃ *om. Nic.*   24 *ante* μετὰ *add.* τὴν A, τῇ *Scaliger*   25 τεταρταίαν A   27 φιλοσοφίας *sec. Nic.* (philosophie [-phye *Nic.*[c]]) *Bas., sed cf. CMG V 10,2, 2 p. 280,21*   πεπεισμένον y   29 ἐπέπειστο MA̤N: ἐπέποιστο LN *(super lineam)*: didicerat *Nic.*: *corr. Cobet*

bath, as did all the others present: only I stayed silent. When he asked
the reason for my silence, I told him that I was not entirely without
suspicion that the beginning of a bout of quartan fever had occurred
on the first day when he asked me to take his pulse. "But since I have 6
not previously known your natural pulse-rate – without which it is
impossible to recognise clearly slight alterations towards the un-
natural – I made no definite statement; just as now I can offer
nothing beyond the suspicion I had then." He had a good bath and a 7
fair meal and then, sending for me about nightfall, he again told me
to take his pulse. He heard the same reply as before his bath, although
made with still greater assurance than before. So he decided to watch 8
more closely on the next date, that would be the seventh day from the
beginning but the fourth from then. He stayed at home, bathed and
had a meal, although several people, as you know, declared that he
was free from fever. When you asked me, I told you my hunch – no 9
doubt you remember this as well – that a very slight attack of
quartan fever would be just beginning, and then I left, having to see
a patient about nightfall who lived some way off. Immediately after 10
his bath Eudemus had a meal and not long after felt a hot sensation
throughout his body, which he ascribed to the drink he had taken –
for he had drunk some old wine – and next day discussed this parti-
cular matter with his regular doctors, who were equally ready to blame
the wine. So, thinking that he would have no further trouble, on the
fourth day after the hot flush he bathed and dined in his normal way.
But when he began to show clear signs of a fever, he was convinced 11
that this was a quartan cycle, and from then on he praised me alone
for having previously taken his pulse accurately, when he had believed
that I had a respectable standing only in philosophical investigation
and dabbled in medicine as a sideline. He had also heard that when my 12
father was introducing me to philosophy, he had been commanded by

προσταχθὲν αὐτῷ δι' ὀνείρων ἐναργῶν ἐκδιδάξαι καὶ τὰ τῆς ἰατρικῆς
οὐχ ὡς πάρεργόν τι μάθημα.
609 13 Τοῦτό μοι γεγονέναι συνέβη τότε κατά τινα τύχην, | ὡς οἶσθα
καὶ αὐτός, νενοσηκότος τινὸς ἀνθρώπου κατὰ τὴν ἀρχὴν τοῦ φθινο-
πώρου νόσον ὀξεῖαν, εἶτα κατὰ τὴν ἀνάληψιν ἀρξαμένου περὶ πέμπ-
την ὥραν πυρέττειν, θεασάμενον τὸν ἄνθρωπον ἀποφήνασθαί σοι
14 παρόντι σαφεστάτην εἰσβολὴν εἶναι τεταρταίου περιόδου. ὁπότε γὰρ
κατ' ἀναλογίαν ἡ διὰ τὴν τετάρτην ἀνταπόδοσις ἐγένετο, πυθόμενος
παρὰ σοῦ τὴν γενομένην πρόρρησιν ὁ Εὔδημος ἔτι μᾶλλον ἐπείσθη
προσέχειν ἐμοί· ὥστ' ἐπειδὴ προὔβαινεν ὁ κατὰ τὴν περίοδον παροξυ-
σμὸς εἰς μέγεθος, ἀθροίσας τοὺς ἀρίστους τῶν κατὰ τὴν πόλιν ἰατρῶν
15 ἠξίωσε σκέψασθαι περὶ τῆς θεραπείας τοῦ νοσήματος. ἐγὼ δ' ἑκὼν
ἀπελείφθην οὐ βουλόμενος ἁμιλλᾶσθαι διὰ λόγων αὐτοῖς· ὡς δὲ τοῖς
ἐνδοξοτάτοις αὐτῶν ἔδοξε τῆς θηριακῆς αὐτὸν πιεῖν ἕωθεν ἐκείνῃ τῶν
ἡμερῶν ἐν ᾗ προσδοκώμενος ἦν ὁ διὰ τῆς τετάρτης παροξυσμὸς ἔσεσθαι,
χωρισθέντων αὐτῶν, ὡς οἶσθα, σοῦ παρόντος ἐπυνθάνετό μου τίνα τὴν
16 ἐλπίδα τῆς τοῦ φαρμάκου χρήσεως ἔχοιμι. γινώσκεις οὖν ὅπως ἀπεκρι-
610 νάμην αὐτῷ μηδὲν ἀμφιβάλλων ὡς οὐ μόνον οὐδὲν ὀνήσει τὸ φάρ|μακον
17 ἀλλὰ καὶ διπλοῦν ἐργάσεται τὸν τεταρταῖον. καὶ τὴν γ' αἰτίαν ἐρωτή-
σαντος αὐτοῦ δι' ἣν οὕτως ἀπεκρινάμην ἄπεπτον ἔφην ἔτ' εἶναι τὸ
νόσημα τό τε φάρμακον τοῦτο κακοχυμίαν ἄπεπτον καὶ μάλιστ' ἐν
χειμῶνος ἀρχῇ μέχρι μὲν τοῦ ταράξαι δύνασθαι προσαγαγεῖν, οὐ μὴν
18 οὔτε πέψαι τελέως οὔτε διαφορῆσαι. ταῦτα μὲν οὖν ἀπεκρινάμην ἐγὼ τῷ
Εὐδήμῳ· κατὰ δὲ τὴν ὑστεραίαν ἕωθεν ἀφικόμενοι πρὸς αὐτὸν οὐδέπω
παρόντων ἡμῶν ἔδοσαν τὸ φάρμακον αἰδεσθέντι διηγήσασθαί τι τῶν
ὑπ' ἐμοῦ λεγομένων αὐτῷ καὶ ἅμα θεασαμένῳ μετ' ἐν[σ]τάσεως [ὡς]
ὑποσχομένους τοὺς ἀφικνουμένους ἰατροὺς ἅπαντας ὀνήσειν αὐτὸν οὐ
19 σμικρὰ τὴν τοῦ φαρμάκου προσφοράν. γενομένου δὲ τοῦ παροξυσμοῦ
κατὰ τὴν αὐτὴν ὥραν ἐνίοτε συμβαίνειν οὕτως ἔφασαν ἐπὶ τῆς πρώτης
πόσεως ὡς κινεῖσθαι καὶ μοχλεύεσθαι τὸ νόσημα· δεύτερον δὲ πιόντ'
ἀπαλλάττεσθαι τελέως εἰ κατὰ τὴν ἡμέραν ἐν ᾗ προσδοκᾶται γενησό-
μενος ὁ διὰ τετάρτης παροξυσμὸς ὁμοίως ἕωθεν αὐτοῦ προσενέγκαιτο.
611 20 ἐκεῖνοι μὲν ⟨οὖν⟩ οὕτως εἰπόντες ἐχωρίσθησαν εὐέλπιδες· οὐ | περιμείνας
δὲ τὴν ἑξῆς περίοδον ὁ τεταρταῖος ἀπροσδοκήτως ἐνέβαλε τὴν ὀγδόην

14–80,5] *exc.* Razes *Kitāb al-ḥāwī* XVI 101,8; 113,6; 123,16 21 ἄπεπτον – 23] *cf.* Gal. In Hipp. Progn. comm. II 31: CMG V 9,2 p. 285,15–23; III 33: CMG V 9,2 p. 357,10–358,23 In Hipp. Epid. I comm. II 14: CMG V 10,1 p. 56,25sq.; II 49: CMG V 10,1 p. 74,19sq.

3 συνέβη *post* Τοῦτό *trsp.* M 5 ἀνάληψιν] anologiam (ana- *Nic.*[a]) *Nic.* 6 θεασάμενον τὸν ἄνθρωπον *om. Nic.* θεάσασθαι yA: *corr. Bas.* 8 *ante* ἀναλογίαν *add.* τὴν M τοῦ τετάρτου L: τοῦ τεταρταίου M: quartam *Nic.*[ac]: quartanam *Nic.*[be] 15 ἦν *om.* A 16 αὐτῶν *om.* M 17 οὖν *iter.* L 18 μηδὲν ἀμφιβάλλων *om. Nic.* 20 ἄπεμπτον A ἔφην *post* εἶναι *trsp.* AP ἔτ' *om.* A, *sscr.* L 21 τε] δὲ A ἄπεμπτον A 23 πέμψαι A τελέως *om. Nic.* 25 τι *om.* y 26 θεασάμενος yA: *correxi* ἐνστάσεως yA: *corr. Kollesch* ὡς *secl. Schöne* 27 ὑποσχουμένους L: ὑπισχνουμένους A 28 μικρῶς A δὲ *om.* y 30 πιόντος L 33 οὖν *sec. Nic.* (igitur) *add. Bas.*

unambiguous dreams to educate me thoroughly in medicine, not just as a hobby.

13 By chance, the following incident happened to occur to me then, as you yourself know. A young man was seized with an acute illness at the beginning of autumn and, during his recovery, he became feverish at the fifth hour. As soon as I saw the man, I told you – for you were present – that the onset of a quartan cycle was very clear. 14 When a corresponding change in his own condition occurred on the fourth day, Eudemus, hearing from you of my other prediction, was even more convinced that he should rely on me. So, when the paroxysm at this period was reaching its height, he collected together the best doctors in the city and determined to discover the treatment for his disease. 15 I was quite willing to be left out since I had no wish to join in a battle of words with them. After the most reputable among them had concluded that he should drink some theriac on the morning of the day on which the fourth-day paroxysm was expected to occur, they went away, as you know. You remained while he asked me what expectation I had of the use of that drug. 16 You remember how I replied to him without prevarication that the drug would not only give him no benefit whatsoever, but on the contrary would double the effect of the quartan fever. 17 When he demanded a reason for my statement, I said that the disease was still unconcocted and that, although the medicine might be able to disturb an unconcocted bad humour, especially at the beginning of winter, it could in no way concoct it completely or disperse it. That was my reply to Eudemus. 18 The next morning they returned to him and administered the medicine in our absence; for he was too embarrassed to tell them my comments and he also noted that every doctor who came earnestly promised that a dose of this medicine would be of no small benefit. 19 Thus when the paroxysm came on at the same hour, they explained that it sometimes happened that at the first dose the disease was moved and dislodged: if he took a second dose, he would be cured completely, if he took it in the same way on the morning of the day on which the fourth-day paroxysm was expected. 20 With these words they went off in high hopes: but the quartan did not wait for the next cycle but attacked unexpectedly at

21 ὥραν, ἰσχυροτέρως ἢ κατὰ τὴν προτέραν ἡμέραν ἐγεγόνει. ἐλθοῦσιν οὖν
ἕωθεν αὐτοῖς, ὡς οἶσθα, δεύτερον ἐδόκει διδόναι τοῦ φαρμάκου. καὶ δὴ
καὶ δόντες ἐπὶ τῆς ἀναλογούσης τῷ προτέρῳ παροξυσμῷ τὸ φάρμακον
ἐχωρίσθησαν. ὅ τε γοῦν ἀνάλογος τῷ προτέρῳ παροξυσμῷ κατ' αὐτὸν
ἀπήντησε καὶ ὁ μετ' αὐτὸν ἐπιγενόμενος δεύτερος· ἐφ' ᾧ κατὰ τὴν
22 ἑσπέραν ἐπυνθάνετό μου τίνα προσδοκίαν ἔχοιμι τῶν μελλόντων. ἐγὼ
δέ, ὡς οἶσθα, καταμαθὼν αὐτοῦ τὴν κίνησιν τῶν ἀρτηριῶν, «νῦν μέν»,
ἔφην, «ἀποκρίνασθαί σοί τι πρὸς τὴν ἐρώτησιν ἀσφαλῶς ἀδύνατος
ὑπάρχω, ἕωθεν δὲ τάχ' ἂν δυνηθείην θεασάμενος ἅπαντα τὰ διὰ
23 τῆς νυκτὸς οὐρηθησόμενα». παραγενόμενος οὖν ὑπὸ τὴν ἕω καὶ
θεασάμενος αὐτὰ σωθῆναί τε κελεύσας αὖθις ἐὰν οὐρήσῃ τι μεταξὺ περὶ
τετάρτην ὥραν ἔφην ἀφίξεσθαι. καὶ μὴν καὶ παραγενόμενος ὡς ἐθεασάμην
τε τὰ οὖρα καὶ τῶν σφυγμῶν ἐπὶ πλέον ἡψάμην ἀπεφηνάμην αὐτῷ
τρίτου τεταρταίου γενήσεσθαι παροξυσμὸν ὡς περὶ τὴν αὐτὴν ὥραν.
612 24 ἐγὼ μὲν οὖν ἐχωρίσθην· ὀλίγον δ' ὕστερον | ἐπισκεψάμενοι τὸν Εὔδημον
ἀφίκοντο Σέργιός τε [καὶ] Παῦλος, ὃς οὐ μετὰ πολὺν χρόνον ἔπαρχος
ἐγένετο τῆς πόλεως, καὶ Φλάβιος ⟨Βοηθός⟩, ὑπατικὸς μὲν ὢν ἤδη καὶ
αὐτὸς ἐσπευκὼς δὲ περὶ τὴν Ἀριστοτέλους φιλοσοφίαν ὥσπερ καὶ ὁ
Παῦλος· οἷς διηγησάμενος ὁ Εὔδημος ἅπαντα τὰ κατ' ἐμὲ λείπειν ἔφη
τὴν τήμερον ἐσομένην πρόρρησιν ἐπὶ τοῦ μέλλοντος παροξυσμοῦ παρα-
25 φυλάττειν δ' ὅπως ἀποβήσοιτο. γενομένου δὲ κἀκείνου περὶ τὴν αὐτὴν
ὥραν τοῖς προγεγενημένοις ὁ μὲν Εὔδημος ἐθαύμαζέ τε καὶ τοῖς ἐπι-
σκοπουμένοις αὐτὸν ἅπασιν ἐδήλου τὰς ἐμὰς προρρήσεις – ἦσαν δ' οὗτοι
σχεδὸν ἅπαντες οἱ κατὰ τὴν Ῥωμαίων πόλιν ἀξιώματί τε καὶ παιδείᾳ
προὔχοντες – ὁ δ' οὖν Βοηθὸς ἀκηκοὼς εἰς ἄκρον ἠσκῆσθαί με τὴν
ἀνατομικὴν θεωρίαν ἔτυχεν ἤδη παρακαλῶν ἐπιδεῖξαί τι περὶ φωνῆς τε
26 καὶ ἀναπνοῆς ὅπως τε γίνοιτο καὶ διὰ τίνων ὀργάνων. ὡς οὖν ἐγνώρισέ

11 θεασάμενος – μεταξὺ] *exc.* Razes *Kitāb al-ḥāwī* XIX 138 paen. 16sq. Σέργιός – πόλεως] *cf.* Gal. Anat. admin. I 1: II p. 218,9–11 K. 25–27] *cf.* Gal. De exam. medico: Meyerhof, p. 77,27–29 26 ἐπιδεῖξαί – 27] *cf.* Gal. Anat. admin. VIII 3: II p. 661,1–666,17 K.; VIII 8: II p. 690,3–693,9 K.

1 ἰσχυρότερος A: fortius *Nic.* ἢ – ἐγεγόνει *om. Nic.* 2 αὐτοὺς L τω φαρμάκω L 3 ἀναλόγου y: ἡμέρας ἀνάλογον *sec. Nic.* (in die proportionali) *coni. Bas.* 4 ἐχωρίσθη y ὅ τε] τε *secl. Bas.* οὖν y ἀνάλογον y πρώτῳ A αὐτὸν] αὐτὰ A 5 ἐπιγενησόμενος A δεύτερον y 6 τῶν μελλόντων *om. Nic.* 8 πρὸς τὴν ἐρώτησιν *om. Nic.* 8sq. ἀδυνα^{T} ὑπάρχειν A 9 ἅπαντα] αὐτὰ P 10 τὴν] τῆς y 11 *post* αὐτὰ *add.* τὰ διὰ τῆς νυκτὸς οὐρηθησόμενα P ἐαθῆναι yAP: dimitti *Nic.*: *sec. Razem (ḥabasa), Rotam, Ludovicum, Iacchinum* (servari) *correxi* οὐρήσει P: οὐρήσῃ *ex* οὐρήσει *corr.* L 12 καὶ παραγενόμενος *om.* P 13 τε *om.* P 14 τρίτον A 15 ἐπισκεψόμενοι A: uisuri *Nic.* 16 τε *om.* A *ante* καὶ *add.* ὁ L, *fort. recte, si hanc formam Graecam cognominis Romani probaueris, post* καὶ M: Sergius et Paulus *Nic.* καὶ *seclusi* πολὺ L 17 Βοηθός *add. Groag, PIR*^{2} *F. 229* ἤδη *om. Nic.* 18 καὶ *om.* A 19 *ante* ὁ *trsp.* ἅπαντα y λυπεῖν M: λυπὴν L: λοῖπον A: *corr. Corn.*: ἐκλείπειν *coni. Schöne* 19sq. λείπειν – πρόρρησιν] hodie dixerunt futuri predictionem (predicationem *Nic.*[a]) *Nic.* 20 τήμερον *scripsi*: σήμερον yA 21 δ' *om.* LA 24 οἱ M 25 προὔχοντο y 26 ἔτυχεν] ἐπεῖχεν A: insistebat *Nic.* ἤδη *om. Nic.* τε *om.* A 27 γίγνοιτο MA ἐγχώρησε L: ἐχώρησα M: que ut nouit cognitus michi factus est *Nic.*

the eighth hour, and with greater vehemence than on the previous day. When they returned in the morning, as you know, they decided to 21 give him a second dose of medicine – which they proceeded to do, giving it him at an hour that corresponded to that of the first paroxysm. They then left. A paroxysm corresponding to the first attacked him, and then a second followed it. As a result, he asked me in the evening what I expected was going to happen. As you know, now that 22 I had discovered the (natural) movement of his arteries, I said, "I cannot give you a safe answer to your question at this moment, but I might possibly be able to do so in the morning when I have inspected the urine you have passed in the night." Having seen it on my return 23 just before dawn, I ordered him to keep again whatever urine he might pass meanwhile and promised that I would come back about the fourth hour. Then on my return, when I had examined his urine and taken his pulse further, I told him that a paroxysm of a third quartan fever would occur at about the same hour. Then I left. A little later 24 there came and saw Eudemus Sergius Paulus, who was made prefect of the city not long after, and Flavius Boethus, who was also himself an ex-consul then and a student of Aristotelian philosophy, like Paulus also. Eudemus told them all about me and said that my prophecy of a coming paroxysm that would occur that day was (still) unfulfilled, and he was watching carefully to see how it would come about. When it too took place at the same time as the 25 previous ones, Eudemus was amazed and revealed my predictions to all his visitors, who included almost all the social and intellectual leaders of Rome. Boethus, who had heard of my excellent training in anatomical theory, happened already to have invited me to demonstrate how speech and breath are produced and by what organs. When 26

μου τὸ ὄνομα καὶ τοῦτ' αὐτὸ τῷ τε Παύλῳ διηγήσατο καὶ μετὰ τὴν πεῖραν ἔφη παρακαλεῖν με δεῖξαί τι καὶ αὐτῷ· πάνυ γὰρ ἔφη δεῖσθαι τῆς
613 27 θέας τῶν κατὰ τὰς ἀνατομὰς φαι|νομένων ὁ Παῦλος. ὁμοίως δὲ καὶ Βάρβαρος ὁ θεῖος τοῦ βασιλεύοντος Λευκίου κατὰ τὴν Μεσοποταμίαν ὀνομαζομένην ὄντος ἐπάρχου ἐδεῖτο τοῦ μαθήματος καὶ αὐτὸς ὥσπερ ὁ Παῦλος. ὕστερον δὲ καὶ Σεβῆρος ὕπατος μὲν ὢν ἐσπουδακὼς δὲ περὶ τὴν Ἀριστοτέλους φιλοσοφίαν.

3. Ὅπως μὲν οὖν τὰ κατὰ τὰς ἀνατομὰς ἐγένετο γινώσκοντί σοι βραχείας ἀναμνήσεως δεήσει μικρὸν ὕστερον ἐσομένης· ἐπὶ δὲ τὰ κατὰ τὸν Εὔδημον ἐπάνειμι. καταπονούμενος γὰρ ὑπὸ τῶν τριῶν τεταρταίων
2 ἀπήλπιστο πρὸς τῶν ἰατρῶν ὄντος ἤδη που μέσου χειμῶνος. ἐγὼ δὲ καὶ οἷα διδασκάλῳ μὲν ἀλλὰ καὶ κατὰ τύχην οἰκῶν αὐτοῦ πλησίον ἀνάγκην
3 εἶχον ὑπακούειν δὶς τῆς ἡμέρας καλοῦντι. καταγελῶν δέ μου κατὰ τὸν καιρὸν ἐκεῖνον Ἀντιγένης, εἷς ⟨ὢν⟩ τῶν Κοΐντου μαθητῶν συγγεγονὼς δὲ καὶ Μαρίνῳ πρωτεύειν τε τῶν ἰατρῶν πεπιστευμένος ἅπαντάς τε τοὺς πολὺ δυναμένους ἰώμενος, οὐκ οἶδ' ὅτι δόξαν αὐτῷ τοῖς ἐπαινοῦσι καταγελῶν ἔφασκεν ὀλίγον ὕστερον αὐτοὺς γνώσεσθαι τίνα τυγχάνου-
614 σιν ἐπαινοῦντες ὅταν ἐκφερόμενον Εὔδημον ἴδωσιν, | καὶ ταῦτα λέγων πρὸς τοὺς παρόντας ἰδιώτας, ἀποστρέφων ἐνίοτε μὲν τὸν λόγον ἀποβλέπων τε πρὸς τοὺς ἰατροὺς ἔφασκεν· «Εὔδημον ἑξηκοστὸν καὶ τρίτον ἔτος ἄγοντα, τρεῖς ἔχοντα τεταρταίους ἐν μέσῳ χειμῶνι θεραπεύειν
4 ὑπισχνεῖται Γαληνός.» σὺ μὲν οὖν, Ἐπίγενες φίλτατε, τάς τε μετὰ ταῦτα γενομένας προρρήσεις ἐπ' αὐτοῦ καὶ τὴν θεραπείαν οἶδ' ὅτι κηρύττων διετέλεσας, ἐμοὶ δ' ἀρχὴ φθόνου τότε πρῶτον ἐγένετο θαυ-
5 μαζόμενος ὡς ἐπί τε βίου σεμνότητος καὶ τοῖς κατὰ τὴν τέχνην ἔργοις. ἐκ γὰρ τῶν τριῶν τεταρταίων τὸν μὲν πρῶτον ἀρξάμενον ἐν τῇδε παύσασθαι τῇ ἡμέρᾳ προειπὼν ἐθαυμάσθην· ἐπεὶ δὲ καὶ τοῦ δευτέρου τὴν προθεσμίαν τῆς λύσεως ἠλήθευσα ἅπαντες μὲν ἐξεπλάγησαν· ἐπὶ τοῦ τρίτου γοῦν ἀποτυχεῖν με τοῖς θεοῖς ηὔχοντο. παυσαμένου δὲ κἀκείνου κατὰ τὴν ὑπ' ἐμοῦ προρρηθεῖσαν ἡμέραν οὐκ ἐπὶ ταῖς προρρήσεσι μόνον ἀλλὰ καὶ τῇ θεραπείᾳ δόξαν ἔσχον οὐ σμικράν.

9 ὕστερον] *v. infra* p. 96,5–100,6 18 ὅταν – ἴδωσιν] *cf.* Martial. XI 71 Anth. Pal. XI 125 24 ἐμοὶ – ἐγένετο] *cf.* Gal. De libr. propr. 1: Scr. min. II p. 96,19sq. Müller = XIX p. 15,15sq. K.

1 μετὰ τὴν πεῖραν] postea *Nic.* 2 ἔφη[I]] ἔφην L πᾶν y 5 *punctum post* ὄντος *add.* y ὑπάρχειν y: *om.* A: ὑπάρχου *coni. Bas.*: *sec. Nic.* (eparchi [ap- *Nic.*[c]]) *correxi* 6 *post* ὥσπερ *add.* καὶ A *Nic.* 7 *ante* περὶ *add.* καὶ M 9 μικρὸν – ἐσομένης *om. Nic.* τὰ *om.* MP 11 που] τοῦ *fort. scribendum* καὶ – 12 καὶ *om. Nic.* καὶ *secl. Bas.* 12 οἷα] ὡς LA, *fort. recte* κατατυχὼν y: κατατυχον[T] A: *sec. Nic.* (secundum fortunam) *corr. Bas.* οἰκεῖν yA: *sec. Nic.* (habitans) *corr. Bas.* 13 μοι L 14 ὢν *sec. Nic.* (unus existens) *addidi* 16 τε] δὲ A 17 αὐτοὶ γνώσονται A: scietis *Nic.* αὐτὸν L 18 ἴδωσιν Εὔδημον M: uideritis Eudimum *Nic.* 19 ἀποστρέφων – λόγον *om. Nic.* μὲν *om.* A 20 ἔφασκον P 21 ἄγοντος A ἔχοντος A τριταίους y χειμῶνος y 22 τάς τε *om.* A 23 γενομένας *ante* μετὰ *(lin. 22) trsp.* A 24 θαυμαζομένῳ τε A 25 ὡς *secl. Bas.* σεμνότητι A 27 καὶ τοῦ *sscr.* L 31 καὶ *om.* A μικράν AP

he discovered my name, he told this too to Paulus, and said that he
was also inviting me after this test-piece to give a demonstration to
him as well; for Paulus agreed that he certainly lacked the opportun-
ity of observing phenomena revealed by dissections. Similarly Bar- 27
barus also, the uncle of the emperor Lucius, who was then ruling
the area called Mesopotamia, requested instruction, like Paulus,
and later also Severus, a consul and an enthusiast for Aristotelian
philosophy.

3. As you know what happened at my dissections, you will
require only a brief reminder, which I shall give a little later, – but I
return to the case of Eudemus. Thoroughly exhausted by the three
quartans, he was given up for lost by his doctors as it was already,
I think, mid-winter. However, since he was my teacher and I happened 2
also to live nearby, I was obliged to attend to his twice daily summons.
On this occasion I was ridiculed by Antigenes, one of the pupils of 3
Quintus and an associate also of Marinus, who was considered to
be the leader of the physicians and who treated all the most influential
people. For some reason or other, he scornfully told my supporters that
they would soon realise whom they were supporting when they saw
Eudemus being carried out. He addressed these remarks to the laity
present, occasionally breaking off his argument and glancing at the
doctors to say, "Look at Eudemus: he is in his sixty third year; he
has had three quartan attacks in mid-winter; and Galen promises to
cure him." I know that you, my dear Epigenes, constantly trumpet- 4
ed my later predictions in this case and my treatment, but here for
the first time there arose jealousy because I was being respected for
my dignified way of life as well as for my professional successes. Thus 5
when I foretold the exact day on which the first of the three quartans
would end, I awakened surprise; when I correctly declared the basis
of the resolution of the second attack, all were astounded; as for the
third, they prayed to the gods for my discomfiture. But when that too
ended on the day that I had predicted, I gained no slight reputation,
not only for my predictions but also for my treatment.

6 Ὁ γοῦν Ἀντιγένης μόνον οὐ κατὰ γῆς ἐδύετο διὰ τὰς προπετῶς
αὐτῷ γενομένας εἰς ἐμὲ βλασφημίας· ὁμοίως δ' αὐτῷ καὶ Μαρτιανός,
615 οὗ καὶ | αὐτοῦ κατά τε τὸν χρόνον ἐκεῖνον ἔτι τε πρότερον ὡς ἀνατο-
μικωτάτου δόξα μεγάλη παρὰ τοῖς ἰατροῖς νεανίσκοις ἦν. ἐσπουδάζετο
7 δὲ δύο βιβλία τῶν ὑπ' αὐτοῦ γεγραμμένων ἀνατομῶν. ἀνιαθεὶς δὲ καὶ
αὐτὸς ἐφ' οἷς Εὔδημος οὐ μόνον ἐπαινεῖσθαι χρῆναί με πρὸς ἁπάντων
δικαίως ἀλλὰ καὶ θαυμάζεσθαι δεῖν ἔφασκεν, οὐκ ἐξ ἰατρικῆς τὰς προρ-
ρήσεις ἀλλ' ἐκ μαντικῆς γίνεσθαι ταύτας ὑπ' ἐμοῦ διέβαλλε· καὶ τήν γε
μαντικὴν ἥντινα λέγοι πυνθανομένων τινῶν ἐνίοτε μὲν οἰωνιστικὴν
8 ἔφασκεν ἐνίοτε δὲ θυτικὴν ἔστι δ' ὅτε συμβολικὴν ἢ μαθηματικήν. ὕστα-
τον δέ τι παρὰ τῷ Εὐδήμῳ τοιοῦτον ἐγένετο· τοῦ τρίτου τῶν τεταρ-
ταίων τῆς ἡμέρας ἐνστάσης ἐν ᾗ τελείαν ἀπαλλαγὴν αὐτῷ προειρήκειν
ἔσεσθαι παραγενόμενος ὁ Μαρτιανὸς πρὸς τὸν Εὔδημον ὥρας ἐνάτης,
οὐ σμικρῷ σφοδρότερον ἀλλὰ καὶ πάνυ πολλῷ τοῦ προγεγενημένου
παροξυσμοῦ τὸν νῦν ὄντα φήσας ὑπάρχειν ἐχωρίσθη παραχρῆμα
φαιδρῷ τῷ προσώπῳ φανερῶς ἐνδεικνύμενος ἐπιχαίρειν ὡς ἀποτετευγ-
9 μένης τῆς προρρήσεως. αἰσθανόμενος δ' ὁ Εὔδημος εὐφορίας ὁποίας |
616 οὔπω πρότερον ᾔσθετο καὶ μέντοι καὶ θαρρῶν ὡς οὐ σφαλησομένῳ μοι
κατὰ τὴν πρόρρησιν ἀνέμεινεν ἀφικέσθαι τινὰ καὶ ἄλλον ἰατρόν. ἀφικο-
μένου δ' οὐχ ἑνὸς μόνον ἀλλὰ καὶ δυοῖν καὶ τριῶν – ἐπετήρουν γὰρ
ἅπαντες ὅπως ἀποβῇ τὰ κατὰ τὴν πρόρρησιν εὐχόμενοι κἂν ἐπί γε τοῦ
τρίτου τῶν τεταρταίων ἀτυχῆσαί με τῆς τε προρρήσεως καὶ τῆς ἐπ'
αὐτοῦ θεραπείας – ὁ μὲν Εὔδημος ἠξίωσε κἀκείνους ἀποφήνασθαι
πῶς ἔχειν αὐτοῖς τὰ κατ' αὐτὸν δοκοίη, τὴν δ' αὐτὴν ἀπόκρισιν ἀκούσας
ἣν ὁ Μαρτιανὸς ἐπεποίητο καὶ προ⟨σ⟩σχὼν ὁμοίως κἀκείνοις ὡς Μαρ-
τιανῷ φαιδροτέροις γεγονόσιν ἐνόησε μὲν καὶ αὐτὸς ἐπιχαίρειν αὐτοὺς
10 ὡς ἀποτετευγμένης τῆς προρρήσεώς τε καὶ θεραπείας. ἐπεὶ δ' ἐχρόνιζον
ἐγὼ παρὰ τὸ ἔθος ἐν ἐπισκέψει τινὶ κατεχόμενος ἔπεμπε συνεχῶς πρός

3 ἀνατομικωτάτου – 5] *cf.* Gal. De libr. propr. I: Scr. min. II p. 94,24–26 Müller = XIX p. 13,9 sq. K. 7 sq. οὐκ – γίνεσθαι] *cf. infra* p. 94,18 sq.; 106,23–26 Gal. De febr. diff. II 7: VII p. 354,4–6 K. De loc. aff. V 8: VIII p. 362,5 sq. K. Syn. de puls. 6: IX p. 447,4–6 K. De crisib. III 8: p. 189,22–190,10 Alex. = IX p. 737,12–738,5 K. In Hipp. Progn. comm. III 42: CMG V 9,2 p. 369,8 sq. De caus. procat. II 18: CMG Suppl. II p. 5,18–23 De nominib. medic. p. 20,31; p. 21,14–18 *exc.* ar-Ruhāwī *Adab aṭ-ṭabīb* fol. 79a: p. 71ª,46–50 Levey

2 γεγενημένας A Μαρτιάλιος *Schöne*: Marcianus *Nic.*ʷ: Martianus *Nic.*ᶜᵉ 3 ἀνατομικωτάτω y 4 ἰατρικοῖς *Schöne* 5 δὲ^II] οὖν A 6 ἅπαντα M: ἅπαντας AL: *sec. Nic.* (ab omnibus) *corr. Schöne* 8 διέβαλε y 9 λέγει A: λέγοιμι L *post* λέγοι *add.* ἂν M πυνθανανομένων L *post* μὲν *add. et del.* ἔτι L 10 ἔστι] ἔτι L ὕστατα A 13 Μαρτιάλιος *Schöne* 14 μικρῷ A 17 αἰσθόμενος A ὁποίας *om.* A 18 καὶ θαρρῶν *om.* A σφαλισομένῳ L 19 ἀνέμεινεν – 21 πρόρρησιν] aduenerunt alii medici *Nic.* ἀναμείνας y 22 τε *om.* A ἀπ' yA: *corr. Corn.* 24 αὐτὴν δὲ A 25 Μαρτιάλιος *Schöne* πεποίηται y προσχὼν yA: *sec. Nic.* (aduertens) *correxi* κἀκείνους yA: *corr. Ald.* *ante* Μαρτιανῷ *add.* τῷ A Μαρτιανοῦ M 26 φαιδρότερον γεγονῶσιν L ἐνενόησε M καὶ αὐτὸς *om. Nic.* καὶ *om.* A 27 δὲ χρονίζων y 28 παρὰ] secundum *Nic.*

Antigenes was completely demolished as a result of the slanders 6
he had so rashly uttered against me. It was the same with Martianus,
who both then and earlier had a great reputation among the young
doctors as an outstanding anatomist. Two of his treatises on anatomy
were especially in vogue. He was annoyed with Eudemus for saying 7
that I rightly deserved not merely praise but admiration from every-
one, and he slanderously maintained that my forecasts derived not
from medicine but from divination. When some people asked him
what sort of divination he meant, he sometimes said that it came from
observing the flight of birds, sometimes from sacrifices, sometimes
from chance happenings or from consulting horoscopes. What finally 8
happened in the case of Eudemus was this. When the day arrived
on which I had predicted his total release from the third quartan,
Martianus visited Eudemus at the ninth hour, and after declaring
that the fresh attack was not just a little stronger but far greater than
the previous paroxysm, he went off immediately with a cheerful
countenance, displaying obvious pleasure at the failure of my predic-
tion. But Eudemus, who was beginning to feel an improvement such 9
as he had not felt before and who was now confident that I would not
fail in my prediction, waited for some other doctor to arrive. So when
not merely one but two or three came – for they were all observing
the outcome of my prediction and praying for me to fail in my forecast
of the third of the quartans at least and in my cure of it –, Eudemus
demanded that they too should tell him how they thought his case was
going. When he heard the same reply as Martianus had made and
noticed that they, like Martianus, had cheered up, he concluded for
himself that they were rejoicing at the failure of my prediction and
treatment. Since I was unusually delayed through being detained on a 10
visit, he persistently sent round to me – for, as I have said, I was a

με πλησίον οἰκοῦντα, καθάπερ ἔφην, ἐπικριθῆναι τὴν εὐφορίαν ἣν εἶχεν
11 ὑπ' ἐμοῦ βουλόμενος. ὡς δ' οὖν ἀφικόμην οὐδὲ καθίσαι με περιμείνας
ἐξέτεινε τὴν χεῖρα κελεύων ἅψασθαι τῶν σφυγμῶν. ἁψαμένου δὲ μετὰ
617 σπουδῆς ἐπυνθάνετο τί ποτ' ἀγγέλλοιμι. | κἀγὼ μειδιάσας, «τί ἄλλο»,
ἔφην, «ἢ ἀγαθά;» «ποῖα», εἶπε, «ταῦτα εἰδικῶς μοι φράσον.» ἐγὼ δέ,
«οὐκ ἀρκέσει», ἔφην, «σοὶ τὸ κεφάλαιον αὐτῶν ἀθρόως ἀκηκοότι χαίρειν
ἐπὶ τοῖς ἐσομένοις;» «οὐδαμῶς», εἶπεν, «ἀκοῦσαι γὰρ ποθῶ καὶ ⟨τὰ⟩ κατὰ
12 μέρος.» «ἄκουε δή· ἀπαλλαγήσῃ τῇ νυκτὶ ταύτῃ τελέως ἁπάσης τῆς νοσώ-
δους διαθέσεως τῶν ⟨τ'⟩ ἐπιγενομένων καὶ τῶν ἐσομένων αὐτῇ συμπτω-
μάτων ἁπάντων ἡ λύσις ἀκολουθήσει. καὶ τοῦτ' ἔφην ἄρτι μοι διὰ τῶν
σφυγμῶν δεδηλωκέναι τὴν διοικοῦσάν σου τὸ σῶμα φύσιν ἐπεγηγερ-
μένην ἤδη καὶ κινουμένην ὡς ἐκβαλεῖν ἐκ τοῦ σώματος ἅπασαν οὖσαν
13 ἔν σοι μοχθηρίαν τὴν ἐν τοῖς κατὰ τὸ σῶμα χυμοῖς.» «πῶς οὖν δὴ παρὰ
τῆς φύσεως τοῦτο λέγεις σοι δεδηλῶσθαι – οὐ γὰρ δὴ φθεγξαμένη γε
ταῦτ' εἶπεν – ἀπόκριναί μοι· πάντως γὰρ οἶσθα παρακολουθήσαντά με
14 τῷ λόγῳ μᾶλλον ἁπάντων τούτων τῶν ἰαλέμων ἰατρῶν.» «ὅτι τὴν
κίνησιν», ἔφην, «τῶν ἀρτηριῶν εἰς ὕψος ἀνήγαγεν ἐπὶ πλέον τῆς ἐφ'
ἑκάτερον διαστάσεως, ὅπερ ἀεὶ ποιεῖν εἴωθεν ἐγχειροῦσα τὸ λυποῦν
618 15 ἐκκρίνειν τοῦ σώματος.» ἐπὶ τούτοις ῥηθεῖσιν ὁ Εὔ|δημος ὑπολαβὼν ἔφη,
«ἀλλ' ἐπεὶ πολλαὶ τῆς ἐκκρίσεως ὁδοὶ τέτμηνται τῇ φύσει – καὶ γὰρ
ἔμετος καὶ γαστὴρ καταρρήξασα, τάχα δὲ καὶ οὔρων πλῆθος ἱδρώτων τε
πολλῶν ἐκκρίσεις αἱμορραγία τε καὶ συνήθης αἱμορροῒς ἀναστομωθεῖσα
κένωσιν ἀθρόαν ἐργάζεται – τῆς σῆς ἂν εἴη τέχνης ἔργον οἰκεῖον ἑρμη-
16 νεῦσαί μοι τὸ τῆς κενώσεως εἶδος.» «αἱμορραγίας μὲν οὖν», ἔφην, «ἐσομένης
τάδε καὶ τάδε προηγεῖται σημεῖα, καθάπερ γε καὶ ἱδρώτων ταυτί.» προσ-
έθηκα δ' ἐν τῷ λόγῳ καὶ τὰ τῶν ἐμέτων προηγούμενα. «τῆς δὲ διὰ τῆς
κάτω γαστρὸς ἀθρόας κενώσεως κριτικῆς οὐδὲν ἔχομεν ἴδιον ἐξαίρετον
σημεῖον ἀλλ' ἐκ τοῦ μηδὲν τῶν ἄλλων παρεῖναι καταλείποιτ' ἂν ἐλπίζειν
ἐπὶ σοῦ γενήσεσθαι τοῦτο.» «διαλεκτικῶς», ἔφη, «συνελογίσω τὴν εὕρεσιν
τοῦ γενησομένου.»

1] *v. supra* p. 82,12 10–29] *exc.* Razes *Kitāb al-ḥāwī* XVII 219,12 10–13] *cf.* Gal. In Hipp. Prorrhet. I comm. III 49: CMG V 9,2 p. 157,2 sq.; III 57: CMG V 9,2 p. 162,20 sq. 20–25] *cf.* Gal. De crisib. III 11: p. 207,1–211,18 Alex. = IX p. 761,12–767,12 K.

4 ἀγγέλοιμι AN 5 ἀγαθόν y: omnia bona *Nic.* ἰδικῶς MA φράστ L ἐγὼ δέ] τὸ δέ L: τόδε M 6 ἀρκέσειν y: ἄρ' A: sufficit *Nic.*: *corr. Ald.* αὐτὸ y ἀθρόως ἀκηκοότι *om.* A, *spatio 16 litt. relicto* 7 τὰ *sec. Nic.* (ea que) *add. Bas.* 9 τῶν^{I} – συμπτωμάτων] quo fiente et sequentium eam sinthomatum *Nic.* τῶν τ'] ὧν yA: *corr. Chart.* ἐπιγενομένων] γενομένων y ἐσομένων] ἐπιγινομένων καὶ τῶν ἐπιγενομένων A συμπτώματα A 10 ἀκολουθῇ L: ἀκολουθεῖ M 10sq. τῶν σφυγμῶν *om. Nic.* 12sq. νόσον ἔν σοι μοχθηρὰν y 13 τὴν] ἣν L: *om.* A δὴ] ἔφη *sec. Nic.* (ait) *coni. Durling, fort. recte* 14 τοῦτο *ante* παρὰ *(lin. 13) trsp.* A γε] τε y 15 εἶπε y 18 ἑκατέρας y: secundum alterutram dimensionem *Nic.* 19 ἔφη *om.* y 20 τετίμενται M: τετίμηνται LN *(e* τέτμηνται *mut.)*: *sec. Nic.* (ordinatae) τετάχαται *Bas.* 21 κατήρξασα y τάχα δὲ *om. Nic.* 22 *ante* αἱμορραγία *add.* καὶ A τε *om.* A 24 αἱμοραγίας L οὖν *om.* y ἔφη L γενομένης y 25 σημεῖα *om. Nic.* γε *om.* A 27 ἀθρόας] repentine *Nic.*: *post* κενώσεως *trsp.* M κινήσεως A 28 καταλοίποιτ' L

neighbour –, wanting me to pass judgement on the feeling of well-being which he had. As soon as I arrived, he did not even wait for me 11
to sit down, but stretched out his hand and ordered me to take his pulse; and when I had done so, he eagerly asked for my opinion. With a smile I said, "Nothing but good." "Tell me", he said, "precisely what it is." "Isn't it going to be enough", I replied, "for you to rejoice at your prospects after hearing a short summary?" "Not at all", he rejoined, "I want to hear a detailed account as well." "Listen then. 12
Tonight you will be completely free of the whole morbid condition, and the resolution of all supervening and future symptoms will follow." I also said that this was just revealed to me through his pulse beats by the nature which governed his body, which was then aroused and active in expelling from the body all that was noxious in his bodily humours. "What do you mean by 'this has been shown by 13
nature'? – for surely it did not tell you so by speaking – answer me that. For you are well aware that I follow your argument far better than all these wretched doctors." "Because it has caused an upward 14
movement of the arteries even more than a lateral expansion", I said, "which it always does when it is trying to discharge an irritant from the body." At this Eudemus interjected, "But since there are many 15
routes of discharge devised by nature – for vomiting, alvine evacuation, possibly also excessive urination and abundant sweats, haemorrhage and normal bleeding piles, all produce wholesale evacuation – it would be the particular task of your art to explain to me the mode of evacuation." "Well now", I said, "this and this group of indications 16
precede an impending haemorrhage, just as these portend sweats." I then added to my argument also those that precede an attack of vomiting. "We have no particular special sign for a wholesale critical evacuation through the lower belly: but since none of the other particular indications is present, it remains to hope that this is what will happen to you." "You have made a truly logical exposition of how you reached this prognosis", he said.

17 Ταῦτα μὲν ἑσπέρας οὔσης ἤδη διελέχθημεν ἀλλήλοις, παραγενόμενος
δ' ἕωθεν ἤκουσας αὐτὸς σὺ τοῦ κεφαλαίου τῆς προρρήσεως, οὐχ ὑπομέ-
νοντος μετρίως φθέγγεσθαι τοῦ φιλοσόφου καθάπερ εἴωθεν κεκραγότος
δὲ πρὸς ἅπαντας ἡμᾶς τοὺς εἰσιόντας φίλους ὡς ὁ Πύθιος 'Απόλλων
619 διὰ τοῦ | Γαληνοῦ στόματος ἐβουλήθη θεσπίζειν τοῖς νοσοῦσι καὶ
μετὰ τοῦτο θεραπεύειν αὐτοὺς ἀπαλλάττειν τε τελέως αὐτοὺς ἐν ἡμέρᾳ
18 προρρηθείσῃ. τὴν γοῦν γεγενημένην λύσιν τοῦ νοσήματος — πέπεισμαι
γὰρ ἤδη τελέως ὑγιαίνειν — ἐπαγγειλάμενος ἐκ πολλοῦ καὶ τῆς θεραπείας
19 καὶ τῆς προρρήσεως ἔτυχεν. ἀπήλλαξε δέ με τριῶν τεταρταίων οἷς ἐξ
ἀκαίρου πόσεως τοῦ θηριακοῦ φαρμάκου περιέπεσον, ὁπότε καιρὸς αὐτῆς
ἐγένετο μηδὲν ἐκείνων φθεγγομένων δοὺς οὗτος ἀπήλλαξέ με, κατα-
γελώμενος ὑπ' αὐτῶν εἴ γε νομίζει γέροντα χειμῶνος ὥρᾳ κάμνοντα τρισὶ
τεταρταίοις ἀπαλλάξειν.

4. Οἱ μὲν ἰδιῶται τῆς ἰατρικῆς τέχνης ἀκούοντες ταῦτα, κοινὸν ἀγαθὸν ἡγούμενοί με τοῖς ἐν 'Ρώμῃ γενήσεσθαι πάντες ἔχαιρον. ὁ δ' οὐκ ἰατρὸς μόνον ἀλλὰ καὶ φιλό⟨σοφο⟩ς εἶναι μαρτυρούμενος Μαρτιανὸς ἀκούσας τήν τε κατὰ τὴν γεγονυῖαν ἡμέραν ἀπόφασίν μου περὶ τῆς ἐν ταῖς ἀρτηρίαις κινήσεως, ἣν ἐκεῖνοι θορυβώδη νομίζοντες, οὐ κριτικήν, ἐδεδίεσαν, εὑρών τε κατὰ φύσιν ἀκριβῶς ἔχοντα τὸν Εὔδημον ἐπαινέσαι μὲν οὐδ' ἄχρι
620 2 ῥήματος | ἑνὸς ὑπέμεινέ με. καταβὰς δ' εἰς τὸ Σανδαλ⟨ι⟩άριον ἀπήντησέ
μοι κατὰ τύχην εὐθέως δὲ μήτε προσαγορεύσας ὡς ἔθος εἶχεν ἐπύθετο πότερον ἀνεγνωκὼς εἴην τὸ δεύτερον τῶν 'Ιπποκράτους Προρρητικῶν ἢ ὅλως ἀγνοοῖμι τὸ σύγγραμμα, κἄπειτ' ἀκούσας ὡς ἀνεγνωκὼς εἴην καί μοι δοκοῖεν ὀρθῶς ἔνιοι τῶν ἰατρῶν οὐκ εἶναι τῶν γνησίων 'Ιπποκράτους βιβλίων αὐτὸ προσηκόντως ἀποφήνασθαι, «πάντως γοῦν γινώσκεις», ἔφη, «τὸ γεγραμμένον ἐν αὐτῷ 'ἐγὼ δὲ τοιαῦτα μὲν οὐ μαν-

22 τὸ δεύτερον τῶν 'Ιπποκράτους Προρρητικῶν] IX p. 7–75 L. 24sq. καὶ – ἀποφήνασθαι] *cf.* Gal. In Hipp. Progn. comm. III 7: CMG V 9,2 p. 115,10–14; III 34: CMG V 9,2 p. 147,28–148,10 In Hipp. Epid. III comm. I 4: CMG V 10,2,1 p. 13, 7–11; III prooem.: CMG V 10,2,1 p. 62,6sq. 26 ἐγὼ – μαντεύομαι] Hipp. Prorrhet. II 1: IX p. 8,2 L. *cf.* Gal. De uteri dissect. 10,11: CMG V 2,1 p. 54,18

1 διηλέχθημεν A παραγενόμενος] aduenienté me *Nic.* 4 ἡμᾶς *om. Nic.*: ἡμᾶς (?) A, *sed forma litterae* υ *magis quam* η *conuenit, fort. melius* ὑμᾶς *scribendum* ὁ Πύθιος 'Απόλλων] deus *Nic.* 5 θεσπίζειν] θεραπεύειν A καὶ *om.* y 6 τοῦτο] τὸ y: cum hoc quod curat *Nic.*: τοῦ *edd.*: τούτου *Scaliger* τελείως A αὐτοὺς *om.* A *Nic.* 7 πέπεισται L 9 ἔτυχον y: prouenerunt *Nic.* δέ με *om.* M 10 περιπεσών yA: *correxi* *post* ὁπότε *sec. Nic.* (quando autem) δὲ *addiderim* 11 μηδὲν – φθεγγομένων *om. Nic.* δοὺς οὗτος] dans iste id *Nic.* 12 νομίζοι *coniecerim* γέροντος A 14 *post* μὲν *sec. Nic.* (igitur) οὖν *add. Bas., inepte* ταὖτο L 15 με τοῖς] μετὰ τῆς A: me in Roma esse *Nic.* ὃ L 16 φίλος yA: *suppl. Schöne* Μαρτιάλιος *Schöne* 17 κατὰ – ἡμέραν *om. Nic.* μου *om.* A περὶ *om.* M 18 ἣν – 19 τε] eum extimans perturbatiuum (-batum *Nic.*[e]) et non creticum, stupuit uidendo *Nic.* εὑρόντες yA: *corr. Corn.* 19 ἀκριβῶς *om.* A 20 Σανδαλάριον yA: *correxi*: Damarium *Nic.*[bc]: Damatium *Nic.*[z] 21 μηδὲ *Schöne, fort. recte* 22 τῶν] τοῦ y Προρρητικὸν y: secundum tractatum proretice *Nic.* 23 τὸ σύγγραμμα] ipsum *Nic.* 24 δοκεῖ ἐν L οὐκ] οὐκέτι y 25 αὐτὸ] αὐτὸν L *post* αὐτὸ *add.* καὶ A προσηκόντως *om. Nic.* πάντως – 90,1 τοῦτο *om. Nic.* 26 τῶν γεγραμμένων y μαντεύσομαι *Hipp.*

We had already discussed this in the evening, and when you 17
arrived next morning, you heard a summary of my prediction. The
philosopher abandoned his normal moderate manner of speaking and
shouted to all of us his friends as we entered the house that Pythian
Apollo deigned to prophesy to the sick through the mouth of Galen,
and then to treat them and cure them completely on the day predicted.
"Galen announced my recovery from this illness long ago: I am con- 18
vinced that I am already fully fit: and he has succeeded both in his
treatment and his forecast. He has cured me of three quartan fevers, 19
to which I succumbed after drinking theriac medicine at the wrong
time. When the time for it was right, although they said nothing, this
man gave it me and cured me, despite being scoffed at by them for
presuming to cure an old man of three quartans in wintertime."

4. When the amateurs of medicine heard this, they were all delight-
ed to think that I was going to be a public benefit to the inhabitants
of Rome. Martianus, on the other hand, who was acknowledged to
be a philosopher as well as a doctor, when he heard my statement of
the previous day about the movement in the arteries – they were
afraid because they thought it indicated a disturbance, not a crisis –,
and when he found Eudemus in perfectly normal health, could not
bear to give me even a word of congratulation. However, he met me 2
by chance as he was on his way down to the street of the Sandal-
makers. Immediately, without even his usual greeting, he asked me
whether I had read the second book of the Prorrhetics of Hippo-
crates or whether I was entirely ignorant of the work. When he heard
that I had read it and that some doctors rightly seemed to me to have
correctly declared that it did not belong to the genuine writings of
Hippocrates, "Then you are well aware", he said, "of the sentence
in it, 'I make no prophecy in these matters'?" "Why have you said

3 τεύομαι';» «πρὸς τί δὲ νῦν», ἔφην, «εἴρηταί σοι τοῦτο;» καὶ ὃς ἄρτι κε-
χωρίσθαι παρ' Εὐδήμου θαυμάζοντος ἔλεγεν ἐπὶ τοῦ χθὲς ἑσπέρας
ἀψάμενόν σε τῶν σφυγμῶν προειπεῖν ἔκκρισιν ἔσεσθαι διὰ τῆς κάτω
4 γαστρὸς ἐφ' ἧς μηκέτι πυρέξειν. εἰπόντος οὖν αὐτοῦ ταῦτα, μόνον ἀπο-
κρινάμενος ἐγώ, «παρ' Εὐδήμου ταῦτ' ἀκήκοας, οὐ παρ' ἐμοῦ», παρῆλθον
αὐτίκα. πορευθείς τε πρὸς τὸν Εὔδημον ἀπήγγειλα τὸ γεγονὸς ἐθαύ-
μαζόν τε τὴν κακόνοιαν τῶν εὐδοκιμούντων ἰατρῶν ἐν τῇ Ῥωμαίων
5 πόλει. ὁ δὲ κατὰ λόγον ἔφη με τοῦτο πεπονθέναι, ἀπεικάζων τοῖς ἐν
621 πατρίδι | τοὺς τῇδε κατὰ πλείους αἰτίας εἰς ἄκρον ἥκοντας κακοηθείας,
6 καὶ διῆλθεν ἁπάσας ἑξῆς ὡδί πως· «μὴ νόμιζε τοὺς ἀγαθοὺς ἄνδρας ἐν
ταύτῃ τῇ πόλει γίνεσθαι πονηρούς, ἀλλ' ὅσοι φθάνουσιν εἶναι πονηροί,
πραγμάτων ὕλην εὑρόντες ἐνταῦθα κέρδη πολὺ μείζονα τῶν ἐν ταῖς
ἔξω πόλεσιν ἔχουσιν. ὁρῶντές ⟨τε⟩ πεπλουτηκότας ὁμοίους ἑαυτοῖς πολ-
λοὺς ἐμιμήσαντο τὰς πράξεις αὐτῶν πολυειδεῖς οὔσας ⟨καὶ⟩ ἐκ πλειόνων
7 αἰτιῶν εἰς ἔσχατον ἥκουσι πονηρίας. ἐρῶ δέ σοί τινας αὐτῶν ὡς ἂν ἐκ
πολλοῦ χρόνου πεπειραμένος. οὐ γὰρ μόνον ἡ φύσις οὐδ' ἡ τῶν κερδα-
λέων πραγμάτων ὕλη τὴν πονηρίαν ηὔξησε τῶν φύσει πονηρῶν ἀλλὰ
καὶ μάθησις ἠκολούθησε πανουργίας ὁδῶν ἃς ἑώρων ὁσημέραι γινομένας
8 ὑπὸ τῶν ὁμοίων ἑαυτοῖς· εἶτ' ἐν τῷ μιμεῖσθαι ταύτας ἐτρίβη⟨σαν⟩. τό τε κἂν
φωραθῶσιν ὑπό τινος πανουργοῦντες ἐπ' ἄλλους ἔχειν ἀγνῶτας ἑαυτῶν
μεταβαίνειν, οἷς ἐκ τῆς πρώτης πείρας ὧν πράττοντες κακῶς ἐγνώσθησαν
622 ἀσφαλέστερον προσφέρονται, οὐ σμικρὰν ἔχει δύναμιν οὐδ' | αὐτὸ πρὸς
9 τὸ μηδέποτε παύεσθαι πανουργοῦντας. οἱ δ' ἐν ταῖς σμικραῖς πόλεσιν
οὐθ' ὑπὸ μεγέθους κερδῶν δελεαζόμενοι καθάπερ οἱ τῇδε γινωσκόμενοί τε
ῥᾳδίως ὑπὸ τῶν πολιτῶν εἰ καὶ μικρὸν ἁμάρτοιεν ἀγύμναστον ἔχουσι
10 τὴν θεωρίαν. ἐνταῦθα δὲ καὶ τὸ μὴ γινώσκεσθαι πρὸς ἁπάντων ἃ πράτ-
τουσιν ἑκάστοτε πανουργοῦντας αὐξάνει τὴν κακίαν τῆς φύσεως αὐτῶν.
ἐπιτίθενται γὰρ τοῖς ἀγνοοῦσιν αὐτοὺς ἀπροοράτως καὶ μάλισθ' ὅταν
ἀντιδακεῖν αὐτοὺς οὗτοι δι' ἁπλότητα γνώμης μὴ δύνανται καθάπερ

6 ἐθαύμαζόν – 8 πόλει] *cf.* Gal. De nominib. medic. p. 21,6–35 19–23] *cf.* Gal. De exam. medico: Dietrich, p. 193,8–10

1 σοῦ L *(corr.* L²*)* M *post* σοι *add.* νῦν y ὡς *Ald.* κεχωρῆσθαι AL, *in* κεχωρέσθαι *mut.* L 2 τοῦ] τῷ A 3 τὸν σφυγμὸν y: pulsum *Nic.* 4 ἧς] ᾗ A 5 παρηλ^θ L: recessit *Nic.* 8 μοι y: *deest* A: *corr. Corn.* ἀπεικάζων – 9 πατρίδι *om. Nic.* ἀπεικάζον^τ L 9 κακοηθίας L 10 ἁπάσας ἑξῆς] quasdam earum *Nic.*^w: quosdam eorum *Nic.*^c 11 φθάνονται L 12 εὑρὼν y: *deest* A: εὗρον N*Ald.*: *sec. Nic.* (inuenientes) *corr. Bas.* *ante* κέρδη *add.* καὶ *sec. Nic.* (et lucra) *Bas.* 13 τε *addidi* ὁμοίως yA: similiter *Nic.*: *corr. Bas.* ἐν αὐτοῖς A: αὐτοῖς M 14 καὶ *sec. Nic.* (et ex aliis) *add. Bas.* 15 ἥκειν yA: ἥκοντας *Ald.*: *corr. Corn. Chart.* 16 ἡ φύσις οὐδ' *om. Nic.* 17 φύσει πονηρῶν] φιλοπονηρῶν A: malignorum *Nic.* 18 πανουργίας *ex* πανούργως *corr.* L ὁδῶν *om. Nic.* 19 ἑαυτῷ L ταῦτα A: *om. Nic.* ἐτρίβη τότε y: ἐτρίβη. τότε A: *om. Nic.*: διετρίβησαν *Bas.*: *correxi* 20 φοραθῶσιν L 22 ἀσφαλέστερον] cautelosius *Nic.* μικρὰν δ' A 23 τὸ *om.* y μικραῖς A 24 τῆσδε yA: hic *Nic.*: *corr. Schöne* 25 ἀγύμναστον] nudam *Nic.* 26 ἐνταυθοῖ y 27 πανουργοῦντες y: κακουργοῦντες A: *correxi* 28 αὐτῶν y ἀπροοράτοις y: ex insperato *Nic.*: *corr. Corn.* 29 ἀντιδακεῖν] cognoscere *Nic.* οὗτοι *scripsi*: οἱ y: *deest* A: οἱ *Bas.* δυνῶνται *Müri, p. 52* καθάπερ – 92,1 ἀδικηθῶσιν *om. Nic.*

that?", I retorted. He answered that he had just left Eudemus, who 3
was amazed that after taking his pulse last night I had predicted an
evacuation through the lower belly, after which he would no longer
have a fever. When he said this, my only reply was, "You heard from 4
Eudemus, not from me", and I immediately passed on. When I
reached Eudemus, I told him what had happened and expressed
surprise at the ill-will of the distinguished doctors in Rome. He said 5
that what had happened to me was entirely reasonable and he com-
pared doctors at home with doctors here, who have plumbed the
depths of malice for many reasons, all of which in turn he proceeded
to enumerate as follows. "Do not imagine that good men become bad 6
in this city: no, those who are already bad, finding a good store of
opportunities, here amass profits far greater than in provincial cities.
Besides, when they see many men like themselves becoming rich, they
imitate their various activities and attain the utmost wickedness, for
several reasons. I shall tell you some of them from my long experience. 7
Not only have nature and a store of valuable opportunities increased
the viciousness of those who are naturally vicious but this has been
accompanied by a knowledge of the ways of crime which they see
trodden daily by their fellows. And they then become practised in
imitating them. One thing especially encourages them never to stop 8
their crimes: even if they are caught red-handed by someone, they can
always move to attack those who do not know them and whom they
assail in greater safety because of their earlier practice of the villainies
they were caught committing. On the other hand, people in small 9
towns, who are not seduced by great gains, as people here are, and
whose slightest mistake is easily noticed by their fellow citizens, keep
their theoretical knowledge of crime still unpractised. Here their 10
ability to escape detection in all their several misdemeanours increases
the vileness of their nature. For they attack unawares people who have
never heard of them, especially when they are prevented by their
simple innocence from retaliating as they do, snapping at each other

11 αὐτοὶ δάκνουσιν ἀλλήλους ἐάν τι καὶ σμικρὸν ἀδικηθῶσιν. ὡς οὖν οἱ παρ'
ἡμῖν λῃσταὶ βοηθοῦσι μὲν ἀλλήλοις ἐπὶ τῇ τῶν ἄλλων ἀδικίᾳ ἑαυτῶν
δὲ φείδονται, κατὰ τὸν αὐτὸν δὴ τρόπον οἱ τῇδε καθ' ἡμῶν ποιοῦνται τὰς
συνωμοσίας μόνῳ τούτῳ διαφέροντες τῶν λῃστῶν τῷ κατὰ τὴν πόλιν,
οὐκ ἐν τοῖς ὄρεσι, κακουργεῖν.»
12 «Ἀλλὰ τό γέ μοι προκείμενον», ἔφη⟨ν⟩, «ἀκήκοας ἤδη πολλάκις,
ὡς ἐπειδὰν ἡ κατὰ τὴν πατρίδα μου στάσις παύσηται παραχρῆμα θεάσῃ
με τῆς πόλεως τῆσδε χωριζόμενον, καὶ ὀλιγοχρόνιον ἔτι ποιήσω τὴν
623 ἐνταῦθα δια|τριβὴν ὥστε θᾶττον ἀπαλλαγῆναι τῆς πανουργίας τῶν
μοχθηρῶν τούτων ἀνθρώπων.»
13 «Ἀλλ' οὔτε γινώσκουσιν», ὁ Εὔδημος ἔφη, «δεδογμένον σοι τοῦτο·
καὶ εἰ γνῶσιν, ὥσπερ αὐτοὶ ψεύδονται, πάντες σε νομιοῦσιν ὁμοίως
14 αὐτοῖς ψεύδεσθαι. καὶ ὥσπερ αὐτοὶ τῶν ἀπόρων τε καὶ ἀπαιδεύτων ὄντες ἐν
ταῖς πατρίσιν οὐ δυνάμενοι ⟨διαμένειν⟩ διὰ τὸ γινώσκεσθαι τἄλλ' ὅσα
προείρηκα πανουργοῦντες [μαθεῖν] εἰς τήνδε τὴν πόλιν ἧκον, οὕτω καὶ
τοὺς ἄλλους οἴονται παραγεγονότας εἰς αὐτὴν οὐκ ἂν ἐθελῆσαι πρὶν
15 ἀθροίσουσιν ἀργύριον ἀπαλλαγῆναι. κἂν ἀκούσωσιν ὑπὸ τῶν πολιτῶν
σου τὸ γένος καὶ τὴν κτῆσιν ὡς οὐκ ἐκ τῶν ἀπόρων εἴης, κατεσκευάσθαι
πάντως ὑπὸ σοῦ φήσουσιν ἕνεκα τῆς τῶν ἀκουσόντων ἀπάτης· ἃ γὰρ
αὐτοὶ πεπράχοιεν περὶ πάντων ὑπονοοῦσιν.»
16 Εἰπόντος οὖν Εὐδήμου ταῦτα καὶ τοιαῦθ' ἕτερα καὶ προσθέντος ὡς
εἰ μὴ ταῖς πανουργίαις ἡμᾶς βλάψαι δυνηθεῖεν ἐπὶ τὴν διὰ τῶν φαρμάκων
ἐπιβουλὴν ἔρχονται· καὶ φάντος γ' ἐν τῇ διηγήσει νεανίσκον τινὰ πρὸ ἐτῶν
624 ὡς δέκα παραγενόμενον εἰς τὴν πόλιν ἐπιδεικνύντα τε δι' | ἔργων ὁμοίως
ἐμοὶ τὴν ἐν τῇ τέχνῃ παρασκευὴν ὑπὸ φαρμάκων ἀναιρεθῆναι μεθ' ὧν
17 ἧκε δυοῖν οἰκετῶν, «χάριν», ἔφην, «γινώσκω σοί, φίλτατε διδάσκαλε,
πάντα μοι διηγησαμένῳ τὰ τῆς πονηρίας αὐτῶν. ἐγὼ γὰρ ἀσφαλῶς
ἐμαυτὸν φυλάξω χωρήσας δ' αὐτοῖς ὁμόσε κατάφωρόν τε τὴν ἀμαθίαν
αὐτῶν ἐργασάμενος ἀπαλλάξομαι τῆς μεγάλης τῆσδε καὶ πολυανθρώπου
πόλεως εἰς τὴν ὀλιγάνθρωπόν τε καὶ σμικρὰν ἐν ᾗ πάντες ἴσμεν ἀλλήλους
ἐκ τίνων τε γεγόναμεν ὅπως τε παιδείας ἔχομεν καὶ κτήσεως καὶ τρόπου
18 καὶ βίου. τραπόμενος οὖν ἐπὶ τοῦτο τὴν ἀμαθίαν αὐτῶν καὶ τὴν πονηρίαν
αὐτῶν ἐλέγχειν οὐκ ἐφρόντισα.»

7sq. ὡς – χωριζόμενον] *cf. infra* p. 116,27 22sq. τὴν – ἐπιβουλὴν] *cf. supra* p. 70,22sq.

1 μικρὸν A 2 ἡμῶν M: *deest* A ἑαυτοῖς M: *deest* A 3 δὴ] δὲ L: *deest* A: quinetiam *Nic.* ποιοῦντες y: *deest* A: *corr. Corn.* 4 τῷ *ex* τῶν *corr.* L^2 6 ἔφη y: *deest* A: *sec. Nic.* (dixi) *corr. Bas.* 8 ὀλιχρόνιον L ποιήσεις y: *deest* A: *sec. Nic.* (faciam) *corr. Bas.* 12 εἰ] ἐὰν *Müri, p. 52* πάντες] πάντως A: omnino *Nic.* σε *om.* y 14 διαμένειν *sec. Nic.* (permanere) *add. Bas.* 15 μαθεῖν] βοηθεῖν N: pati *Nic.*: *secl. Bas.* 16 *ante* οὐκ *add.* καὶ A 17 ἀκούσουσιν y 18 κατασκεύασθαι A 19 πάντα A: *om. Nic.* ἀκουσάντων A: qui audiunt *Nic.* 20 πεπράχασι A πάντων] aliis *Nic.* 21 καὶ^{II} *om.* A 24 ἐπιδειγνύντα L: ἐπιδεικνύναι A 25 ὑπὸ φαρμάκων *om. Nic.* ἀναιρεθέντα y 26 ἱκετῶν y 27 μοι *om.* y 28 χωρήσας – ὁμόσε] cedens enim eis *Nic.* χωρίσας L δ' *om.* y 28sq. κατάφωρόν – ἐργασάμενος *om. Nic.* 29 αὐτὴν L 33 αὐτῶν *om. Nic.* ἐλέγχων L

for even a slight offence. Robbers in our own country band together 11
to harm others and spare themselves: similarly those here combine
against us, the only difference from bandits being that these men
operate in the city, not in the mountains."

"At any rate", I said, "you have already heard many times my 12
professed resolve that you will see me leave this city as soon as the
turmoil at home has died down: indeed, I shall make my stay here
short so that I am the more quickly rid of the evil of these criminals."

"But they are not aware of your decision", Eudemus said, 13
"and, even if they are, being liars themselves, they all will believe you
to be as big a liar as them. Besides, since they come from a background 14
of poverty and ignorance in their own cities, and have come to town,
being unable to stay there because of the notoriety of their crimes, as
I have said, so they imagine that anyone else who comes here could
not wish to depart before he has made his pile. Even if they are told 15
by your fellow townsmen that you come from a not undistinguished
family and that your wealth is not inconsiderable, they will claim that
it is all a fabrication designed by you to deceive your audience. They
suspect everyone of acting as they would have done themselves."

This was the general outline of Eudemus' message, and he added 16
the further warning that, if they could not harm me by their intrigue,
they would resort to poison plots. He told in his discourse of a young
man who had arrived in the city some ten years earlier and who had
been poisoned, together with the two servants who accompanied him,
because, like me, he had given a practical demonstration of his pro-
ficiency in the art of medicine. "I am grateful to you, my dear teacher", 17
I said, "for telling me all this about their villainy. I shall take good
care of myself and, now that I have joined issue with them and un-
covered their ignorance, I shall leave this great and populous city for
that small town where we all know one another, our parentage, our
education, wealth and way of life. Having come to this decision, I do 18
not intend to expose their ignorance and villainy further."

5. Ἀλλὰ τόν γε προειρημένον νεανίσκον ᾧ παραγενόμενος εὐθέως
κατὰ τὴν πρώτην ἡμέραν ἔφην εἰσβολὴν παροξυσμοῦ τεταρταίου πυρετοῦ
γεγονέναι παραλαβὼν ἐθεράπευσα, τὴν προθεσμίαν τῆς λύσεως τοῦ
2 νοσήματος ὡς ἐπ' Εὐδήμου προειπών· ὑπὸ σοῦ τε παρακληθεὶς ἄν-
θρωπόν τινα Χαριλάμπους τοῦ κοιτωνίτου μέν, ὡς ἅπαντες οἱ νῦν
625 Ἕλληνες ὀνομάζουσι, σωματοφύλακος δέ, ὡς οἱ περιέρ|γως ἀττικί-
ζοντες, νευρότρωτον γενόμενον ἐθεράπευσα μηδενὸς τῶν κατὰ τὴν αὐλὴν
3 ἰατρῶν δυναμένου τοῦτο ποιῆσαι· καὶ μετ' αὐτὸν ἐν τῷ Σανδαλ⟨ι⟩αρίῳ
ῥήτορος Διομήδους, οὗ μηδ' αὐτοῦ τῶν ἐκ τῆς αὐλῆς οἱ εὐδοκιμώτατοι
τὴν διάθεσιν τοῦ νοσήματος ηὕρισκον ἀλλὰ διὰ τῶν ἐναντίων ἢ προσῆκεν
ἐποιοῦντο τὴν θεραπείαν, ἡμέραις ὀλίγαις προνοησάμενος ⟨ἰασάμην⟩ τε-
4 λέως χρόνιον τὸ νόσημα. καὶ τοῦ θέρους ἐπιστάντος ἐπὶ τῶν πρωτευόν-
των ἐν τῇ Ῥώμῃ προρρήσεις τε καὶ θεραπείας ἐποιησάμην ἀξίας ἐπαίνου
μεγάλου καὶ πολλὴ δόξα παρὰ πᾶσιν ἦν, ὡς οἶσθα, καὶ μέγα τοὔνομα
5 Γαληνοῦ. συνηυξάνετό τε τῇ δόξῃ φθόνος ἐκ τῶν οἰομένων εἶναί τι καὶ
αὐτῶν ὡς ἂν ἐν παντὶ μέρει τῆς τέχνης ὑπ' ἐμοῦ νικωμένων ἔλεγόν τε
περιθέοντες τὴν πόλιν ἄλλος ἄλλο τι διαβάλλων, ὁ μὲν ὡς κατὰ τύχην
ἰασάμην τόνδε τινὰ ῥιψοκινδύνῳ τρόπῳ θεραπείας χρησάμενος, ὁ δ' ὡς
6 ἐκ μαντικῆς αἱ προρρήσεις καὶ οὐκ ἐκ θεωρίας ἰατρικῆς γίνοιντο. προσ-
εγένετο δὲ καὶ τὸ κατὰ τὴν ζήτησιν ἣν πρὸς τοὺς Στωϊκούς τε καὶ
626 Περιπατητικοὺς ἐποιησάμην | ἀθροίσαντος αὐτοῦ τοῦ Βοηθοῦ,
καὶ μετὰ ταῦτα ⟨τὰ⟩ τῆς Ἰούστου γυναικός, ἧς συντηκομένης ἄνευ
τοῦ φαίνεσθαί τι μόριον πεπονθέναι ἐξεῦρον οὐ μόνον ἐρῶσαν ἀλλὰ καὶ
7 τίνος ἤρα· καὶ μικρὸν ὕστερον ὅθεν εὗρον τοῦτο λεχθήσεται. τῶν δὲ
κατὰ τὸν πρὸς τοὺς Στωϊκούς τε καὶ Περιπατητικοὺς ἀγῶνα παρ-
όντων καὶ ἄλλων τινῶν ἅμ' αὐτοῖς ἰατρῶν τε καὶ φιλοσόφων, ἀναμνήσω
σε πρότερον ὅθεν ἤρξατο διελθὼν ἵν' εἰ καί τινι τῶν ἀξίων κοινωνίας
τοιούτων λόγων ἐθελήσαις μεταδοῦναι τουτὶ τὸ γράμμα, τὴν ἀκολου-
θίαν ἅπασαν ἴδοι τῶν γενομένων· καὶ μὴ διὰ παντὸς ἀσχολίαν ἔχοις
αὐτὸς διηγούμενος ὅσα διά τε τῶν ἔργων τῆς ἰατρικῆς τέχνης ἀνατομῶν τε

1 νεανίσκον] *v. supra* p. 78,4–7 4sq. ὡς – κοιτωνίτου] *cf.* ar-Ruhāwī *Adab aṭ-ṭabīb* fol. 81a: p. 72ᵃ,55–72ᵇ,3 Levey 12–15] *cf.* Gal. De loc. aff. V 7: VIII p. 362,4–6 K. 22 τὰ τῆς Ἰούστου γυναικός] *v. infra* p. 100,7–104,23

1 Ἀλλὰ] Ut nosti autem *Nic.* γε] τε y: *deest* A: *correxi* 5 Χαριλαμπῶς L: Χαριλαμποῦς M κοινωνητοῦ y: κιν *(spatio 4 litt. relicto)* οῦ A: *corr. E. Rohde, Der griechische Roman (Leipzig 1876), p. 331, et Cobet* 5sq. μέν – ἀττικίζοντες *om. Nic.* 6 σωματοφύλακα L 7 νεωτέρωτον L 8 Σανδαλιαρίῳ *scr. H. Jordan, C. Hülsen, Topographie der Stadt Rom, I (Berlin 1907), p. 329, n. 17*: Σανδαλαρίῳ yA: Sandalario *Nic.* 9 Δημώδους A δοκιμώτατοι M 11 ἰασάμην *sec. Nic.* (sanaui) *add. Bas.* 13 τῇ *om.* M 14 πολλὴ – τοὔνομα] in magna gloria, ut nosti, eram et magnum erat nomen (... nomen erat *Nic.*[b]) *Nic.* 18 τῶνδε L ὁ] ᾧ A 21 περιπατικοὺς L 22 τὰ *addidi* Ἰούστου] *deest* A: Iustini *Nic.* 24 τῶν δὲ] τὸν δὲ y: *deest* A: *corr. Schöne* 25 περιπατητικοὺς *ex* -πατικ- *corr.* L 27 πρότερον] πρῶτον M: *deest* A τίνων y: *deest* A: *sec. Nic.* (alicui) *corr. Corn.* 28 ἐθελήσης L 29 ἤδη y: *deest* A: ἴδιοι *sec. Nic.* (uideat) *Bas.*: ἴδοις *Chart.*: *corr. Corn., Morel, nisi* ἴδῃ *praetuleris* ἔχεις y: *deest* A: *sec. Nic.* (habeat) *corr. Ald., nisi* ἔχῃς *praetuleris* 30 ἔργων] ὀργάνων y: opera *Nic.*

5. However, I took up and cured the young man I have already
mentioned. As soon as I came to him on the first day I said that this
was the beginning of an attack of a paroxysm of quartan fever and I
forecast the same basic conditions for the removal of the disease as in
the case of Eudemus: I was also summoned by you to treat a servant 2
of Charilampes, the chamberlain – as all the modern Greeks call
him – or the bodyguard – as the over-sophisticated Atticists prefer –,
who had an injured tendon which none of the palace doctors could
cure: after that there was Diomedes, an orator from the street of 3
the Sandalmakers, the constitution of whose illness the most
famous of the palace doctors failed to discover, proceeding to employ
completely the wrong treatment. Having considered the case first for
a few days, I was able to cure his chronic illness entirely. Indeed, by 4
high summer I had made many praiseworthy predictions and cures in
cases involving leading Romans: my reputation stood high among
all, as you know, and great was the name of Galen. But envy grew 5
apace with fame, especially among those who thought they were some-
body and were vanquished by me in every aspect of their art. They ran
round the city spreading various rumours; one that I had cured this
or that man by good luck, using a highly dangerous method of treat-
ment; another that my predictions derived from divination, not medi-
cal theory. There was also what happened at the enquiry I held with 6
the Stoics and Peripatetics that Boethus had assembled, and
after that the case of Iustus' wife, who was wasting away without
displaying any diseased part. I discovered not only that she was in
love, but also whom she loved – I shall tell you shortly how I did it.
As for my debate with the Stoics and Peripatetics in the presence 7
of some other doctors and philosophers, I shall first remind you how
it began, giving many details so that, should you wish to share this
story with someone worthy of participation in such arguments, he
may see the whole sequence of events; and also so that you will not
have to spend all your time in telling what I did in my practice of
medicine, in my dissections and in the subsequent debates to refute

καὶ τῶν ἐπ' αὐταῖς λόγων ἐπράχθη μοι τοὺς φθονεροὺς ἰατρούς τε καὶ
8 φιλοσόφους ἐλέγχοντι. προπηλακιζόμενος γὰρ ὑπ' αὐτῶν ἐπὶ τοῦτ'
ἦλθον Ὁμήρου με παιδεύσαντος
«ἄνδρ' ἐπαμύνασθαι ὅτε τις προτέρως χαλεπήνῃ».
627 9 τοιαύτην οὖν ἀρχὴν ἔσχεν ἡ πρὸς αὐτοὺς συνουσία. Φλά|βιος Βοηθὸς
ὑπατικὸς ἀνὴρ ὅπως μὲν ἦν φιλόκαλός τε καὶ φιλομαθὴς οἶσθα καὶ σύ, διδασκάλῳ δ' ἐχρῆτο τῶν Περιπατητικῶν δογμάτων Ἀλεξάνδρῳ
τῷ Δαμασκηνῷ γινώσκοντι μὲν καὶ τὰ Πλάτωνος ἀλλὰ τοῖς Ἀριστο-
10 τέλους προσκειμένῳ μᾶλλον. ὁπότ' οὖν παρεκάλεσέ με διδάξαι διὰ
τῶν ἀνατομῶν ὅπως ἀναπνοή τε καὶ φωνὴ γίνεται παρεσκεύασεν ἐρίφους τε καὶ χοίρους πλείονας· πιθήκων γὰρ οὐδὲν ἔφην δεῖσθαι τὴν ἀνατομήν, ὁμοίαν γε τὴν κατασκευὴν ἐχόντων οὐ μόνον τούτων τῶν ζῴων ἀλλὰ καὶ τῶν πεζῶν σχεδὸν ἁπάντων· ὅσα φωνὴν ἔχει μεγάλην ἐπιτηδειότερα τῶν μικροφώνων εἶναι παρασχεῖν ἀποδεικτικὰ λήμματα
11 πρὸς τὴν τοῦ προκειμένου πίστιν. παρῆσαν δ' ἐν τῇ μελλούσῃ γενήσεσθαι δείξει καὶ ἄλλοι μέν τινες ἀτὰρ οὖν καὶ Ἀδριανὸς ὁ ῥήτωρ, οὔπω σοφιστεύων ἀλλ' ἔτι συνὼν τῷ Βοηθῷ, καὶ Δημήτριος Ἀλεξανδρεύς, ἑταῖρος Φαβωρίνου δημοσίᾳ λέγων ἑκάστης ἡμέρας εἰς τὰ
12 προβαλλόμενα κατὰ τὴν ἰδέαν τῆς Φαβωρίνου λέξεως. ἐμοῦ δὲ πρὶν
628 ἀνατέμνειν εἰπόντος ὡς αὐτὸς μὲν δείξαιμι τὰ ἐκ τῆς ἀνατομῆς φαι|νόμενα, συλλογίσασθαι δὲ τὰ ἐξ αὐτῶν περαινόμενα οὐκ ἐμοῦ μόνον ἀλλὰ καὶ τῶν ἁπάντων μᾶλλον ἐλπίζοιμι δύνασθαι τὸν διδάσκαλον Ἀλέξανδρον, οἱ μὲν ἄλλοι πάντες ὡς ἐπιεικῆ τὸν λόγον ἀπεδέξαντο, τιμὴν εἰς τὸν Ἀλέξανδρον ἔχοντες καὶ ἅμα προτροπὴν εἰς τὸ τὴν ὅλην ⟨συν⟩-
13 ουσίαν ἄνευ φιλονεικίας γενέσθαι. γινώσκεις γὰρ ὡς ἐπὶ τούτῳ τῷ πάθει πρὸς ἁπάντων Ἀλέξανδρος ἐγινώσκετο, καθάπερ καὶ τότε σαφῶς ἐδή-
14 λωσεν. δεῖξιν γὰρ ὑποσχομένου μου νευρίων λεπτοτάτων ὡς εἶναι τρι-

3sq. Ὁμήρου – χαλεπήνῃ] Il. Ω 369 Od. π 72; φ 133 6 διδασκάλῳ – 9] *cf.* Gal. Anat. admin. I 1: II p. 218,6–8 K. 25–98,4] *cf.* Gal. Anat. admin. VIII 7: II p. 689,8–17 K.; XI 4: p. 81,31–87,31 Duckworth; XI 11: p. 104,27–107, 23 Duckworth; XIV 6–8: p. 203,7–208,18 Duckworth De usu part. XVI 4: II p. 386,10–389,5 Helmr. = IV p. 278,3–282,1 K. De loc. aff. I 6: VIII p. 49,16–55,14 K.; IV 9: VIII p. 266,12–272,14 K.

1sq. τε καὶ φιλοσόφους *om. Nic.* 2 ἐλέγχονται L: ἐλέγχονται ⸆ A: ἐλέγχοντα M: *corr. Ald.* 4 ἄνδρ'] ἂν δ' y πρότερος *Hom. cod.* A, *fort. recte*: prius *Nic.* 5 συνουσία] iniquitas *Nic.* 7 περιπατικῶν L 8 *ante* Πλάτωνος *add.* τοῦ M 9 με] μοι A 11 πλέονας A πιθήκους yA: *corr. Bas.* 12 ὁμοίως M γε] τε yA: *corr. Schöne* 13 σχεδὸν ἁπάντων] multis *Nic.* ὅσα – 14 εἶναι *om. Nic.* *post* ὅσα *add.* δὲ *Bas.* ἔχουσι A 14 λείμματα L 15 γενήσεσθαι *iter.* M 16 *ante* Ἀδριανὸς *add.* ὁ L, *del.* L[2] 18sq. δημοσίᾳ – λέξεως *om. Nic.* 19 ἐμοῦ – 22 Ἀλέξανδρον] dicente me quoniam per ea que (quo *Nic.*[a]) ex anathomia (ano- *Nic.*[c]) omnia que sillogistice (sil- *Nic.*[c]) concluduntur non a me solum sed (etiam *add. Nic.*[z]) aliis omnibus spero posse doctori Alexandro *Nic.* 21 συλλογίσεσθαι L αὐτοῦ y: *sec. Nic.* (ea que) *corr. Bas.* 24 καὶ – 25 γενέσθαι] totam disceptationem attribuerunt (atrib- *Nic.*[b]) *Nic.* τὸ *deletum in* L: *om.* M: *restit. Corn. Schöne* συνουσίαν *suppl. Corn. Schöne* 27 δείξειν yP: ostendere *Nic.*: *corr. Schöne* ὡς *secl. Baumgarten, Galen, Über die Stimme (Göttingen 1962), p. 102*

these jealous doctors and philosophers. For I did this only when they 8
really slung mud at me; for I follow the precept of Homer that

> "a man should defend himself when someone else
> becomes angry first".

My meeting with them began like this. You well remember the 9
great interest in art and learning of Flavius Boethus, the ex-consul:
he also had as his tutor in Peripatetic doctrine Alexander of
Damascus, an expert also in the teachings of Plato but who inclined
more to those of Aristotle. When he invited me to show him by dis- 10
sections how breath and speech are produced, he got several kids and
pigs ready. I had said that there was no need to dissect apes since not
only these but almost all other land animals are similar in structure:
those with loud voices are much better at providing a convincing
demonstration to prove the point at issue than those with soft. The 11
prospect of the demonstration attracted some others, including
especially Adrian the orator – he was not yet a sophist but still
attached to Boethus – and Demetrius of Alexandria, a follower
of Favorinus, who used to lecture daily on suggested themes in the
style of Favorinus' discourse. Before dissecting, I said that I would 12
demonstrate what was revealed by dissection and that I rather hoped
that Alexander could be my guide, indeed the guide of all of us, in
drawing the logical conclusions from what was thereby achieved.
Everybody else accepted this suggestion as reasonable, for they
respected Alexander and were eager that the whole meeting should
pass off without acrimonious disputation. As you recall, Alexander 13
was renowned among all for this failing, as he then revealed clearly.
I promised a demonstration of the minutest nerves, and to show how 14

χοειδῆ συζυγίαν τινὰ τοῖς τοῦ φάρυγγος μυσὶν ἐμφυομένην, τοῖς μὲν ἐκ
τῶν ἀριστερῶν μερῶν τοῖς δ' ἐκ τῶν δεξιῶν, ἐφ' οἷς βρόχῳ διαληφθεῖσιν
ἢ τμηθεῖσιν ἄφωνον γίνεσθαι τὸ ζῷον οὔτ' εἰς τὴν ζωήν τι βλαπτόμενον
οὔτ' εἰς τὴν ἐνέργειαν, ὁ Ἀλέξανδρος ὑποτυχὼν πρὶν δειχθῆναι,
«τοῦτο πρῶτον», ἔφησεν, «ἂν σοι συγχωρηθείη τοῖς διὰ τῶν αἰσθήσεων
15 φαινομένοις πιστεύειν ἡμᾶς δεῖν;» ἀκούσας δ' ἐγὼ ταῦτα, καταλιπὼν αὐ-
τοὺς ἐχωρίσθην ἓν μόνον φθεγξάμενος, ὡς ἐσφάλην οἰόμενος οὐκ εἰς τοὺς
ἀγροικοπυ⟨ρ⟩ρων⟨ε⟩ίους ἥκειν ἢ οὐκ ἂν ἀφικνεῖσθαι. |
629 16 Ἐμοῦ δὲ χωρισθέντος οἵ τ' ἄλλοι τοῦ Ἀλεξάνδρου κατέγνωσαν
ὅ τ' Ἀδριανὸς καὶ ὁ Δημήτριος, ἐχθρῶς ἀεὶ διακείμενοι πρὸς τὴν
17 φιλονεικίαν αὐτοῦ, πιθανὴν ἀφορμὴν εἶχον ἐπιτιμῆσαι σφοδρῶς. ἐπεὶ δὲ
καὶ τοῖς φιλολόγοις ἅπασιν ὅσοι κατὰ τὴν τῶν Ῥωμαίων πόλιν ἦσαν
ἐγνώσθη τοῦτο καὶ τῷ Σεβήρῳ καὶ τῷ Παύλῳ καὶ τῷ Βαρβάρῳ,
πάντες οὖν σφοδρῶς ἐπετίμησαν αὐτῷ καὶ παρόντων ἑαυτῶν ἠξίωσαν
γενέσθαι τὰς ἀνατομάς, ἀθροίσαντες εἰς ⟨τ⟩αὐτὸ τοὺς ἄλλους ἅπαντας
18 ὅσοι κατὰ τὴν ἰατρικήν τε καὶ φιλοσοφίαν ἦσαν ἔνδοξοι. γινομένης δὲ
πλείοσιν ἡμέραις τῆς συνουσίας καὶ δείξαντος ἐμοῦ τὴν μὲν εἰσπνοὴν
γίνεσθαι διαστελλομένου τοῦ θώρακος τὴν δ' ἐκπνοὴν συστελλομένου,
δείξαντος δὲ καὶ τοὺς μῦς ὑφ' ὧν τε δια⟨στέλλεται καὶ συ⟩στέλλεται καὶ
πρὸς τούτῳ γε τὰ εἰς αὐτοὺς κατεσχισμένα νεῦρα τὴν ἔκφυσιν ἐκ τοῦ
νωτιαίου μυελοῦ ποιούμενα καὶ ὡς ἡ μὲν ἀβίαστος ἔξω φορὰ τοῦ πνεύ-
ματος ἐκπνοὴν ἄψοφον ἐργάζοιτο, βιαίαν δ' εἶναι τὴν ἑτέραν αὐτῆς γι-
19 νομένην μετὰ ψόφου, ἣν ἐκφύσησιν ὀνομάζομεν· ἐπιδείξαντος δὲ καὶ ὡς
630 ἡ | τοιαύτη μόνη κατὰ τὴν διὰ τοῦ φάρυγγος ἔξοδον ὑπὸ τῶν κατ' αὐτὸν
χόνδρων πληττομένη τὴν φωνὴν ἐργάζοιτο καὶ ὡς ὑπὸ μυῶν οὗτοι κινοῖντο
καὶ ὡς τὰ νεῦρα τὰ τούτους κινοῦντα κακωθέντα τὴν ἀφωνίαν ἐργάζοιτο
καὶ τῶν παραφθεγξαμένων ὁπότ' ἐδείκνυον ταῦτα πάντων ἐλεγχθέντων ὁ
20 Βοηθὸς ἐδεήθη μου σχεῖν αὐτῶν ὑπομνήματα. καὶ πέμψαντός γ' αὐτοῦ
τοὺς διὰ σημείων ἠσκημένους ἐν τάχει γράφειν ὑπηγόρευσα πάντα τά τε

17 δείξαντος – 21 ποιούμενα] *cf.* Gal. Anat. admin. VIII 2: II p. 657,3–660,19 K.; VIII 6: II p. 683,15–684,12 K. 28 Βοηθὸς – ὑπομνήματα] *cf.* Gal. Anat. admin. I 1: II p. 215,5–216,7 K. De libr. propr. I: Scr. min. II p. 94,18–21 Müller = XIX p. 13,3–6 K.

1 ἐμφυομένην P: ἐκφυομένην y: coniugationem ... implantatam *Nic.*: ἐμφυομένων *Baumgarten* τοῖς[II]] τοῦ yP: *corr. Ald.* 2 τοῖς] τοῦ P 3 τμημηθεῖσιν L: τμηθήσιν P γίνεται MP, *fort. recte* τὴν ζωήν] alios actus *Nic.* βλαπτόμενον P: βλαπτομένου y 4 ὑπολαβὼν *Bas., inepte* 5 ἔφη *edd.* συγχωρηθῇ y: *corr. Schöne* 6 δ' *om.* L 7 ἐχωρίσθη L οὐκ] ὡς y: *corr. Bas.* 8 ἀγροικοπυρωνίους y: *corr. Chart.* ἢ – ἀφικνεῖσθαι *om. Nic.* ἀφικόμην *maluerim* 11 αὐτῷ y, *qui et punctum post* φιλονεικίαν *colloc.*: *corr. Corn.* 12 φιλολόγοις] amatoribus bonorum *Nic.* 13 Σευήρῳ M 14 ἑαυτῶν *scripsi*: αὐτῶν y 15 αὐτὸ y: *sec. Nic.* (idem) *correxi* 18 *ante* γίνεσθαι *add.* οὐ y: *non hab.* P 19 διαστέλλονται y: διαστέλλοιτο P: a quibus constringitur *Nic.*: *corr. et suppl. Baumgarten* 20 τούτῳ P: τοῦτο y κατεσχισμένα P *Corn.*: κατεχημένα M: κατισχημένα L: ἐσχεμμένα *Schöne* 21 ὡς *om.* M 24 κατ' αὐτὸν P: κατὰ τὸν y: κατὰ τοῦτον *coni. Baumgarten* 26 τούτους P: τούτοις y 28 ἐδεήθην L 29 ἠσχημένους L: ἐσχημένους M: qui exercitati erant *Nic.*: *corr. Ald.*

there is a hairlike pair implanted in the muscles of the larynx, on both
left and right, which if ligated or cut render the animal speechless
without damaging either its life or its functional activity. Alexander
intervened before I could show this and said, "Should we agree with
you on this primary point, that we should all believe in the evidence of
the senses?" When I heard this, I left them and went off, saying only 15
that I was mistaken in thinking that I was not coming to meet boorish
sceptics; otherwise I should not have come.

On my departure, the others condemned Alexander; and 16
Adrian and Demetrius, who were always ill-disposed to his con-
tentiousness, had a plausible occasion to censure him severely. When 17
this was made known to all the intellectuals living in Rome and to
Severus, Paulus and Barbarus, they all roundly reproached him
and demanded that the dissections be performed in their presence
when they had assembled together all others distinguished in medicine
and philosophy. The meeting lasted several days, in which I showed 18
that an intake of breath is produced by the dilation of the thorax, an
exhalation by its contraction, and displayed the muscles by which it is
dilated and contracted, and also the nerves branching to them which
have their origin in the spinal cord. I also demonstrated how an un-
forced release of breath produces a soundless exhalation and the
alternative, forced release is accompanied by sound and we call it
efflatus. I also revealed how this efflatus by itself, when, in its passage 19
along the larynx, it strikes against the cartilages there, produces voice:
these cartilages are activated by muscles and damage to the nerves
that activate the latter results in loss of voice. My detractors were all
put to confusion when I showed this, and Boethus begged me to give
him my lecture notes on it. He even sent trained shorthand writers to 20

δειχθέντα καὶ λεχθέντα μὴ προορώμενος εἰ μέλλοι δώσειν αὐτὰ πολλοῖς.
21 καὶ μέχρι γε νῦν, ὦ Ἐπίγενες, οὐδεὶς ἐτόλμησεν ἀντειπεῖν αὐτοῖς ἐτῶν
ἐν τῷ μεταξὺ γεγονότων πεντεκαίδεκα καίτοι γε διαβουλευομένων [γε]
πολλῶν ἀντειπεῖν ὅπως ἀκουσθῶσιν αὐτὸ τοῦτο μόνον, ὡς ἀντειρήκασιν,
οὐ μὴν τολμώντων γ' εἰς κρίσιν ἐπὶ φιλολόγων ἀνδρῶν ἀγαγεῖν τὰ
γραφέντα.

6. Λοιπὸν οὖν ὅπερ ὑπεσχόμην ἐφεξῆς σοι διηγήσομαι, ἣν λέξιν
καὶ προσθῆναι δεῖ τῷ παρόντι λόγῳ, μάλιστ' ἐπειδὴ καὶ τῶν σοφιστῶν
ἰατρῶν ἔνιοι, ἀγνοούμενοι τίνι λόγῳ τὸν ἔρωτα τῆς παλλακῆς τοῦ πα-
631 τρὸς Ἐρα|σίστρατος ἐγνώρισεν, ἔγραψαν τὰς ἀρτηρίας [τοὺς σφυγ-
μοὺς] τοῦ νεανίσκου σφυζούσας ἐρωτικῶς ἐξευρεῖν αὐτόν, οὐκέθ' ὑπομεί-
ναντες εἰπεῖν ἐκ τῶν σφυγμῶν εὑρεθῆναι [καὶ ὅτι τῆς πατρὸς παλλακῆς].
ἐγὼ δ' ὅπως μὲν Ἐρασίστρατος ἔγνω τοῦτο λέγειν οὐκ ἔχω· ὅπως
δ' αὐτὸς ἔγνων ἤδη σοι φράσω.

2 Παρεκλήθην μὲν εἰς τὴν ἐπίσκεψιν τῆς γυναικὸς ὡς ἀγρυπνούσης ἐν ταῖς
νυξὶ καὶ μεταβαλλούσης ἑαυτὴν ἄλλοτ' εἰς ἄλλο σχῆμα κατακλίσεως, εὑρὼν
δ' ἀπύρετον ἐπυθόμην ὑπὲρ ἑκάστου τῶν κατὰ μέρος αὐτῇ γεγονότων
3 ἐξ ὧν ἴσμεν ἀγρυπνίας συμβαινούσας. ἡ δὲ μόγις ἢ οὐδ' ὅλως ἀπεκρίνετο,
ὡς μάτην ἐρωτωμένην ἐνδεικνυμένη[ν], καὶ τὸ τελευταῖον ἀποστραφεῖσα
τοῖς μὲν ἐπιβεβλημένοις ἱματίοις ὅλῳ τῷ σώματι σκεπάσασα πᾶσαν
ἑαυτὴν ἄλλῳ δέ τινι μικρῷ ταραντινιδίῳ τὴν κεφαλὴν ἔκειτο καθάπερ
4 οἱ χρῄζοντες ὕπνου. χωρισθεὶς οὖν ἐγὼ δυοῖν θάτερον αὐτὴν ἐνόησα

7 ὑπεσχόμην] *v. supra* p. 94,24 ἣν—104,23] *eandem curam brevius narrat Galenus:* In Hipp. Progn. comm. I 8: CMG V 9,2 p. 218,14–219,5 In Hipp. Epid. II comm. II: CMG V 10,1 p. 208,17–29 *cf.* Gal. In Hipp. Epid. VI comm. VIII: CMG V 10,2,2 p. 494,10–21; 494,42–495,2 10 Ἐρασίστρατος] *cf.* Gal. In Hipp. Progn. comm. I 4: CMG V 9,2 p. 206,16–207,2 *Haec fabula saepissime narratur a scriptoribus antiquis:* Valer. Max. V 7 ext. 1 K. Plut. Demetr. 38 Appian. Syr. 59sqq. Lucian. De dea Syr. 17,18: III p. 347,28–349,8 Jacobitz Icarom. 15: II p. 410,30sq. Jacobitz Iulian. Misopogon: II p. 446–448 Wright Stephan.: I p. 74,20–76,26 Dietz Suda s. v. Ἐρασίστρατος *cf.* ar-Ruhāwī *Adab aṭ-ṭabīb* fol. 82a: p. 72ᵃ,45–72ᵇ,28 Levey Ibn abī Uṣaibiʿa, *ʿUyūn al-anbāʾ*: II p. 128,15 Müller *Haec versio Galeni cum fabula de Hippocrate facta* (Sor. Vita Hipp. 5: CMG IV p. 176,4–11 Marcellin. De pulsib. 29–32 Schöne) *contaminata esse videtur* 10sq. ἔγραψαν – αὐτόν] *cf.* Gal. In Hipp. Progn. comm. I 8: CMG V 9,2 p. 218,19 15 Παρεκλήθην – 104,23] *cf.* ar-Ruhāwī *Adab aṭ-ṭabīb* fol. 79b: p. 71ᵃ,50–55 Levey Ibn abī Uṣaibiʿa, *ʿUyūn al-anbāʾ*: II p. 128,15–22 Müller

1 προορώμενα y: *sec. Nic.* (prouidens) *corr. Bas.* 2 ὦ Ἐπίγενες *om. Nic.* οὐδὲν ἐτόλμησέ τις M 3 ιε' y: *numerum plenius scripsi* γε *seclusi* 6 γραφέντα] que dixerunt *Nic.* 7 λέξαι y: enarrare *Nic.*: *corr. Bas.* 8 προσθεῖναι M 9 διηγούμενοι y: *sec. Nic.* (ignorantes) *corr. Bas.* 10 γράψαι y: querunt *Nic.*: *corr. Bas.* 10sq. τῶν ἀρτηριῶν τοὺς σφυγμοὺς ... σφυζουσῶν y: arteriarum pulsu (pulsibus *Nic.*ᵛ) pulsantibus hiis *(om. Nic.*ᵇ*)* amatiue inuenit *Nic.*: *hunc locum difficillimum uerbis Galeni in Commentario I In Hippocratis Prognosticum (CMG V 9,2, p. 218,19) collatis correxi* 12 καὶ – παλλακῆς *om. Nic.*, *sec. quem secl. Guinther, Bas.* παλακῆς L 15 Παρεκλήθην μὲν] παρεκλήθημεν y: *sec. Nic.* (uocatus fui) *corr. Schöne* ἐπίσχεσιν y: *sec. Nic.* (ut uisitarem) *corr. Bas.* 16 κατακλήσεως y: *sec. Nic.* (accubitus) *corr. Ald.* εὗρον y: *corr. Corn.* 17 αὐτὴν L 18 συμβαινούσης M 19 ἐνδεικνυμένην y: se ostendens *Nic.*: *corr. Chart.* 20 σκεπάσασαν L

whom I dictated all my demonstration and argument without troubl-
ing to see whether they were going to be widely distributed. To this 21
very day, Epigenes, no one has dared to contradict them, although
fifteen years have elapsed: many have schemed to contradict them
simply for the fame of contradicting them, although they have not
dared to defend their writings in a trial before intellectuals.

6. My next story fulfils the promise I made earlier and also fits my present argument, especially since some of the sophistic doctors, not knowing on what grounds Erasistratus discovered the young man's love for his father's concubine, have suggested that he found the arteries pulsating madly with love, although they cannot yet bear to say that this was discovered through his pulse beats. Just how Erasistratus found this out I cannot say: but I shall tell you how I did so.

I was called in to see a woman who was said to lie awake at night, 2
constantly tossing from one position to another. When I found that
she was not suffering from fever, I asked about each of the details that
had happened to her from which we know the presence of insomnia.
She replied hesitantly or not at all, as if to show the folly of such 3
questions, and finally turned over, buried herself completely deep in
the blankets, covered her head with a small wrap and lay there as if
wanting to sleep. On my departure I decided she was suffering from 4

πάσχειν, ἢ μελαγχολικῶς δυσθυμεῖν ἤ τι λυπουμένην οὐκ ἐθέλειν
5 ὁμολογεῖν. εἰς τὴν ὑστεραίαν οὖν ἀνεβαλ[λ]όμην ἀκριβέστερον διασκέ-
632 ψασθαι περὶ | αὐτῶν καὶ πορευθεὶς τὸ μὲν πρῶτον ἤκουσα τῆς παραμε-
νούσης οἰκέτιδος ὡς ἀδύνατον αὐτὴν ἄρτι θεάσασθαι· δεύτερον δ' ἐπανελ-
6 θὼν ὡς ἤκουσα πάλιν ταὐτό, τρίτον αὖθις ἧκον. εἰπούσης δέ μοι τῆς
θεραπαίνης ἀπαλλάττεσθαι, μὴ βούλεσθαι γὰρ ἐνοχλεῖσθαι τὴν γυναῖκα,
καὶ γνοὺς αὐτὴν ἐμοῦ χωρισθέντος λελουμένην τε καὶ τῶν συνηθῶν
προσενηνεγμένην ἧκον τῇ ὑστεραίᾳ καὶ μόνος διαλεχθεὶς τῇ θεραπαίνῃ
πολυειδῶς ἔγνων σαφῶς τινι λύπῃ τειρομένην, ἣν ἐξεῦρον κατὰ τύχην,
7 ὁποίαν οἶμαι καὶ Ἐρασιστράτῳ γενέσθαι. προεγνωσμένου γάρ μοι
τοῦ μηδὲν εἶναι κατὰ τὸ σῶμα πάθος ἀλλ' ἀπὸ ψυχικῆς τινος ἀηδίας
ἐνοχλεῖσθαι τὴν γυναῖκα συνέβη κατὰ τὸν αὐτὸν καιρὸν ὃν ἐπεσκόπουν
αὐτὴν βεβαιωθῆναι τοῦτο παραγενομένου τινὸς ἐκ τοῦ θεάτρου καὶ
8 φάντος ὀρχούμενον ἑωρακέναι Πυλάδην· ἠλλάγη γὰρ αὐτῆς καὶ τὸ
βλέμμα καὶ τὸ χρῶμα τοῦ προσώπου, κἀγὼ θεασάμενος τοῦτο, τῷ
καρπῷ τῆς γυναικὸς ἐπιβαλὼν τὴν χεῖρα, τὸν σφυγμὸν εὗρον ἀνώμαλον
ἐξαίφνης πολυειδῶς γενόμενον, ὅστις δηλοῖ τὴν ψυχὴν τεθορυβῆσθαι· ὁ
633 9 αὐτὸς οὖν καὶ τοῖς ἀγωνιῶσι περί τι πρᾶγμα | συμβαίνει. κατὰ τὴν
ὑστεραίαν οὖν εἰπὼν ἀκολούθῳ τινὶ τῶν ἐμῶν, ὅταν ἐπισκεψάμενος
ἔλθω πρὸς τὴν γυναῖκα, μετ' ὀλίγον ἀφικόμενον ἀναγγεῖλαί μοι Μόρφον
ὀρχεῖσθαι τήμερον, εἶθ' ὡς ἤγγειλεν ἄτρεπτον εὗρον τὸν σφυγμόν.
10 ὁμοίως δὲ καὶ κατὰ τὴν ἑξῆς ἡμέραν ποιήσας ἀγγελθῆναι περὶ τοῦ τρίτου
τῶν ὀρχηστῶν, ὁμοίως μείναντος ἀτρέπτου τοῦ σφυγμοῦ, κατὰ τὴν
τετάρτην ἠκρίβωσα νύκτα πάνυ παραφυλάξας, ἡνίκα Πυλάδης ὀρχού-
μενος ἠγγέλθη παραχρῆμα ταραχθέντα πολυειδῶς ἰδὼν αὐτὸν εὗρον
οὕτως ἐρῶσαν τοῦ Πυλάδου τὴν γυναῖκα καὶ τοῦτο παραφυλαχθὲν
ἀκριβῶς ἐν ταῖς ἐφεξῆς ἡμέραις εὑρέθη βεβαίως, καθάπερ γε καί τινος
ἄλλου τῶν πλουσίων δοῦλος οἰκονόμος ὁμοίως κάμνων ἐγνώσθη μοι.
11 Λυπούμενος γὰρ ἐν τῷ μέλλειν ἀποδιδόναι λογισμοὺς ὧν διῴκησεν,
ἐν οἷς ἠπίστατο λεῖπον οὐκ ὀλίγον ἀργύριον, ὑπὸ τῆς φροντίδος ἠγρύπ-
νει τε καὶ λυπούμενος ἐτήκετο, προειπὼν δ' αὐτοῦ τῷ δεσπότῃ μηδὲν
εἶναι σωματικὸν πάθημα τῷ πρεσβύτῃ σκέψασθαι συνεβουλευσάμην ὅτι
634 φοβοῖτο μέλλοντος αὐτοῦ τοὺς λόγους ὧν ἐνεχείρισεν | ἀπαιτεῖν, καὶ διὰ

16 τὸν – 18] *cf.* Gal. Introd. in puls. 11: VIII p. 473,4–7 K. De caus. puls. IV 1–5: IX p. 156,1–161,9 K. In Hipp. Progn. comm. I 4: CMG V 9,2 p. 207, 5–14 27 καθάπερ – 104,8] *exc.* ar-Ruhāwī *Adab aṭ-ṭabīb* fol. 105b: p. 90[a],35–47 Levey

2 ἀνεβαλλόμην y: *sec. Nic.* (distuli) *correxi* 3 πρότερον M 4 οἰκεδίδος L 5 αὖθις] πάλιν M ἥκων L μου y: *corr.* N[2] *Morel* 6 *ante* ἀπαλλάττεσθαι *add.* ἰδὼν L, *del.* L[2] 7 τὰ συνηθῶς y: *correxi* 9 ἔγνως M 12 ἐσκόπουν M 15 βλέμα L 17 ὥς τις L 19 εἶπον *Schöne, fort. recte* ἐπισκεψάμενος] *sec. Nic.* (uisitaturus) -όμενος *scr. Corn. Chart., fort. recte* 20 ἀνάγγειλόν M 21 σήμερον y: *correxi* 24 νύκτα] die *Nic.* 25 παραχρῆμα *om.* M ἰδὼν *om.* M 26 οὕτως *om. Nic.* 30 ὑγρυπνεῖ L 32 σωματικὸν *om. Nic.* τῷ πρεσβύτῃ *om. Nic.* *si p. 104,2 conferas, fort.* συνεβούλευσα μὲν *scripserim; sed cave ne Galenus hac forma uerbi utatur ad hiatum euitandum* 33 φοβεῖτο L ἐγχειρίσαι L

one of two things: from a depression caused by black bile or from some
worry she was unwilling to confess. I thus postponed a further in- 5
vestigation until the next day and, on my arrival, I was first told by
the maid in attendance that it was impossible to see her just then.
I was told the same thing on my second visit, but I came yet a third
time. Then the maid ordered me to go away, for her mistress did not 6
wish to be disturbed. Knowing full well that she had bathed and eaten
a normal meal after I had left, I returned the next day and in a private
conversation with the maid on one subject and another I discovered
beyond doubt that she was racked with grief. Exactly what this was I
found out only by chance, as I believe Erasistratus did. After I had 7
diagnosed that there was no bodily illness and that the woman was
troubled by some psychological disturbance, I happened to receive
some information at the time of my visit which confirmed my sus-
picions. A man coming from the theatre remarked that he had seen
Pylades dancing. Her expression and facial colour changed, and 8
observing this and putting my hand on her wrist, I found that her
pulse had suddenly become irregular in several ways, which indicates
that the mind is disturbed: the same happens to those who are entering
any sort of contest. The next day I told one of my followers to arrive 9
just after I had come and seen the woman and to announce that
Morphus is dancing today. When he did so, I found that her pulse
was unaffected. Similarly also on the following day, when I had an 10
announcement made about the third member of the dancing troupe,
her pulse stayed steady. On the fourth evening I kept a very careful
watch when it was announced that Pylades was dancing and I saw
that her pulse became immediately wildly disturbed. Thus I discovered
that the woman was in love with Pylades, and by careful watch on
subsequent days my discovery was confirmed. I made a similar
diagnosis in the case of a rich man's slave steward who suffered a
similar indisposition.

He was disturbed because he was about to render an account of 11
the money he administered, in which he knew that there was a consider-
able sum missing. He was kept awake by the thought of this and was
worn out by anxiety. I told his master that the old man suffered from
no physical ailment and I advised him to observe that he was scared
because an account was going to be demanded of all he administered

τοῦτο λυποῖτο, γινώσκων οὐκ ὀλίγον ἐν αὐτοῖς εὑρήσεσθαι λεῖπον.
12 ἐπεὶ δὲ καλῶς ἔφη με στοχάζεσθαι τοῦτο, συνεβούλευσα βεβαίας ἕνεκεν
διαγνώσεως εἰπεῖν αὐτῷ ὅσον ἔχει παρακείμενον ἀργύριον αἰτῆσαι
τοῦτο, μή πως ἐξ αἰφνιδίου τελευτήσαντος ἀπόληται μεταστάσης εἰς
ἄλλον οἰκέτην τῆς διοικήσεως οὗ μήπω πεῖραν ἔχοι· παρὰ γὰρ ἐκείνου
13 μὴ χρῄζειν ἀπαιτήσεως λογισμῶν. ὡς δ' ὁ δεσπότης αὐτῷ ταῦτα διελέχθη
πεισθεὶς οὐκ ἐξετασθήσεσθαι καὶ διὰ τοῦτο γινόμενος ἄλυπος ἐν τῇ
τρίτῃ τῶν ἡμερῶν τὴν κατὰ φύσιν ἕξιν τοῦ σώματος ἀνεκτήσατο.
14 Τί δή ποτ' οὖν ἐλάνθανε τοὺς ἔμπροσθεν ἰατροὺς τήν τε προειρη-
μένην γυναῖκα καὶ τὸν προειρημένον οἰκέτην ἐπισκοπουμένους; ἐκ γὰρ
κοινῶν ἐπιλογισμῶν εὑρίσκεται τὰ τοιαῦτα κἂν βραχεῖαν ἐπιστήμην
15 ἔχῃ ⟨τις⟩ τῆς ἰατρικῆς θεωρίας. ἐγὼ μὲν ἡγοῦμαι διότι μηδεμίαν ἔχουσι
διάγνωσιν ὧν τὸ σῶμα διὰ τῆς ψυχῆς πάθη πάσχειν εἴωθει, ἴσως δ'
οὐδ' ὅτι διὰ τοὺς ἀγῶνας καὶ τοὺς φόβους ἐξαίφνης τὴν ψυχὴν ταρά-
ξαντας οἱ σφυγμοὶ τρέπονται γινώσκουσιν· ὅπερ Ἐρασίστρατος
635 ἐπι|στάμενος ἐπὶ τῆς αὐτῆς οἰκίας τῷ νοσοῦντι τῆς γυναικὸς ὑπαρχούσης
εὐκολώτερον ἐξεῦρεν ὡς ἂν δυναμένης αὐτῆς συνεχέστερον ὁρᾶσθαι
⟨ὑπὸ⟩ τοῦ νεανίσκου, μὴ διὰ πλειόνων ἡμερῶν καθάπερ ὁ Πυλάδης,
ὃς [οὖν] οὐδὲ τότε φαινόμενος ἀλλ' ἀκουόμενος ἐξετάραττε τὴν γυναῖκα.
16 λῆρος οὖν μακρὸς ἐρωτικῶς κινούμενοι σφυγμοὶ τῶν οὐ γινωσκόντων
ἔρωτος μὲν οὐδένα δηλωτικὸν σφυγμὸν εἶναι, θορυβουμένης δὲ ψυχῆς
ἐφ' ὅτῳ δή ποτε τοὺς σφυγμοὺς ἀλλοιοῦσθαι μήτε τὴν κατὰ φύσιν
ὁμαλότητα μήτε τὴν τάξιν ἀποσῴζοντας.
7. Ἓν οὖν ἔτι προσθεὶς ἐφ' οὗ παραχρῆμα μὲν ἐξεπλάγη Βοηθὸς
ἀκούσας δ' ὅπως εὑρέθη θαυμάζειν οὐκέτι ἔφασκεν ἀλλὰ τῶν ἀγνοούν-
των τὸ θεώρημα καταγινώσκειν ὡς ἀμαθῶν, ἐπ' ἄλλο τι μεταβήσομαι.
2 νοσήσαντος γὰρ αὐτῷ θατέρου τῶν υἱῶν εἶτα ῥωσθέντος ὑποστρέψαν-
τός τε τοῦ νοσήματος εἶτ' αὖθις παυσαμένου καὶ μετὰ ταῦτα πάλιν
ἐπιπυρέξαντος τοῦ παιδὸς ἐμοῦ τε λέγοντος ἐσθίειν αὐτὸν λάθρᾳ — τὰ
636 γὰρ ἐν τῷ φα|νερῷ διδόμενα πρὸς τῷ ταῖς ποιότησιν ὑπάρχειν ἐπιτήδεια
καὶ τῇ ποσότητι σύμμετρα εἶναι — τὴν μητέρα τοῦ παιδὸς ὑποσχομένην
ἀκριβῶς αὐτὸν φυλάξαι ἐπέστησε φύλακα παρακαθημένην τε δι' ὅλης

9 sq. τήν — οἰκέτην] *v. supra* p. 100,15–102,28; 102,29–104,8

1 ἐν αὐτοῖς *om. Nic.* 2 ἐπεὶ δὲ] ἐπειδὴ y: *sec. Nic.* (ut autem) *corr. Corn.* 2 sq. βεβαίας – εἰπεῖν *om. Nic.* 4 *post* τοῦτο *sec. Nic.* (querat eam solam) μόνον *addiderim* 5 οὐ L ἔχει M 6 διειλέχθη M 7 ἐξαιτασθήσεσθαι M 8 τοῦ σώματος *om. Nic.* 10 ἐπισκοπούμενος y: *sec. Nic.* (qui uisitabant) *corr. Bas.* 12 ἔχει y: *corr. Chart.* τις *sec. Nic.* (aliquis) *addidi* ἰατρικῆς θεωρίας] artis medicine (medicatiue *Nic.*[v]) *Nic.* δι' ὅτι μὴ δὲ μίαν L 13 *ante* τῆς *addiderim* τὰ 14 ὅτι οὐδὲ y: *ordinem uerborum sec. Nic.* (neque quoniam) *mutaui* 16 αὐτὴν L 17 sq. δυναμένου αὐτοῦ ... τὸν νεανίσκον y: *sec. Nic.* (utpote potente ea frequentius uideri a iuuene) *correxi* 18 sq. ὁ Πυλάδης οὐδ' οὖν οὐδὲ τότε φαινομένου ἀλλ' ἀκουομένου ἐκταράττειν y: τοῦ Πυλαδοῦ ... ἐκταράττοντος *Corn.*: *sec. Nic.* (qui neque tunc apparens sed auditus exagitabat mulierem) *correxi* 20 μακρὸς *om.* M *ante* ἐρωτικῶς *addiderim* οἱ 22 μηδέποτε M 25 sq. ἀλλὰ – ἀμαθῶν *om. Nic.* 27 *ante* θατέρου *add.* τοῦ L 32 ἐπέστησα L

and was thus worried as he knew that a considerable sum of money
would be found to be wanting. When he declared that that was a good 12
guess, I instructed him, in order to make my diagnosis certain, to tell
the slave that he was only asking him for the money he had in hand,
lest it be lost in the event of the slave's sudden death when the admi-
nistration passed to another servant as yet untried: for he did not
require a full statement of accounts from him. When his master told 13
him this, he was convinced that he would not have to undergo an
audit, he thus stopped worrying and in three days recovered his
natural physical condition.

Now what was it that escaped the notice of earlier doctors who 14
examined the aforesaid woman and slave? For such discoveries are
made from common inductions, even if one has only the slightest
acquaintance with medical science. I think that it is because they have 15
no clear conception of how the body tends to be affected by mental
conditions, possibly they do not know also that the pulse is altered
by strivings and fears that suddenly upset the mind. Erasistratus
knew that, although his discovery was made with less difficulty
because the woman was in the same house as the patient and so could
be seen more often by the young man, not just occasionally, like
Pylades, whose name, let alone whose appearance, was enough to
disturb the woman. 'Erotically motivated pulses' are the nonsensical 16
idea of those who do not know that there is no pulse indicative of love,
and that the pulse rate changes, retaining neither its natural evenness
nor its order, when the mind is in any way disturbed.

7. I shall pass on after I have related yet one further incident, at
which Boethus was at once dumbfounded and then, when he heard
how I discovered the truth, said that he was no longer surprised but
now condemned as ignoramuses those who did not know the theory I
used. One of his sons fell ill, then he recovered, then the illness return- 2
ed, then it stopped, and then the boy had another feverish attack.
I said that he was taking food surreptitiously, for that which was
openly given him was appropriate in quantity as well as suitable in
quality. Boethus set the boy's mother on guard as she promised to
keep a close watch on him, sitting by him all day and stopping his

τῆς ἡμέρας ἀποκωλύουσάν τε τοὺς εἰς [τὸν οἶκον] ἐκεῖνον εἰσιόντας, κατὰ
τὸν οἶκον αὐτοῦ κοιμωμένην ἀποκεκλεισμένον ἔνδοθεν ἀκριβῶς ὑπ' αὐτῆς.
3 ἐπεὶ δὲ τέτρασιν ἡμέραις οὕτω φυλαττόμενος ἐθερμάνθη διὰ τῆς νυκτός, ὁ
Βοηθὸς ἀναρτήσας με καὶ παραλαβὼν ἦγεν εἰς τὴν οἰκίαν ἐπὶ τὸν παῖδα
συνηκολούθησαν δ' αὐτῷ καὶ οἱ κατὰ τὴν ὁδὸν ἀπαντῶντες, ἐν οἷς ἦσθα
4 καὶ σύ. κατέλαβον δ' ἐκ [μὲν] τοῦ κοιτῶνος ἅμα τῇ μητρὶ προεληλυθότα
τὸν παῖδα πρὸς ἕτερον οἴκημα ἐν ᾧ καὶ κλίνη καθ' ἧς ἡ μήτηρ τοῦ
παιδὸς ἐκαθέζετο· σκίμπους δέ τις ἔζευκτο μικρὸν τῶν μέσων αὐτοῦ
κατωτέρω καθ' οὗ τὸν παῖδα κατακλίνασα παρεφύλαττεν ὡς μηδεὶς
5 αὐτῷ προσέρχοιτο. καθέδρα δ' ἦν μία † τοῦ σκίμποδος, οἷα σύμμετρον
ἐφ' ἑαυτῇ ἐπ' αὐχένι ἔχουσι † κατάντικρυς δὲ τοῦ σκίμποδος πρὸς τοῖς
637 ἄνω πέρασι τῆς κλίνης ἐφεξῆς ἀλλήλων ἔκειντο δύο βάθραι | καθ' ὧν ὁ
Βοηθὸς ἡμᾶς καθίσας, αὐτὸς τῇ γυναικὶ παρακαθεσθείς, «ἤγαγον»,
ἔφη, «Γαληνὸν τοῦτον ὅπως ἀκούσῃ παρὰ σοῦ περὶ τῆς ἀκριβοῦς
φυλακῆς ἐν ταύταις ταῖς ἡμέραις γεγενημένης τοῦ παιδὸς ὡς οὐδὲν ἐν τῇ
διαίτῃ πλημμελοῖτο· θεασάμενός τε π[ρ]ότερον ὄντως ἐπύρεξε διὰ τῆς
νυκτὸς ἢ σὺ φάσκουσά μοι θερμότερον αὐτὸν γεγονέναι παρελογίσθης
ὑπὸ δειλίας ὡς οἰηθῆναι πυρετὸν εἶναι τὴν θερμότητα δι' ἄλλην ἴσως
αἰτίαν γενομένην, ὅπως διάγει σαφῶς ἡμῖν δηλώσειεν, ἅμα δὲ καὶ τὰ τῆς
διαίτης αὐτοῦ πάντα σε διδάξειεν.»
6 Ἀψάμενος οὖν ἐγὼ τῆς κατὰ τὸν καρπὸν ἀρτηρίας τοῦ παιδὸς
ἀπύρετον μὲν αὐτὸν ἔφην εἶναι, παρέχειν δέ μοι σκωμμάτων ἀρχὴν τοῖς
7 ὀνομάζουσί με μάντιν. ὑποτυχὼν οὖν ὁ Βοηθὸς ἔφη· «κἀγὼ πρὸς
ἐκείνους, ὡς οἶσθα, καλεῖν εἴωθά σε μάντιν ὄντα ὅταν τοιοῦτον εἴπῃς
ὁποῖον οἱ ἀντίτεχνοί σου φάσκουσιν ἀδύνατον εἶναι διὰ τῶν τῆς ἰατρικῆς
8 θεωρημάτων γνωσθῆναι.» «ἀλλά τοι μέχρι δεῦρο πάντα», ἔφην, «ἔδειξά
σοι τὰ τοιαῦτα διὰ θεωρίας ἰατρικῆς εὑρισκόμενα καί τινάς γε τῶν
638 9 ἰατρῶν | αὐτὰ γεγραφότων.» λέγειν οὖν ἐκ[κ]ελεύετέ μοι πάντες ἤδη τὸ
μάντευμα· κἀγὼ δεηθεὶς ὑμῶν ἅπαξ ἔτι συγχωρήσειν μοι τῶν σφυγμῶν
ἅψασθαι τοῦ παιδός, ἐπειδὴ τοῦτ' ἔπραξα, «μαρτυρήσεις», ἔφην, «ὦ
Βοηθέ, μηδένα μοι παραγινομένῳ μετὰ σοῦ διαλεγομένων ἡμῶν δι'
ὅλης τῆς ὁδοῦ προσεληλυθότα τὸ μέλλον λέγεσθαι μάντευμα μεμηνυκέ-
10 ναι.» φάντος οὖν αὐτοῦ μαρτυρήσειν οἶσθ' ὅπως γελάσας ἐγὼ προσέχειν

1 ἀποκωλύουσάν – 2 αὐτῆς] excludentem eas que in illa domo ingrediebantur ut non dormirent ibi de nocte et claudentem ab intra (intus *Nic.*[c]) diligenter *Nic.* τὸν οἶκον *seclusi* 2 αὐτοῦ] αὐτῶν L κοιμωμένου M: κοιμωμένω L: *correxi* ἀπ' M 3 ἐπεὶ δὲ] ἐπειδὴ M 4 ἀγανακτήσας y: *sec. Nic.* (requirens) *corr. Bas.* *post* παραλαβὼν *add.* αὐτὸν L 5 συνηκολούθησε L ἦσθα *ex* οἶσθα *corr.* L 6 μὲν *seclusi* 7sq. τοῦ παιδὸς *om. Nic.* 10 ἑαυτῶν L καθέδρα – 12 ἀλλήλων *om. Nic.* 11 ἐπ' αὐχένι] ὑπαυχένιον *coni. Kontos, 'Αθηναῖον 6, 1877, p. 110* 14 ἔφη *post* Γαληνὸν *trsp.* M περὶ] παρὰ L 16 θεασάμενός – 17 νυκτὸς *om. Nic.* πρότερον y: *corr. Morel Chart.* 18 θερμότητα] debilem caliditatem *Nic.* 20 αὐτῷ M πάντα *om. Nic.* 21 τῆς – ἀρτηρίας] pulsum *Nic.* 22 σκωμμάτων] occasionis *Nic.* 23 μάντην L ὑπολαβὼν *Bas., inepte* 24 μάντην L *ante* τοιοῦτον *sec. Nic.* (aliquid) *addiderim* τι 26 πάντα] proculdubio *Nic.* 27 τε y: *corr. Kollesch* 28 ἐκκελεύετε M: ἐκκελεύεται L: poscebat *Nic., sec. quem in mg.* ἐκέλευε *coni. Bas.*: *corr. Morel Chart.* πάντες] omnino *Nic.* 29 ὑμῶν *om. Nic.*: *secl. Bas.*

visitors and sleeping in his room, which she locked carefully on the
inside. When after four days of such surveillance the boy became hot 3
in the night, Boethus seized me and took me along home to see the
boy. People who met us in the street, of whom you were one, also came
with him. I found that the boy had left the bedroom with his mother 4
to go to another room where there was a couch on which his mother
sat; a camp bed was attached, a little below the middle of it, on which
she had laid the boy, and now she was watching to see that no one
came near him. There was one chair . . . and, on the side opposite the 5
camp bed, by the head of the couch, two stools placed together.
Boethus sat us on them, then seating himself by his wife, he began.
"This is Galen. I have brought him to hear from you of your careful
watch over the last few days to prevent any excess in our son's diet.
Then, when he has seen whether he really had a fever during the night
or whether, when you informed me that he had become hotter, you were
frightened into the false belief that this hot sensation was a fever,
although it may have been caused by something else, I hope that
Galen will clearly indicate to us his condition and, at the same time,
give you full instructions on his diet."

As soon as I touched the boy's artery at the wrist, I said that he 6
was not feverish and that this was going to be a source of great amuse-
ment to those who called me a prophet. Boethus interrupted to say, 7
"Indeed, as you know, I too used to call you a prophet in their presence
– as indeed you were when you declared what your opponents denied
could be known through medical theories." "At any rate", I said, 8
"until now I have shown you that everything like that has been
revealed through medical theory and I have mentioned some at least
of the doctors who have described this." You all began telling me to 9
declare my prophecy: I asked your further permission to take the boy's
pulse once again, and when I had done this, "You are prepared to
testify, Boethus", I said, "that no one has approached me on my
way here during the course of our conversation along the road and
revealed the prophecy I am about to deliver." When he agreed that 10
he would testify, you remember how I laughed and told you to listen

τε καὶ ἀκούειν ὑμᾶς ἐκέλευσα τὸ τοῦ μάντεως θέσπισμα τοιόνδε τι φήσας
εἶναι· «τῷ Κυρίλλῳ τούτῳ κατὰ τὸν οἶκον τοῦτον ἀποκέκρυπταί τι τῶν
ἐδωδίμων ὅπως ὅταν εἰς τὸ βαλανεῖον ἡ μήτηρ αὐτοῦ πορευομένη
κλείσῃ τὸν οἶκον, εἶθ' ὑπὲρ ἀσφαλείας εἰς γλωττόκομον ἐμβάλλουσα τὴν
κλεῖν κατασημήνηται — τοῦτο γὰρ ἀκούω ποιεῖν αὐτὴν ἑκάστοτε — ⟨τὸ⟩
κατακεκρυμμένον ἀνελόμενος ὁ υἱὸς αὐτῆς οὕτως προσενέγκηται.»
11 Ταῦτ' ἀκούσας Βοηθὸς εὐθέως ἐξορμήσας πρὸς τὸν παῖδα συναρ-
πάζει τε καὶ μετακομίσας ἐπὶ τὴν κλίνην, στορεσθῆναι τὸν σκίμποδα
κελεύσας, ἐπειρᾶτο ⟨τὸ⟩ κατακεκρυμμένον ὡς αὐτίκα φανησόμενον.
12 ἐπεὶ δὲ τά τ' ἐπιβλήματα πάντα καὶ τὸ ὑπεστορεσμένον αὐτοῖς ἀνετινάχθη
639 τὸ γνάφαλον ἑξῆς | ἀνετίναξεν, εἶτα τὴν καθέδραν ἐπάρας ἐπεσκοπεῖτο
μή τι κατακεκρυμμένον ὑπ' αὐτῇ φανείη. ὡς δ' οὐδὲν οὐδ' οὕτως ἐφάνη,
μετακομίσας ἀπὸ τῆς κλίνης τὸ παιδίον ἐπὶ τὸν σκίμποδα, τὴν κλίνην
13 ὅλην ἀναστορέσας, ἐκέλευσεν αὖθις στρών⟨ν⟩υσθαι. γελάσας τε, «τί»,
φησίν, «ὁ μάντις λέγει;» θαυμάσας δ' ἐγὼ διότι μηδὲν εὗρεν ἐφ' ὧν ᾤετο
κατακεκρυμμένον, ὃ μόνον ἦν ἀζήτητον ὡς οὐδενὸς ὑποπτεύοντος ἐν
αὐτῷ περιέχεσθαι τὸ ζητούμενον ἐπάρας ἀνέσειον. ἦν δὲ τοῦτο παντελῶς
σμικρὸν τῆς μητρὸς αὐτοῦ ταραντινίδιον ἐπικείμενον τῇ καθέδρᾳ.
σεισθέντος δ' αὐτοῦ μέρος ἄρτου τὸ περιεχόμενον ὑπ' αὐτοῦ κατὰ γῆς
ἔπεσε καὶ ὑμεῖς πάντες ἀνακεκράγατε μέγιστον ἅμα τῷ Βοηθῷ γελῶντες
14 καὶ τὴν μαντικὴν ἐπαινοῦντες. ὁ δ' οὖν Βοηθὸς ὑπὲρ πάντας γελῶν
ἐθαύμαζε πῶς ὁ σφυγμός, εἰ καὶ τὸ κατακεκρυμμένον ἐδώδιμον ἱκανός
ἐστι δηλοῦν, ἀλλά τό γε μέλλον ὑπὸ τοῦ παιδὸς ἔσεσθαι λουομένης τῆς
μητρὸς ἐμήνυσε· κἀγὼ πρὸς αὐτὸν ἔτ' ἔφην, «ὦ δριμύτατε, μὴ δηλωσάν-
15 των τοῦτο τῶν σφυγμῶν ὁ Γαληνὸς ἐτεκμήρατο. κλεισθείσης γὰρ
640 ἀκριβῶς | τῆς θύρας κατὰ πολλὴν σχολήν, τὴν ἐδωδὴν αὐτοῦ τῷ παιδὶ
γενέσθαι δυναμένην ἀδεῶς οὐ χαλεπὸν ἦν τεκμήρασθαι, ἀλλὰ καὶ ὅτι
κατακέκρυπταί τι καὶ τὸ κατακεκρυμμένον ἐδώδιμόν ἐστιν ὁ μὲν σφυγμὸς
οὐκ ἤγγειλέ μοι. τεταραγμένον δ' αὐτὸν θεασάμενος ἐνόησα καθάπερ ἐπὶ
τῆς ἐρώσης γυναικὸς καὶ τοῦ φοβουμένου δούλου τὴν ταραχὴν ἐπὶ
16 ψυχικῷ τινι πάθει γενέσθαι, ἀπυρέτου τελέως γ' ὄντος τοῦ παιδός. ἐρω-
τήσεις οὖν ἴσως ἐκ τίνος ἐτεκμηράμην ἐδώδιμον εἶναι τὸ κατακεκρυμ-

22 σφυγμός — 24 ἐμήνυσε] *cf.* Marcellin. De pulsib. 20sq. Schöne 29sq. καθάπερ — δούλου] *v. supra* p. 100,15–102,28; 102,29–104,8

4 ἐμβάλλουσι L 5 τὸ *addidi* 6 ἀνεχόμενος L 8 στορευθῆναι L: στορεθῆναι M: *correxi*: *sec. Nic.* (transuerti) ἀναστορεθῆναι *coni. Bas.* 9 τὸ *add. Chart.* ὡς — φανησόμενον *om. Nic.* 10 ἐπεὶ δὲ] ἐπειδὴ y: cumque *Nic.*: *corr. Corn.* ἐπιβλήματα *sec. Nic.* (amicta) *coni. Bas.*: ἐπιβλαστήματα y 13 ἐπὶ *iter.* M 14 στρώννυσθαι *scr. Bas.* 16 ἦν *om.* M 17 *post* τοῦτο *addiderim* τὸ 17sq. παντελῶς σμικρὸν *om. Nic.* 18 ταραντινι^δ y: ταραντινίδιον N: ταραντινίδος *edd.* 19 μέρους L ὑπ' αὐτῷ *sec. Nic.* (in eo) *coni. Durling* ὑπ' *om.* L 20 ὑμεῖς *ex* ἡμεῖς *corr.* M: ἡμεῖς L 22 εἰ *om. Nic.*: *secl. Schöne* ἱκανόν y: *corr. Chart.* 24 ἐμήνυσα y: sic coniecturaui *Nic.*: *correxi* κἀγὼ — 25 ἐτεκμήρατο *om. Nic.* αὐτὴν y: *corr. Ald.* δριμύτητε M δηλωσάντων] γινωσκόντων y: *corr. Chart.* 25 κλειθείσης L 26 αὐτοῦ *om. Nic.*: αὐτῷ *Bas.* 27 χαλεπὸν *ex* χαλεπῶν *corr.* M 30 φοβουμένου *om. Nic.* 31 τελέως *om. Nic.* 32 ἴσως *om. Nic.*

closely, saying that the prophet's utterance was like this. "Cyrillus here has some food hidden in this room: so, when his mother goes to the bathroom and locks the door, and then makes this clear by pushing the key into the lock for safety's sake – I am told that she does this each time – her son can take out his hidden food and eat it."

11 On hearing this, Boethus instantly rushed to the boy, grabbed him, moved him over to the couch, ordered the camp bed to be shaken out, and tried to find the hidden food at once. When all the coverlets 12 and the underlay had been shaken out, he next shook the pillow and then lifted up the chair to see if anything was hidden underneath. When he found nothing at all, he transferred the boy from the couch to the bed, shook the whole couch and then ordered it to be shaken again. With a laugh, he said, "What does our prophet say now?" 13 I was surprised that he had not discovered the food where he had thought it hidden, and so I picked up the one thing that had escaped scrutiny because none suspected that what we were looking for was contained there, and began to shake it. This was a very small wrap, belonging to his mother, that lay on the chair. As I shook it, the piece of bread enveloped in it fell to the ground, and you all gave a great cheer, laughing with Boethus and praising my powers of divination. Boethus, who laughed loudest, was amazed that, if the pulse 14 could show that there was some hidden food, it could also reveal what the boy was going to do when his mother was in the bathroom. My reply was: "My dear chap, Galen didn't declare all this because the pulse beats showed him. It was not difficult to conclude that when the 15 door was carefully locked for a long time, the boy could eat his food without any fear. But the pulse beat did not tell me that there was something hidden and that what was hidden was edible: no, when I saw him worried, as in the case of the woman in love and the frightened slave, I conjectured that his distress had some psychological cause, since the boy was entirely free from fever. You will possibly ask how I 16 concluded that what was hidden was edible: listen then and I shall tell

μένον· ἄκουε δὴ καὶ περὶ τοῦδε· τὴν ταραχὴν τῆς ψυχῆς οὔτε δίκην
μέλλων ἐρεῖν ὁ παῖς οὔτε παλαίειν ἢ παγκρατιάζειν ἢ ὅλως ἐπιδείκνυσθαι
πλεονέκτημά τι σωματικὸν ἢ ψυχικὸν οὔθ' ὁ ἐγκαλούμενός τι διαμένου-
17 σιν ἴσχειν.» ἀκούσας οὖν ὁ Βοηθὸς ταῦτα, νὴ τοὺς θεοὺς ἔφη θαυμά-
ζειν εἰ οὕτως εὔγνωστα φάρμακα τῶν ἰατρῶν οὐδεὶς οἶδεν. εὔδηλον γὰρ
ὅτι μήτ' αὐτοὶ τοιοῦτον ἔργον ἐπεδείξαντο πώποτε καὶ σὲ πάντα μᾶλλον
18 ἢ ἐξ ἰατρικῆς τέχνης αὐτὰ πράττειν φασίν. «ἐοίκασι δ'», ἔφη, «μὴ μόνον
641 ἀγνοεῖν ὁποῖός ἐστι τῶν ἀγωνιώντων ὁ σφυγμὸς ἀλλὰ μηδ' εἴπερ | ἔγνω
τις αὐτῶν κατὰ τύχην ἃ προσελογίσω προσεπιλογίσασθαι δύνασθαι διὰ
τὸ μήτε φῦναι συνετοὶ μήτε μαθήσει γεγυμνάσθαι τὸν λογισμόν.»
«ἀλλὰ τά γε τῆς κακοηθείας», ἔφην, «ἔργα γεγυμνασμένοι τ' εἰσὶ καὶ
σοφοί.»

8. Τούτων μὲν οὖν, ὦ Ἐπίγενες, αὐτὸν ἔχω μάρτυρά σε, πολλῶν
δ' ἄλλων ἑτέρους ἁπάντων τῶν πραχθέντων μοι κατὰ τὴν πρώτην
ἐπιδημίαν, ἤκουες δ' αὐτὸ⟨ς⟩ παρ' αὐτῶν τῶν ὑπ' ἐμοῦ θεραπευθέντων.
ἓν οὖν ὄντως θαυμάσιον πραχθὲν ὃ οὐ μόνον με παραδοξολόγον ὡς
ἔμπροσθεν οἱ πολλοὶ τῶν ἰατρῶν ὠνόμαζον ἀλλὰ καὶ παραδοξοποιὸν
2 ἐποίησε κληθῆναι. ἡ γὰρ τοῦ Βοηθοῦ γυνὴ τῷ καλουμένῳ ῥῷ γυναι-
κείῳ περιπεσοῦσα κατ' ἀρχὰς μὲν αἰδουμένη τοὺς ἀξιολόγους ἰατρούς,
ὧν εἷς ἤδη κἀγὼ πᾶσιν ἐδόκουν εἶναι, ταῖς συνήθεσι μαίαις ἀρίσταις
οὔσαις τῶν κατὰ τὴν πόλιν ἑαυτὴν ἐπέτρεπεν· ὡς δ' οὐδὲν ὠφελεῖτο,
3 πάντας ἡμᾶς ὁ Βοηθὸς ἀθροίσας ἐπεσκοπεῖτο τί χρὴ ποιεῖν. ὡς δὲ
642 συν|ωμολογήθη κατὰ τὴν γεγραμμένην ὑφ' Ἱπποκράτους τε καὶ τῶν
ἀρίστων μετ' αὐτὸν ἰατρῶν θεραπείαν ἅπαντα πράττειν, ἀξιώσαντος
αὐτοῦ συνεχῶς ἐπιφαίνεσθαί με ταῖς ὑπηρετούσαις αὐτῇ γυναιξὶν ὁρᾶν
τε τὰς ὕλας τῶν κατὰ μέρος βοηθημάτων πρὸς τὸν καθόλου σκοπὸν
ἀποβλέποντα, κεφάλαιον ἔχοντα ξηραίνειν μὲν οὐ μόνον τῆς μήτρας τὰ
χωρία ἀλλὰ καὶ σύμπαν τὸ σῶμα, προσφέρειν δὲ καὶ ἀλειμμάτων στυ-

1–4] *cf.* Gal. De praes. ex puls. I 1: IX p. 219,17sq. K. De crisib. II 13: p. 162,4–8 Alex. = IX p. 696,17–697,6 K. In Hipp. Epid. VI comm. VIII: CMG V 10,2,2 p. 494,25–42 16 με – 18 κληθῆναι] *cf.* Gal. Quod opt. med. sit etiam phil. 1: Scr. min. II p. 2,11 Müller = I p. 55,1 K. De exam. medico: Meyerhof, p. 80, 8–13 Ibn abī Uṣaibiʿa, *ʿUyūn al-anbāʾ*: I p. 85,14–18; 97,23–25 Müller 18–116,12] *cf.* Gal. De purg. med. fac. 5: XI p. 341,12–15 K. *exc.* Razes *Kitāb al-ḥāwī* IX 3,1 18–112,22] *exc.* Maimonides Aphor. XVI 28: p. 356,15–357,6 ed. Basil. 1579 27 κεφάλαιον – 112,2] *exc.* Razes *Kitāb al-ḥāwī* IX 53,5

1 τούτου M τὴν – 4 ἴσχειν] exagitatio quidem anime pueri cum neque in iudicio (-tio *Nic.*[c]) deberet respondere neque luctari (-are *Nic.*[ba]) neque agonizare in aliqua superhabundantia (super- *om. Nic.*[c]: superab- *Nic.*[a]) corporali magis quam animali consistit *Nic.* 3 ὁ] ὅλως y: *correxi* 6sq. πάντα μᾶλλον ἢ] aliunde quam *Nic.* 7 τέχνης *om.* M 11 τά *om.* M 14 ἑτέρους *om. Nic.* τῶν *secl. Schöne* 15 αὐτὸς *scripsi*: αὐτὸ y θεραπευθέντων *ex* θεραπευομένων *corr.* L 16 ἓν – 18 κληθῆναι] unum tamen admirandum actum a me monet (mouet *Nic.*[av]) non tacere *Nic.* 18 ἐποίησα y: *corr. Bas., quae et post* κληθῆναι *add.* σιοπήσω (σιωπήσω *Chart.*: οὐ σιωπήσω *W. Herbst, Galeni de studiis Atticissantium testimonia [Leipzig 1911], p. 158*) 25 *ante* συνεχῶς *add.* καὶ *Bas.* μοι y: *corr. Bas.* 27 *ante* κεφάλαιον *add.* καὶ *Bas.* 28 *ante* δὲ *add.* τε M

you. No boy can continue to check his mental anxiety when he is about
to speak in court or wrestle or perform the pancration on the sports
field or make any display of physical or mental prowess – and certainly
not when he is accused of something." When he heard this, Boethus 17
said that, by Jove, he was surprised that none of the doctors knew
these simple prescriptions: for it was obvious that they themselves had
never displayed any achievement like this and that they insisted that
I had succeeded in this by every means but medicine. "They seem", 18
he said, "not only to be ignorant of the particular pulse beat of men
under stress but also, if one of them happens to know your conclusions,
they cannot reason them out for themselves because they are not
naturally intelligent and have not trained their logical faculty by
learning." "At any rate", I said, "they are well trained and learned
in deeds of malice."

8. I have you to corroborate these tales, Epigenes, and other
people can attest all the many other achievements of my first stay, and
you yourself heard of them from those who were treated by me. But
there is one really remarkable case which gave me earlier the title of
'wonderworker' to go with that of 'wonderteller', as many doctors
called me. Boethus' wife suffered from the so-called female flux. 2
She was ashamed at first to tell this to the top doctors, of whom I
was universally acknowledged to be one, but put herself in the care of
her usual midwives, who were the best in Rome. When no improve-
ment took place, Boethus called us all together and asked us what to
do. When it was agreed to act entirely according to the treatment 3
prescribed by Hippocrates and the best of his medical successors,
he decided to introduce me often to her attendants and asked me to
examine the composition of individual remedies, always keeping the
general aim in view, with the intention, in short, of drying her whole
body instead of only the area of the womb, and also of applying

4 φόντων τοῖς γυναικείοις τόποις, ἐποίουν οὕτως. ἐπεὶ δὲ ταῦτα †πράττων†
ἐφαίνετο καὶ χείρων ἡ διάθεσις ἀποτελουμένη, κατὰ τὸ εἰκὸς ἀπορία
πᾶσιν ἡμῖν ἐγίνετο καὶ ζητοῦσιν ἑτέραν ἀγωγὴν θεραπείας ἐφ' ἣν
μεταβῶμεν οὔτ' ἐκ λογισμοῦ τις ηὕρισκεν οὔτ' ἐκ πείρας ἀνεμιμνῄσκετο
5 βέλτιον τῆς ὑπὸ τῶν ἀρίστων ἰατρῶν ὁμολογουμένης. ἐν τούτῳ δὲ καὶ
ὄγκος τις ὤφθη κατὰ τὴν γαστέρα παραπλήσιος τῷ γινομένῳ ταῖς
κυούσαις, ὃν ἔνιαι τῶν θεραπευουσῶν αὐτὴν γυναικῶν ᾠήθησαν ὄντως
ἐπὶ κυήσει γενέσθαι, οὐ μὴν τῶν γ' ἄλλων ἰατρῶν τις ἐπίθετο. τὰ γὰρ
ἐκκρινόμενα γνωρίσματα τοῦ γυναικείου ῥοῦ καθ' ἑκάστην ἡμέραν |
643 6 ἀντεμαρτύρει τῇ δόξῃ ταύτῃ. τῆς φυλαττούσης οὖν αὐτήν, ἣν ἐπεπι-
στεύκειμεν ἀρίστην εἶναι, τά τ' ἄλλα πραττούσης ὡς ἐπὶ κυούσης λυούσης
τε καθ' ἑκάστην ἡμέραν συνέβη κατὰ τὸν πρῶτον οἶκον τοῦ βαλανείου,
σφοδροτάτης ὠδῖνος γενομένης οἷαι ταῖς τικτούσαις εἰώθασι συμπίπτειν,
ὑδατῶδες ὑγρὸν ἐκκενωθῆναι τοσοῦτον ὡς λειποθυμήσασαν ἐξενεχθῆναι
7 τοῦ βαλανείου τὴν γυναῖκα. κλαιουσῶν δὲ καὶ κεκραγυιῶν τῶν ἀμφ'
αὐτὴν οὐδεμιᾶς δ' οὐδὲ πόδας οὐδὲ χεῖρας οὐδὲ τὸ στόμα τῆς γαστρός,
ὃ δὴ καὶ στόμαχον ὀνομάζουσι κατὰ τὸ σύνηθες, ἀνατριβούσης ἐγὼ κατὰ
τύχην ἑστὼς πρὸ τῆς ἔξω θύρας τοῦ βαλανείου, κραυγῆς ἀκούσας,
εἰσεπήδησα καὶ θεασάμενος ἀπεψυγμένην αὐτήν, εἰς χεῖρας λαβὼν
ναρδίνου μύρου τὸν στόμαχον ἀνέτριβον ἐγκελευσάμενος ταῖς παρούσαις
μὴ μάτην ἑστάναι κεκραγυίας ἀλλὰ τὰς μὲν τοὺς πόδας ἐκθερμαίνειν τὰς
8 δὲ τὰς χεῖρας ἐνίας δ' ὀσφραντὰ προσφέρειν τῇ ῥινί. τότε μὲν ἀνεκτη-
σάμεθα ταχέως αὐτήν· ἥδετο δὲ μεγάλως ἡ μαῖα προσ⟨σ⟩ταλείσης ἐπὶ
τῇ κενώσει τῆς γαστρός, οὐχ οὕτως ἐπὶ τῷ σφαλῆναι ἐπὶ τῇ τοῦ τίκτειν |
644 δόξῃ ἀλλ' ἐπὶ ⟨τῷ⟩ τὸ διατεταγμένον ἀπιστοῦσιν ἡμῖν ἀντιλέγειν ὡς
ἐπιστημονικῶς εἰδυῖα τὸ πρᾶγμα.
9 Ἀποροῦντος δ' ἑκάστου ὅ τι δεῖ[ν] πράττειν καὶ μή⟨τε⟩ κατὰ τὸν
αὐτὸν σκοπὸν τῷ πρόσθεν ἰᾶσθαι τὴν γυναῖκα κατατολμῶντος ⟨μήτ'⟩
ἐφ' ἕτερον μεταβῆναι, φροντίζοντί ⟨μοι⟩ νύκτωρ ἐπῆλθε τοιόνδε τι.

17 ὃ – σύνηθες] *cf.* Gal. Meth. med. VIII 5: X p. 573,8sq. K. De venae sect. adv. Erasistr. Rom. deg. 9: XI p. 242,15sq. K. De comp. med. sec. loc. VIII 1: XIII p. 121,17–122,3 K. In Hipp. Epid. VI comm. VII: CMG V 10,2,2 p. 438,9sq. 20 ἐγκελευσάμενος – 23] *exc.* Razes *Kitāb al-ḥāwī* XVI 217,3

1 τοῖς – οὕτως *om. Nic.* πράττων] his gestis *Nic.*: πραττόντων *Bas.*, *fort. recte* 2 χεῖρον L 3 ζητ^{οῦ} L 4 οὔτ' ἐλογισμοῦ L ἀνεμιμνῄσκετο *om. Nic.* 5 *ante* τῆς *add.* τι *Corn.*, *fort. recte* 6 γιγνομένῳ L 7 ὃν *ex* ὧν *corr.* L 8 ἐπύθετο M: putabat *Nic.*: ἐπείθετο *Corn. Chart.* 9 τοῦ – ῥοῦ] τοῦ ῥοῦ τοῦ γυναικείου M: existentia muliebri fluxus *Nic.*, *sec. quem* ὄντα *add. Bas.* 10 ἐπεπιστεύκει μὲν y: *sec. Nic.* (confidebamus) *corr. Ald.* 13 ὠδίνης M 15 καλουσῶν y: *sec. Nic.* (plorantibus) *correxi* 17 ὀνομάζεται L: nominatur *Nic.* ἀνατριβούσης *ex* -τριψάσης *corr.* L 20 ἀνατρίβειν y: fricare iussi *Nic.*: *corr. Corn.* 21 κεκραγυίας] clamans *Nic.* 23 ἠδεῖτο y: ἡδεῖτο *Ald.*: *corr. Chart.* προσταλείσης y: *sec. Nic.* (contracto) *correxi* 24 οὐχ – 26 πρᾶγμα *om. Nic.* 25 τῷ *add. Corn.* διατεταγμένως L 27 δεῖν y: *corr.* N *in mg.*, *Bas.* μὴ y: *corr. Corn.* 28 *ante* κατατολμῶντος *add.* καὶ L μήτ' *add. Corn.* μήτ' – 29 τι] et (tunc *Nic.*^{z}) me sollicito existente per noctem (et – noctem *om. Nic.*^{b}) et non (non *om. Nic.*^{cev}) audente ad aliquid (-quod *Nic.*^{cev}) aliud transire aduenit quid (quidem *Nic.*^{c}) tale *Nic.* 29 μοι *addidi*

styptic ointments to her genital region. That is what I did: but since 4
her condition was obviously deteriorating under this (treatment), we
were all understandably at a loss and we looked for another method of
treatment to follow. But neither could we find one by reasoning nor
did our experience suggest anything better than what had been agreed
by the best doctors. Meanwhile a swelling also became visible in the 5
belly similar to that found in pregnant women, which indeed some of
her nurses thought was really caused by pregnancy. None of the other
doctors believed this, for the daily excretion of traces of the female
flux disproved this idea. Her chief nurse, whom we considered an 6
excellent woman, acting as if she was pregnant, gave her a daily bath.
One day, as she was in the first room of the bath, she happened to feel
a great pain such as usually afflicts women in childbirth and she
evacuated so much watery fluid that she was carried from the bath
in a dead faint. Her attendants screamed and shouted, but not one 7
began to rub her feet and hands and the entrance to the stomach,
what we usually call *stomachos*. By chance I was standing before the
outer door of the bathroom and, hearing a shriek, I rushed in and saw
her frozen stiff. Grabbing some nard ointment, I began to rub her
stomach, telling the women present to stop standing uselessly about,
just screaming, and to warm her feet and hands or apply smelling
substances to her nose. We then quickly revived her: but the midwife 8
was highly delighted when the abdomen contracted at the evacuation,
not so much because she was wrong in her diagnosis of labour as because, through knowing her stuff well, she had spoken against us when
we had refused to trust the accepted treatment.

As we each wondered what to do, for we dared neither continue 9
treating the woman with the same intention as before nor change to
another method, an idea came to me one night as I considered the case.

10 λειποψυχίας αὐτῇ γεγενημένης, ὡς ἔφην, ὁπότε καὶ τὰς γυναῖκας εἶπον
οὐδὲν μὲν βοηθεῖν ἑστάναι δὲ κλαιούσας ἐμαυτόν τε μύρον νάρδινον εἰς
τὰς χεῖρας λαβόντα τό τε στόμα τῆς γαστρὸς καὶ τὸ ὑποχόνδριον παρα-
τρίβειν, ἀνεμνήσθην ὅτι τοσαύτην εὗρον ἐν τοῖς χωρίοις τούτοις μαλακό-
τητα τῶν καθ' ὑποχόνδρια μυῶν ὡς ἐμὲ γοῦν ἐν ἀρχῇ βιαιότερον ἀνατρί-
βειν αὐτὰ διεγνωκότα, φοβηθέντα μὴ θλίψας τὴν σάρκα πελιδνὸν
11 ἐργασαίμην τι μόριον, ἀποστῆναι τοῦ βιαίου. ὡς γὰρ ἄν τις ἄκρως
εἰκάσαι βουληθείη παραπλήσια γάλακτι μὲν πηγνυμένῳ εἰς τυροῦ
γένεσιν οὐ μὴν ἤδη γε πεπηγότι κατεφάνη μοι τὰ κατὰ τὸ ὑποχόνδριον
12 ἅπαντα. τοῦ μὲν οὖν ξηραίνειν τὴν ἄμετρον ὑγρότητα τοῦ πάθους
ὑδατώδους ὄντος [τυροῦ] πάντες ἔχεσθαι διεγνώκαμεν, ἐξευρεῖν δὲ τρόπον
645 ἰάσεως | οὐ ⟨διὰ⟩ ξηραινούσης ὕλης μόνον ἀλλὰ καὶ θερμαινούσης [δέον]
ὅπως μὴ τήκοιτο τὸ σῶμα ψυχρᾶς κράσεως ἀμέτρως ὑπάρχον. καὶ
μάλιστ' ἐπειδὴ θέρους ὥρᾳ κατ' ἐκεῖνον τὸν καιρὸν ἡμεῖς τοὐναντίον
13 ἐπράττομεν, ἐν θαλαττίᾳ ψάμμῳ θερμῇ κατακλίναντες αὐτήν· λογισά-
μενος δέ τι καὶ ἄλλο κοινότερον ἁμάρτημα κατὰ τὰ πλεῖστα τῶν παθῶν
ἑκάστοτε γιγνόμενον ὑπὸ τῶν ἰατρῶν κενούντων μὲν τὸ περιττὸν ὅπως
δὲ μὴ γεννῷτο παραπλήσιον τῷ κενωθέντι παραλειπόντων ἐνενόησα
τὸν σκοπὸν τῆς διαίτης ποιήσασθαι διά τε πόματος ἐλαχίστου καὶ
τρίψεως ὅλου τοῦ σώματος ἔτι τε χρίσεως οὕτω σκευαζομένης, οὐ διὰ
πίττης τε καὶ ῥητίνης ἀλλὰ διὰ μέλιτος μόνου μέχρι πλείονος μὲν ἑψηθέν-
τος ἀποψυχθέντος δ' εἰς τοσοῦτον ὡς τούτῳ δὴ τῷ κατὰ τὰς κρήνας
14 ὕδατι θέρους ὥρᾳ παραπλήσιον εἶναι. καθάπερ δὲ διὰ τοῦ δέρματος
ἔγνων ἄμεινον εἶναι διαφορεῖν τὴν περιττὴν ὑγρότητα, τὸν αὐτὸν
τρόπον οὐρητικοῖς τε φαρμάκοις ἐπὶ τὴν κύστιν αὐτὴν ποδηγεῖν
15 ἐπιμελεῖσθαι δὲ τοῦ καὶ διὰ ⟨τῆς⟩ κάτω γαστρὸς ὑπάγεσθαι. πειρα[σ]-
646 θεὶς δ' ἐν ταῖς μετὰ | τὴν ἀθρόαν ἔκκρισιν ἡμέραις ἐφεξῆς ὡς ἑπτά, καθ'
ἃς ὁ μὲν Βοηθὸς ἅπαντας ἡμᾶς ἰδίᾳ τε καὶ κοινῇ παρεκάλει σκοπεῖσθαί
τινα θεραπείας τρόπον, ⟨ἐγὼ δ'⟩ ἀπαγαγὼν αὐτὸν ἀπὸ τῶν παρόντων
οἰκετῶν τε καὶ φίλων ἐπὶ τῆς οἰκίας ἰδίᾳ ὧδε διελέχθην, «οὐδέν», εἰπών,
«ἄχρι τήμερον οὐδὲ καθ' ἓν με σφαλέντα τῶν ἰατρικῶν ἔργων ἐπιστάμε-
νος ἐπίσκεψαι κατὰ σαυτὸν εἰ συγχωρεῖς δέκα ταῖς πάσαις ⟨ἡμέραις ὡς⟩
βούλομαι πρᾶξαι περὶ τὴν γυναῖκά σου· κἂν μὲν ἄμεινον ἴσχειν ἑκάστοτε

1 ὡς ἔφην] *v. supra* p. 112,14–20 9 κατεφάνη – 116,18 χρυσοῦς] *exc.* Maimonides Aphor. XVI 28: p. 357,8–18 ed. Basil. 1579 20 τρίψεως – 23] *exc.* Orib. Syn. ad Eustath. IX 46: CMG VI 3 p. 306,8–10 Paul. Aeg. III 62: CMG IX 1 p. 279,5–8 21 sq. ἀλλὰ – τοσοῦτον] *exc.* Razes *Kitāb al-ḥāwī* VII 185,7 sq.

3 τό τε] tunc *Nic.*: τὸ M 4 ἀνεμνήσθην – τοσαύτην *om. Nic.* 5 καθ' ὑποχόνδρια] ὑποχονδρίων M 11 τυροῦ] super *Nic.*[x]: *secl. Nic.*[v] *Corn.* 12 διὰ *sec. Nic.* (per) *add. Bas.* δέον *secl. Bas.* 13 καὶ – 15 ἐπράττομεν *om. Nic.* 16 τι *om. Nic.* 18 τῷ κενωθέντι *om. Nic.* ἐνενόησα *ex* ἐνο- *corr.* L 20 *ante* τοῦ *add.* τε L χρίσεως *ex* χρήσ- *corr.* MN[2]: χρήσεως L σκευαζομένου L 24 τὴν] τε y: *corr. Bas.* 26 τῆς *add. Schöne* πειρασθεὶς y: *corr. Ald.* 29 ἐγὼ δ' *sec. Nic.* (ego autem) *addidi* 30 ἰδίᾳ ὧδε *om.* M διελέχθην N: διειλ- M: διελέγχθην L εἶπον *Schöne, fort. recte* 32 συγχωρῆ L ἡμέραις ὡς *sec. Nic.* (diebus ut) *add. Bas.*

As I have said, when she fainted, I shouted that the women were no 10
use but simply stood around screaming, and I took some nard oint-
ment into my hands and proceeded to rub the entrance to the sto-
mach and the hypochondrium. I recalled that when I did this I found
in these areas such a softness of the muscles of the hypochondrium
that, although I had decided to rub rather hard at first, I eased the
pressure from fear that I might bruise some part by pressing too hard
on the flesh. All the region of the hypochondrium appeared to me, 11
if one may use the comparison, like milk which is being curdled into
cheese but which has not yet set firm. We had all decided to continue 12
drying the excess moisture of her watery ailment and to find a
method of treatment that included both drying and calefacient ma-
terial so as to prevent the body from being worn away through
an excess of cold temperament: especially since at that time, in sum-
mer, we were trying to achieve the opposite effect by laying her down
in a bed of warm sand from the sea shore. When I reflected that 13
one of the more common errors regularly perpetrated by doctors in
very many cases is that of causing an excessive evacuation and then
not preventing a recurrence of a condition similar to that which was
purged, I decided to alter my treatment to giving a very small po-
tion, rubbing her whole body and then anointing it as follows: not
with a mixture of pitch and resin, but only with honey cooked for
a long time and then cooled to about the summer temperature of
spring water. I decided that it was better to disperse the excessive 14
moisture through the skin as well as channelling it to the bladder
by using uretic drugs, and also seeking to remove it through the lower
belly. I tried this for seven successive days after she had had her mas- 15
sive evacuation, and then **Boethus** invited us, severally and collec-
tively, to consider a method of treatment. Taking him on one side,
away from the servants and friends who were with him in the house,
I had the following private conversation. "Since you know", I said,
"that until today I have never failed in even one of my medical
duties, ask yourself whether you are prepared to let me take whatever
action I see fit in the case of your wife for all the next ten days. If there

φαίνηται, μετὰ ταῦτα ἄλλαις τοσαύταις ἐπιτρέψεις μοι πράττειν τι περὶ
αὐτήν· εἰ δὲ μή, τότε κἀγὼ χωρισθήσομαι τελέως αὐτῆς.»
16 Ἑτοίμως δέ μοι συγχωρήσαντος αὐτοῦ πρῶτον μὲν ὑδραγωγῷ
φαρμάκῳ διὰ τῆς κάτω γαστρὸς ἐκένωσα, μετὰ ταῦτα δὲ πίνειν ἐδίδουν
17 ὕδωρ ἐναφεψηθέντος ἀσάρου τε καὶ σελίνου. ἐπεὶ δὲ ταῖς πρώταις
ἡμέραις δύο τούτων γενομένων οὐδὲν ἐφάνη τοῦ ῥοῦ, κατὰ τὴν τρίτην
ἔδωκα πάλιν οὐ πολὺ τοῦ διὰ τῆς κάτω γαστρὸς ἐκκενοῦντος τὸ ῥέπον
ἔμπροσθεν εἰς τὴν μήτραν, οὐ μόνον δι' οὔρων ἀλλὰ καὶ διὰ τῆς κάτω γα-
647 18 στρὸς παροχετεύειν βουλό|μενος. καὶ μετ' αὐτὸ ἔχριόν τε τῷ μέλιτι καθ'
ἑκάστην ἡμέραν ἀνέτριβόν τε τὸ σῶμα, τὰ μὲν πρῶτα διὰ σινδόνων
μαλακωτάτων, εἶτα καὶ διὰ σκληροτάτων, ἐδίδουν τε κρέα τῶν ὀρείων
19 ὀρνίθων ἰχθύων δὲ πετραίων. ὡς δὲ διὰ τούτων ἡμέραις πεντεκαίδεκα
τῆς θεραπείας γινομένης οὐδὲν ὅλως ἐφάνη τοῦ πάθους γνώρισμα,
γνοὺς ὁ Βοηθὸς μεῖζον ἢ κατὰ τὴν ὑπόσχεσιν εἰργασμένον με, τελέως
ἐκθεραπεῦσαι τὴν διάθεσιν ἐδεῖτο ὑποθήκας τε δοῦναι πρὸς τὸν λοιπὸν
20 χρόνον ὅπως μηκέθ' ὁμοίως νοσήσειεν. ἐπεὶ δὲ πληρωθέντος τοῦ μηνὸς
εὔχρους τ' ἦν ἀκριβῶς ὡς μηδὲν ἀποδεῖν τῆς κατὰ φύσιν ἕξεως οὐδὲν δὲ
τοῦ ῥεύματος ἐπεφάνη, τετρακοσίους μὲν ἔπεμψέ μοι χρυσοῦς ηὔξησέ τε
τὸν φθόνον τούτων τῶν γενναίων ἰατρῶν ἐφ' οἷς ἐτύγχανεν ἐπαινῶν με.
21 καὶ μέντοι καὶ αὐτὸς ἕτοιμος ἦν ὥσπερ ὁ [τε] Σεβῆρος τὸ μηνῦσαι τὰ κατ'
ἐμὲ τῷ τε κατὰ τὴν τῶν Ῥωμαίων πόλιν ὄντι Μάρκῳ Αὐρηλίῳ
Ἀντωνίνῳ αὐτοκράτορι. Λεύκιος γὰρ ἀπεδήμει τῆς πόλεως ἕνεκα τοῦ
Παρθικοῦ πολέμου γενηθέντος ὑπὸ Βολογαίσου. |
648 9. Κἀγὼ θεασάμενος αὐτῶν τὴν ὁρμὴν καὶ δείσας μὴ φθασάντων τι
πρᾶξαι κωλυθῶ τῆς ἐς Ἀσίαν ἐπανόδου παρεκάλεσα βραχὺν ἐπισχεῖν
χρόνον. ἐγὼ γὰρ ἔφην ἐρεῖν αὐτοῖς τὸν καιρὸν ὁπόταν βουληθῶ τοῦτό
2 μοι γενέσθαι. καὶ τοίνυν ὅτ' ἀνεπυνθανόμην πεπαῦσθαι τὴν στάσιν,
ἄφνω τῆς Ῥωμαίων πόλεως ἐξῆλθον ὡς δῆθεν εἰς Καμπανίαν ἀπιών,
ἕνα καταλιπὼν οἰκέτην φυλάττοντα τὰ κατὰ τὴν οἴκησιν· ᾧ προσέταξα
πλοῖον ἐπιτηρήσαντι τῶν εἰς Ἀσίαν ἐξιόντων ἡμέρᾳ μιᾷ τῶν ἐκ τῆς
Σιβούρας κερκώπων παραλαβόντα τινὰ πωλῆσαί τε τὰ κατὰ τὴν

3 πρῶτον – 10 σινδόνων] *exc.* Razes *Kitāb al-ḥāwī* VII 185,1–7 πρῶτον – 5] *exc.* Orib. Syn. ad Eustath. IX 46: CMG VI 3 p. 306,10–12 Paul. Aeg. III 62: CMG IX 1 p. 279,8–10 Razes *Kitāb al-ḥāwī* IX 3,2 5–12] *exc.* Razes *Kitāb al-ḥāwī* IX 53,5 12 sq. ὡς – γνώρισμα] *exc.* Razes *Kitāb al-ḥāwī* IX 3,1 20–23] *cf.* Gal. De loc. aff. III 3: VIII p. 144,5–7 K. 24–118,8] *cf.* Gal. De libr. propr. 1: Scr. min. II p. 96,17–19 Müller = XIX p. 15,13–16 K.; p. 97,6–8 Müller = XIX p. 16,6–8 K.; p. 98,11 sq. Müller = XIX p. 17,15 sq. K.

1 τοσαύταις] tot diebus *Nic.* 4 ἐδίδουν *om.* M 5 σελήνου y: *corr. Chart.* 7 τοῦ] τὸ y: *corr. Ald.* 7 sq. ἐκκενοῦντος – γαστρὸς *om. Nic.* 9 αὐτοῖς L 11 καὶ *om.* M 12 ιε' y: *numerum plenius praeb. Chart.* 16 νοσήσειε M: νοσεῖεν L: *correxi* πληρωθέντος] non completo *Nic.* 17 ἀκριβῶς *ante* τῆς *iter.* M 19 ἰατρῶν – ἐτύγχανεν *om. Nic.* 20 τε *seclusi* 21 τε *fort. secludendum* τῶν *om.* L Μάρκῳ – 22 αὐτοκράτορι] Marco Antonino (Antonio *Nic.*[ze]: Anthonio *Nic.*[c]) et etiam Abrilio (Amb- *Nic.*[c]: Abilio *Nic.*[z]) *Nic.* Αὐριλίῳ L 23 Βολογαίσου *scripsi*: βολογέσου y 27 ὅταν ἐπυνθανόμην y: *corr. Schöne* 30 sq. ἐκ τῆς Σιβούρας *om. Nic.* 31 Βηβούρας y: *corr. Cobet, nisi* Συβούρας *praeferas*

is a steady improvement, you will permit me to continue my cure
for a further ten days: if not, then I will leave her completely."
As he readily agreed, I first purged her through the lower belly 16
with a hydragogic drug and then gave her a drink of water in which
asarabacca and celery had been boiled. When after the first two 17
days of this treatment there was no sign of the flux, on the third
day I again gave her a small dose of something that would purge
through the lower belly what had formerly flowed into the womb,
wishing to channel it through the lower belly as well as through her
urine. Next I daily anointed her with honey and massaged her 18
body, first with very soft cloths, then also with some very rough
ones, and gave her mountain birds and rock fish to eat. When after 19
fifteen days of this treatment there was not a trace of her affliction,
Boethus realised that I had done more than I had promised and begged
me to cure her condition completely and to give him instructions
to prevent its future recurrence. When at the end of the month she 20
had recovered her colouring and her natural condition and there was no
sign of the flux, he sent me four hundred gold pieces, but he increas-
ed the jealousy of these honourable doctors before whom he hap-
pened to praise me. Besides, like Severus, he was eager to tell every- 21
thing about me to Marcus Aurelius Antoninus, the emperor,
who was then in Rome – Lucius was abroad fighting the Parthians
under Vologaeses.

9. As soon as I discovered their desire, I was afraid that, if
they moved first, I should be prevented from returning to Asia,
and so I asked them to hold back for a little while, saying that I
would tell them the moment when I wanted this done for me. So, 2
when I heard of the ending of the disorder at home, I immediately
left Rome as if to visit Campania, keeping one servant behind to
look after the house, with instructions to wait for a boat going to Asia
and then, all in one day, engage an auctioneer from the Subura to

οἰκίαν ἐξελθεῖν τε παραχρῆμα καὶ τῆς νεὼς ἐπιβάντα κατὰ τὸν ἐπὶ
3 Σικελίας πλοῦν εἰς τὴν πατρίδα παραγενέσθαι. ταῦτα μὲν οὖν ὀλίγον
ὕστερον ἐπράχθη· ἐγὼ δ' ἐν Καμπανίᾳ γενόμενος, εἶτ' ἐκεῖθεν ἔσπευσα μὲν
εἰς τὸ Βρεντήσιον, ἀφικόμενος δ' ὥρισα κατὰ τὴν πρώτην ἀναγομένην
ναῦν εἴτ' ἐς Δουρράχιον εἴτ' ἐπὶ τῆς Ἑλλάδος πλέοι διαπεραιωθῆναι,
649 δεδιὼς μή | τις ἄρα τῶν πολὺ δυναμένων ἀνδρῶν ἢ καὶ αὐτὸς ὁ αὐτο-
κράτωρ γνούς μου τὴν ἔξοδον ὡς δραπέτου πέμψας στρατιώτην εἰς
4 Ῥώμην ἐπανελθεῖν κελεύσειεν. ἐγὼ μὲν οὖν οὕτως μετὰ μίαν ἡμέραν
εἰς Κασ⟨σ⟩ιόπην ἔπλευσα. ζητοῦντες δέ με οἱ ἐν Ῥώμῃ φίλοι παρά
τε τοῦ καταλειφθέντος οἰκέτου πυνθανόμενοι ποῦ ποτ' εἴην, ἀκούοντες
δ' ἐν τῇ Καμπανίᾳ διατρίβειν με, τὸ μὲν πρῶτον ὑπώπτευον τὸ γε-
γονὸς προϊόντος δὲ τοῦ χρόνου μήθ' ὁρῶντές ⟨με⟩ μήτε τὸν ἐμὸν ἄνθρωπον
ἐν Ῥώμῃ, ἔγνωσαν πεποιηκότα με τὰ ἐξ ἀρχῆς λεγόμενα· καὶ τότε μόγις
ἐπείσθησαν ἅπαντες οἱ πρόσθεν ἀπιστοῦντες ὄντως προ[σ]κεῖσθαί μοι
καταλιπεῖν τὴν Ῥώμην ὅτι μὴ ψευδῶς ἀλλ' ἀληθῶς ἔφασκον τοῦτο.
5 Μετὰ χρόνον δ' οὐ πολὺν ἐπανεληλυθότος τοῦ Λευκίου, πολέμου
[δ'] ἑτέρου τοῦ πρὸς Γερμανοὺς πολεμηθέντος αὐτοῖς ἀρχὴ καθεστήκει.
γενομένου ⟨δὲ⟩ λόγου περὶ τῶν ἔργοις οὐ λόγοις ἐπιδεικνυμένων ἰατρικήν
τε καὶ φιλοσοφίαν, οὐκ ὀλίγοι τῶν περὶ αὐτοὺς ὠνόμαζον ἐμὲ τοιοῦτον
6 ὑπάρχειν. ἐξωρμηκότες οὖν ἤδη τῆς πόλεως ὡς ἐπὶ τὸν πόλεμον ὡρικότες
650 τε τοῦ | χειμῶνος ἐν Ἀκυληίᾳ διατρῖψαι παρεσκευακότες τε καὶ συγκρο-
τοῦντες τὸ στράτευμα, πέμπουσιν εἰς ἐμὲ κελεύοντες ἥκειν ὡς αὐτούς. ἀλλὰ
τοῦ Λευκίου κατὰ μέσον τὸν χειμῶνα μεταστάντος εἰς θεοὺς ὁ ἀδελφὸς
αὐτοῦ κομίσας εἰς Ῥώμην τὸ σῶμα καὶ ποιήσας ἀμφ' αὐτῷ τὰ νομι-
ζόμενα, τῆς ἐπὶ τοὺς Γερμανοὺς ὁδοιπορίας εἴχετο κελεύων ἕπεσθαι
7 κἀμέ. χρηστὸν δ' ὄντα καὶ φιλάνθρωπον αὐτὸν ἐδυνήθην, ὡς οἶσθα,
πεῖσαι καταλιπεῖν ἐν τῇ Ῥώμῃ με· καὶ γὰρ διὰ ταχέων ἐπανήξειν. παντὶ
δ' οὖν τῷ τῆς ἀποδημίας αὐτοῦ χρόνῳ μεμνημένος τῆς συνήθους κα-
κοηθ⟨ε⟩ίας τῶν κατὰ τὴν πόλιν ἰατρῶν τε καὶ φιλοσόφων ἔγνων ἀνα-
χωρεῖν αὐτῆς ἄλλοτε εἰς ἄλλο χωρίον ἐν ᾧπερ ἂν ὁ υἱὸς αὐτοῦ Κόμ-
⟨μ⟩οδος, ὑπὸ Πειθολάῳ τρεφόμενος ἐντολὰς ἔχοντι παρ' αὐτοῦ τοῦ
αὐτοκράτορος Ἀντωνίνου καλεῖν πρὸς τὴν ἐπιμέλειαν τοῦ παιδὸς εἰ
8 νοσήσειέ ποτε. παρὰ προσδοκίαν δ' αὐτοῦ χρονίσαντος ἐν τῷ Γερμανικῷ

20–120,3 ἔδωκα] *cf.* Gal. De libr. propr. 2: Scr. min. II p. 98,12–100,2 Müller = XIX p. 17,16–19,18 K. 25 τῆς – 27] *cf.* Gal. De antidot. I 1: XIV p. 4,11–13 K.

3 Καμπανίᾳ N: Καμπύῃ y: in Campaniam *Nic.* ἐσπεύσαμεν M: ἐσπευσάμεν L: festinaui *Nic.*: *corr. Chart.* 4 Βρεντίσιον L ἀναγομένην *ex* ἀναν- *corr.* N: ἀναγενομένην y 5 Δυρράχιον *in* Διρρ- *mut.* M 9 Κασιόπην y: *corr. Chart.* 10 καταλειφθέντος] admisso *Nic.*, *unde* amisso *conieci* 12 με *sec. Nic.* (me) *addidi* 14 ἀπιστοῦντος L προσκεῖσθαι y: dicebam *Nic.*: *corr. Chart.* 15 Ῥωμαίων L 17 δ' *seclusi* αὐτοὺς L 18 δὲ *sec. Nic.* (autem) *add. Bas.* οὐ λόγοις] paucis *Nic.* ἐπιδειγνυμένων L 20 ἐξωρμηκότες N: ἐξορμηκότες y 21 Ἀλυκηίᾳ y: Akilea *Nic.*[v]: alkilea *Nic.*[b]: allilea *Nic.*[z]: alkileta *Nic.*[c]: Εἰκυληίᾳ *Bas.*: *corr. Corn. Chart.* 22 πέμπουσιν] misit *Nic.* εἰς] ὡς M αὐτούς] eum *Nic.* 23 τοῦ χειμῶνος M 26 ὡς οἶσθα *om. Nic.* 27 πεῖσθαι M 29 κακοηθίας y: *corr. Bas.* 30 ἂν] ἦν *Corn.* Κόμοδος y: *corr. Chart.* 33 νοήσειεν L

sell the house, depart at once, and embark for Sicily, coming home that
way. This indeed happened soon afterwards. I went off to Campania, 3
then hurried from there to Brindisi and, once arrived there, I deter-
mined to cross on the first boat to weigh anchor, whether it was sail-
ing for Durazzo or Greece; for I was scared that one of the very
influential men (in Rome), or even the emperor himself, might
discover my escape like a runaway slave and send a soldier to order
my return to Rome. So, one day later, I sailed for Cassiope. My 4
friends in Rome searched for me, and, when they asked the servant
I had left behind of my whereabouts, they were told that I was stay-
ing in Campania. At first they merely suspected what had happen-
ed: but, as time went on and they saw neither me nor my man in Rome,
they realised that I had done what I had threatened at the beginning.
Only then were all those who doubted that I had really intended to
leave Rome convinced, albeit with difficulty, that my professions
were true, not false.

Lucius returned not long after, but then a second war broke 5
out, this time with the Germans. When there was a general discus-
sion about those who had demonstrated medicine and philosophy by
deeds as well as by words, not a few of the emperors' friends mentioned
my name. So, although they had already left Rome on campaign 6
and had decided to winter at Aquileia preparing and assembling
the army, they sent a message to me, commanding me to appear
before them. But at mid-winter Lucius was translated to his place
among the gods and his brother (Marcus) brought his body to Rome and
performed all the customary rites for him. He still continued with his
German campaign, telling me to accompany him as well. But since he 7
was a good and charitable man, I was able, as you know, to persuade
him to leave me behind in Rome; for, indeed, his return would not
be long delayed. During the whole of his absence, remembering the
usual malice of the doctors and philosophers in the city, I decided to
retire at different times to the various spots where his son Commodus
resided. He was under the tutelage of Peitholaus, who had instruc-
tions from the emperor Antoninus himself to call me to attend his
son, should he ever fall ill. The emperor's involvement in the German 8

πολέμῳ, παντὶ τούτῳ τῷ χρόνῳ πολλὰς πραγματείας ἔγραψα φιλοσόφους
τε καὶ ἰατρικάς, ἃς ὑποστρέψαντος εἰς τὴν Ῥώμην τοῦ βασιλέως αἰτήσασι
651 τοῖς φίλοις ἔδωκα, παρὰ μόνοις ἐκείνοις ἐλπίσας | αὐτὰς ἔσεσθαι· ὡς εἴ γ'
ἠπιστάμην ἐκδοθήσεσθαι τοῖς ἀναξίοις οὐκ ἂν οὐδ' ἐκείνοις ἔδωκα. καλῶ
δ' ἀναξίους ὅσοι μοχθηροὶ τὴν ψυχήν, οὐχ ἕνεκα τοῦ μαθεῖν τι πρὸς
τὴν ἀνάγνωσιν ἥκουσιν ἀλλ' ὅπως ἐπηρεάσαι τινὰ δυνηθῶσιν ἐξ αὐτῶν.
9 ἐν τούτοις οὖν τοῖς βιβλίοις ἡ θεωρία πᾶσα γέγραπται τῆς τε διὰ
10 τῶν σφυγμῶν προγνώσεως καὶ τῶν ἄλλων προγνωστικῶν σημείων. ἣν
οὖν πρόγνωσιν ἐποιησάμην ἐπὶ θατέρου τῶν Κοϊντι[α]λίων υἱῶν
Ἕξστου βουληθέντι σοι μαθεῖν ἐκ τίνος θεωρίας ἐγένετο, ῥᾳδία καὶ καταφανὴς τὴν Περὶ κρίσεων πραγματείαν ἀναγνόντι, γεγυμνασμένῳ τὸν
λογισμὸν ἐκ παιδὸς ἐν γεωμετρίᾳ τε καὶ διαλεκτικῇ· τοῖς πολλοῖς δὲ
τούτοις ἰατροῖς, ὅσοι τῆς μὲν ἐν τοῖς ἔργοις γυμνασίας ἀπέστησαν, εἰς
πανουργίαν δ' ἐκτραπόμενοι τὴν ἐπ' αὐτῇ τέχνην ἤσκησαν, οὔτε
γνωσθῆναί τι τῶν γεγραμμένων δύναται οὔτ' ἀσκηθῆναι.

10. Ἕξστος οὖν ἤρξατο μὲν ὀξύτατα νοσεῖν ὡς μὴ δύνασθαι τὴν
652 ἑβδόμην ἡμέραν | ὑπερβαλεῖν ἄνευ κρίσεως. ἥτις δ' αὐτοῦ τούτου πρόγνωσίς ἐστι διὰ τῶν Περὶ κρίσεως ὑπομνημάτων γέγραπται, δι' ὧν καὶ
ὅτι προεκρήγνυται πολλάκις ἡ κρίσις οὐ περιμείνασα τὴν πιστῶς κρί-
2 νουσαν δεδήλωται. συμβῆναι δὲ τοῦτο τῷ Ἕξστῳ δυνάμενον ἔγνων
κατὰ τὴν τετάρτην ἡμέραν, ὡς προεῖπον ἐρομένῳ Πειθολάῳ τῷ κοιτωνίτῃ ὅ τι θεσπίζοιμι περὶ τῶν μελλόντων. ἤρετο γὰρ οὗτος ἐπειδὴ
προεπειρᾶτό μου πολλὰ τῶν δοκούντων τοῖς σοφωτάτοις ἰατροῖς ἀδυ-
3 νάτων εἶναι προειρηκότος. ἀπεκρινάμην οὖν αὐτῷ γελάσας, τῆς μὲν ἑβδόμης ἡμέρας ἐξωτέρω μὴ δύνασθαι προελθεῖν τὸ νόσημα· κριθήσεσθαι
δὲ πάντως ἢ ἑκταῖον ἢ ἑβδομαῖον. ἑκταῖον μὲν οὖν κριθὲν ὑποστρέφειν
αὐτό· ἑβδομαῖον δὲ βεβαίαν ἕξει⟨ν⟩ τὴν κρίσιν· ἔσεσθαι μέντοι τὴν κρίσιν
4 ἐξ ἀνάγκης δι' ἱδρῶτος. ἐπεὶ δὲ κατὰ τὴν ἕκτην ἡμέραν οὕτως γ' ἐκρίθη,
φιλόνεικος ὢν ἐσχάτως ὁ Ἕξστος, ὅπως ἐλέγξῃ ἐμὲ μὴ γενομένης ὑπο-

3sq.] *cf.* Gal. De dign. puls. I 1: VIII p. 773,16–774,2 K. 7sq.] *cf.* Gal. De libr. propr. 5: Scr. min. II p. 110,1–111,8 Müller = XIX p. 32,1–33,13 K. 8sq. ἣν ... πρόγνωσιν] *v. infra* l.16–126,2 11 Περὶ κρίσεων] p. 69–212 Alex. = IX p. 550–758 K. 15 οὔτ' ἀσκηθῆναι] *cf.* Gal. In Hipp. Progn. comm. I 8: CMG V 9,2 p. 218,6–10 17–20] Gal. De crisib., *in primis* III 10: p. 195,7–196,12 Alex. = IX p. 745,18–748,14 K. 28–122,9 πυρέττειν] *exc.* Razes *Kitāb al-ḥāwī* XVII 96,9; XVIII 218,10

2 ἰατροὺς y: ἰατρικοὺς *sec. Nic.* (medicinales) *Ald.*: *corr. Chart.* τοῦ βασιλέως *ante* εἰς *trsp.* M 5 οὐκ L 8 καὶ – σημείων *om. Nic.* 9 πρόγνωσιν *om. Nic.* Κοιντιαλίων (Κυιντ- M) y: Quintiliani *Nic.*: *correxi* 10 Ἕξστου] ἐξ αὐτοῦ y: ex hoc *Nic.*: *correxi* καὶ καταφανὴς *om. Nic.* καταφανῆ L 11 *ante* τὴν *add.* ἔσται *sec. Nic.* (erit) *Bas.* ἀναγνῶντι L 14 αὐτῇ] eis *Nic.* 15 ἀσκησθῆναι L: ἀκουσθῆναι M: exerceri *Nic.*: *corr. Schöne* 16 *post* οὖν *add.* Antonii filius *Nic.* 17 ζ' y: *numerum plenius praeb. Chart.* 18 κρίσεως] crisibus *Nic.* ὧν *ex* ὢν *corr.* L[2] 20 τοῦτο *ex* τούτῳ *corr.* M: τούτῳ L 21 ὡς *om. Nic.* προειπεῖν y: *correxi* ἐρωμενῳ L: *om. Nic.* τῷ κοιτωνίτῃ *om. Nic.* 22 οὕτως *Corn.*: ipse *Nic.* 23 ἀδύνατον L 24 ζ' y: *numerum plenius praeb. Chart.* 27 αὐτόν L ἕξει y: *corr. Ald.* 28 οὕτως γ' *om. Nic.* 29 ἐμὲ] με *scripserim*

war lasted unexpectedly long, and during this time I wrote many
philosophical and medical treatises, which, on the emperor's return
to Rome, I gave to my friends who asked for them, expecting that
they would remain in their possession; for, if I had known that they
would be distributed to the unworthy, I would not have given them
even to my friends. – By unworthy I mean those who, corrupt at
heart, approach the reading of a tract, not in the hope of learning
something from it, but of disparaging some of its points. – In these 9
works I have described all the theory of prognosis through the pulse
and other prognostic signs. Thus if you want to learn upon what 10
theory I based my prognosis in the case of Sextus, one of the
younger Quintilii, you will find it easy and obvious if you read
my tract 'On crises', since your mind has been trained from childhood
in geometry and dialectic. On the other hand, most of these doctors
have abandoned education in these subjects and have turned to exercising their skill in crime: thus they can neither understand nor put
into practice anything I have written there.

10. Now Sextus began to be so acutely ill that he could not
pass the seventh day without a crisis. The prognosis in this very case
has been described in my books 'On crises', where I have shown that
a crisis often occurs prematurely, without waiting for the real critical
day. I realised that this could have happened on the fourth day to 2
Sextus, as I told Peitholaus the chamberlain when he asked my
forecast of the future – he made this enquiry when he already had
much previous experience of the predictions I had made which had
seemed impossible to the wisest doctors. I replied with a laugh that 3
the disease could go no further than the seventh day, but would come
to a crisis either on the sixth or on the seventh day: if on the sixth,
it would recur: if on the seventh, a definite crisis would take place,
which would necessarily take the form of a sweating bout. When a 4
crisis came in this way on the sixth day, Sextus, who was extremely
stubborn, in order to prove me wrong by not having a relapse, took

στροφῆς, ἐλούετο μὲν καθ' ἑκάστην ἡμέραν οὔτε δ' οἶνον ἔπινεν οὔτε
προσηνέγκατό τι πλὴν χυλοῦ πτισάνης ἢ αὐτὴν καθ' ἑαυτὴν ἢ μετὰ ψιχῶν
653 ἄρτου· πολλάκις | δὲ καὶ αὐτὸς τὸν ἄρτον ἐν ὕδατι βρέξας ἠρκεῖτο μόνον.
5 ταῦτα ποιήσας ἄχρι τῆς δωδεκάτης ἡμέρας ἐκαυχήσατο κατ' αὐτὴν
νενικηκέναι μου τὴν πρόρρησιν. ἔπιε δὲ κατὰ τὴν τρισκαιδεκάτην ἡμέραν
ὑδατώδους οἴνου βραχύ τι σὺν τῷ καὶ τὴν ὅλην δίαιταν ἁδροτέραν βραχὺ
ποιήσασθαι τῆς ἔμπροσθεν, ἔτι μέντοι φυλάττων λεπτήν· ἀλλὰ κατά
τε τὴν ἑξῆς ἡμέραν ἀπὸ τῆς πρώτης κατακλίσεως τετταρεσκαιδεκάτην
οὖσαν ἀρξάμενος πυρέττειν ἐκέλευσε μηδένα μοι δηλῶσαι, νομίζων μηδὲ
σφοδρὸν ἔσεσθαι τὸν πυρετὸν μηδ' ⟨ἐπὶ⟩ πλέον ἡμέρας μιᾶς ἐκταθήσεσθαι
6 αὐτόν. ἐπεὶ δὲ προϊούσης τῆς ἡμέρας ἀεὶ καὶ μᾶλλον ἐσφοδρύνετο,
Κλαύδιος Σεβῆρος ὑποστρέφων εἰς τὴν ἑαυτοῦ οἰκίαν πλησίον οὖσαν
τῆς ἐκείνου, πυθόμενος αὐτὸν πυρέττειν ⟨ἐπορεύθη πρὸς αὐτὸν⟩ εὑρών
τε σφοδρῶς ἤδη πυρέττοντα, πρῶτον μὲν ἐπύθετο τίνα γνώμην ἐγὼ
περὶ τῆς ἀρχῆς τοῦ γεγενημένου νῦν αὐτῷ πυρετοῦ φαινοίμην ἔχων,
ἀκούσας τε παρ' αὐτοῦ τὸ ἀληθές, ὡς διὰ φιλονεικίαν οὔτ' ἐδήλω-
σε⟨ν οὔτ' εἴασε⟩ πορευθῆναί τινα πρός με, καὶ κελεύσας παρακαλεῖν ⟨μ'⟩
εἰς τὴν ἐπίσκεψιν τοῦ Ἔξστου καὶ μετὰ ταῦτα πρὸς αὐτὸν ἀφικέσθαι,
654 τούτων | γενομένων, ἐπυνθάνετο τί μοι δοκεῖ περὶ τῆς ὑποστροφῆς τοῦ
7 νοσήματος. ἀπεκρινάμην οὖν αὐτῷ ὅπερ καὶ τῷ Ἔξστῳ προειρήκειν,
μετὰ τρεῖς ἡμέρας λυθήσεσθαι τὴν ἐπιβολὴν ταύτην ἱκανῶς θερμοῦ γενο-
μένου τοῦ πυρετοῦ κατ' αὐτάς, εἶτα κριθησομένου κατὰ τὴν ἑπτακαι-
8 δεκάτην ἀπὸ τῆς ἀρχῆς ἡμέραν. Ἔξστος οὖν ἡδέως ἀκούσας τὴν ἐν
τάχει γενησομένην λύσιν ἑτοίμως ἐπίστευσεν· ὃ γὰρ ἕκαστος βούλεται
δηλονότι τοῦτο καὶ οἴεται γενήσεσθαι.

9 Σεβῆρος δ' ὅτι οὐκ ἂν σφαλείην ὑπὲρ τοῦ σωθήσεσθαι τὸν Ἔξστον
ἐπίστευσέ μοι· τὸ δὲ τῆς ἡμέρας ἐν ᾗ τελέως ⟨ἂν⟩ ἀπαλλαγείη τοῦ νοσήματος
οὐκ ἐπίστευε, δύσκολον εἶναι νομίζων ἄνευ τοῦ περιμεῖναι κἂν τὴν ἑξῆς
ἡμέραν ἀποφήνασθαί τι βέβαιον ὑπὲρ τῶν εἰς τετάρτην ἡμέραν ἐσο-
10 μένων. ἅτε δ' οὕτως διακείμενος ἔπεμψεν ὄρθρου βαθέος ἐπὶ τὴν οἰκίαν

24sq.] *cf.* Gal. In Hipp. Epid. VI comm. IV 8: CMG V 10,2,2 p. 198,25

1 ἑκάστης ἡμέρας L 2 ἑαυτήν] αὐτὴν y: *correxi* ψίχας y: *sec. Nic.* (cum panis micis) *corr. Corn.* 4 ιβ' y: *numerum plenius praeb. Chart.* 5 πρόγνωσιν M *post* ἡμέραν *sec. Nic.*[wv] (tercia hora) *add.* τρίτῃ ὥρᾳ *Bas.* 7 τῆς] τοῖς y: *corr. Chart.* φυλάττειν y: *om. Nic.*: *corr. Bas.* 8 τε *secluserim* ιδ' y: *numerum plenius praeb. Chart.* 10 ἐπὶ *sec. Nic.* (ad plus) *add. Durling* 11 αὐτόν] τὸν πυρετόν L: *om. Nic.* ἐφαιδρύνετο M 13 ἐπορεύθη πρὸς αὐτὸν *sec. Nic.* (adiuit ipsum [iuit ad ipsum *Nic.*[v]]) *add. Bas.* εὑρών] uidens *Nic.* 15 πυρετοῦ *ante* νῦν *trsp.* M 16 φινεικίας *ex* φην- *mut.* L 16sq. οὐκ ἐδήλωσε y: *corr. et suppl. Schöne*: dixit non enumptiari (enunciari *Nic.*[c]) quid michi *Nic.* 17 καὶ κελεύσας] dixitque (quoque *Nic.*[z]) Claudio me *(om. Nic.*[c]*)* ad uisitationem ipsius Esti (est *Nic.*[b]) *Nic.* παρακαλεῖν *ex* παραβαλεῖν *corr.* L: παραβαλεῖν M μ' *sec. Nic.*[wv] (me) *addidi* 22 πυρετοῦ] πῦ L 23 ἡμέρας L 24 ἑτοίμως *ante* οἴεται *(l. 25) indic. Nic.* (prompte credit) 27 ἂν ἀπαλλαγείη *scripsi*: ἀπαλλαγοῖτο y 28 ἐπίστευε *ex* ἐπίστευσεν *corr.* L 30 οὕτως *om. Nic.* βάθεως y: *corr. Chart.*

a daily bath and abstained from wine and food except for barley gruel,
either on its own or with small pieces of bread. Often bread dipped
in water would be enough for him. When he had kept this up until the 5
twelfth day, he boasted that he had thus defeated my prediction. On
the thirteenth day he took a little diluted wine, at the same time making
his diet also a little stronger than before, although still keeping it
light. But on the next day – that is, the fourteenth from when he
first took to his bed – he began to be feverish, but refused to let
anyone tell me, assuming that the fever would not be severe or last
more than a day. But as the day wore on and the fever increased yet 6
more, he was visited on his way home, which was close by, by Clau-
dius Severus, who had heard that he was in a fever. Finding him
already in the grip of a high fever, he first asked what opinion I had
given at the onset of this new attack, and, when he heard the truth
from him, that through obstinacy he had neither shown me his con-
dition nor allowed anyone to go and inform me, he ordered me to go
and visit Sextus and then to come to him. This done, he asked me
my views on the recurrence of the disease. My reply was the same as I 7
had predicted to Sextus: that the attack would be over in three days
when the fever had reached a sufficient degree of warmth, and then
the crisis would occur on the seventeenth day from the beginning.
Sextus, who had heard with pleasure that the end would come 8
quickly, readily believed this; for what a man wants, he always
thinks will happen.

Although Severus believed that I was correct in saying that 9
Sextus would be saved, he doubted the day on which he would be
totally free of the disease, for he thought it difficult to make a definite
statement about what was to happen on the fourth day without
even waiting for the second. With this in mind, at crack of dawn he 10

τοῦ Ἕξστου περιμένοντά τε καὶ πρὸς αὐτὸν ἄξοντά ⟨με⟩ μετὰ τὴν
11 ἐσομένην ἐπίσκεψιν. ὡς δὲ θεασάμενος τὸν Ἕξστον ἐπορεύθην πρὸς
αὐτόν, «ἀντιφήσεις», ⟨ἔφη⟩, «οἷς χθὲς εἶπες, ἢ διαμενεῖς ἐπὶ τῶν αὐτῶν;»
655 ἐπεὶ δὲ νῦν μᾶλλον ἔφην ἢ χθὲς ἀποφήνασθαί μοι | ταὐτά, μετ' ἄριστον
αὖθίς με καλέσας ἤρετο πάλιν εἰ βεβαίως εἴην πεπεισμένος Ἕξστῳ ἐσο-
12 μένην κρίσιν. ἤκουεν οὖν παρ' ἐμοῦ μᾶλλον ἢ χθὲς ἔχειν διατείνασθαι. ⟨...⟩
πότερον φυλάττομεν τὴν αὐτὴν γνώμην ἐπὶ τοῖς προειρημένοις ἤ τι καὶ
μετακινοῖμι τῶν ῥηθέντων, ἤκουσεν οὐδὲν μὲν ἐκείνων κινεῖν, προστί-
13 θεσθαι δέ τι τοῖς εἰρημένοις ἔχειν. καὶ ὃς αὖθις ἤρετο, «τί τοῦτό ἐστιν;»
ἤκουσεν ὅτι διελθούσης τῆς ἑπτακαιδεκάτης ἡμέρας ἄρξασθαι τὸν ἱδρῶτα
14 περὶ δευτέραν ὥραν νυκτερινήν. «ἆρ' οὖν», ἔφη, «καὶ Πειθολάῳ ταῦτ'
εἶπας;» εἰρηκέναι τ' ἔφην αὐτῷ καὶ πεπεῖσθαί γ' ἐκεῖνον ὡς οὐκ ἂν σφα-
15 λείην ἐν τῇ προρρήσει καὶ θεραπείᾳ. πάντως οὖν ἔφη καὶ τῷ αὐτοκράτορι
δεδηλωκέναι τὸν Π⟨ε⟩ιθόλαον. «ἴσως», ἔφην, «οὗτος ἔφη. ἐμοὶ δ' οὐ μέ-
λ[λ]ει τῆς ἐπὶ τοῖς τοιούτοις δόξης· οὐ γὰρ περιέρχομαι κηρύττων τὰς ἐμὰς
προγνώσεις τε καὶ θεραπείας ἵνα μᾶλλον οἱ ἰατροί τε καὶ φιλόσοφοί με μι-
16 σῶσι, γόητά τε καὶ μάντιν ἕτερά τε κατ' ἐμοῦ τοιαῦτα θρυλοῦντες. ὑμῖν
656 δὲ τοῖς φίλοις ὅσοι κατεγνώκατε | τῆς ἰατρικῆς τέχνης ἐκ τῆς τούτων
ἀμαθίας ἐπιδείκνυμι τὴν μὲν τέχνην ἀξίαν Ἀπόλλωνός τε καὶ Ἀσκλη-
πίου, τοὺς δ' ἰατροὺς τούτους ὑβρίζειν αὐτήν· ὥσπερ καὶ τοὺς φιλοσό-
φους φιλοσοφίαν οἵ γε μηδενὸς ἰδιώτου βέλτιον βιοῦντες ὀνομάζουσιν
ἑαυτοὺς ὀνόματι σεμνῷ τῷ τῆς φιλοσοφίας.»
17 Ταῦτα μὲν εἶπον τῷ Σεβήρῳ· σὺ δέ, ὦ Ἐπίγενες, [ὡς] ἔγνως
τὴν κακοήθειαν τῶν ἰατρῶν σχεδὸν ἁπάντων εὐχομένων φανερῶς ἀπο-
τυχεῖν με πεμπόντων τε δι' ὅλης ἡμέρας τοὺς γνωσομένους τε καὶ ἀγ-
18 γέλλοντας αὐτοῖς τὸ γενησόμενον. ἐπεὶ δὲ περὶ τὴν ἑβδόμην ὥραν ἐπι-
παροξυνθέντα τὸν Ἕξστον ἐπύθοντο, καταγελῶντες καὶ φανερῶς ἐπι-
χαίροντες ἅπασι τοῖς ἀπαντῶσιν ἔλεγον κερτομοῦντες ὡς ἡ θαυμαστὴ
μαντεία τοῦ Γαληνοῦ κατὰ τοὐναντίον ἀπέβη. οὐ γὰρ ᾔδεσάν με τῷ
Σεβήρῳ καὶ Πειθολάῳ προειρηκότα δείλης ὄψεσθαι ἐσομένην τὴν
19 ἀρχὴν τῆς κρίσεως. γενομένης μέντοι τῆς κρίσεως ὡς προειρήκειν κατὰ

15–17] *cf. supra* p. 70,14

1 τοῦ Ἕξστου] Σέξστου M   περιμένοντά – 3 αὐτόν] dicens expectare eum me; post uisitationem uero redirem ad ipsum *Nic.*^{w}: dicens expectare eum ut uisitaturum (se *add. Nic.*^{v}) uocet Estus *(om. Nic.*^{v}*)* deinde mittar ad eum *Nic.*^{cev} με *addidi*   3 ἔφη *sec. Nic.* (ait) *add. Bas.*   4 ἀποφήνεσθαί L   5 με *om. Nic.* 5sq. ἐσομένης κρίσεως y: *corr. Bas.*   6 *post* κρίσιν *add.* ut dixeram *Nic.*   ἔχειν *om. Nic.*   *lacunam indicavi*: ut autem et secundo die interrogabat (intero- *Nic.*^{c}) *Nic.*: ὡς δὲ τὴν (*ante* τὴν *addiderim* καὶ) δευτέραν ἡμέραν ἐπύθετό μου *sec. Nic. add. Bas.*   7 φυλάττοιμι *Bas.*   9 ὃς] qui *Nic.*: ὡς *Corn.*   10 ἤκουσεν] scias, dixi *Nic.*   11 νυκτερινήν *om. Nic.*   13 αὐτοκρατόρη L   14 Πιθόλαον y: *corr. Ald.* ἴσως – ἔφη] ille, dixi, ut uult faciat *Nic.*   μέλλει y: *sec. Nic.* (cura est) *corr. Ald.* 18 τέχνης] ὅλης L: *om. Nic.*   *post* τέχνης *add.* et desperauistis (dis- *Nic.*^{c}) *Nic.* 19 Ἀπόλωνος L   22 αὐτοὺς y: *correxi*   23 ὡς *om. Nic.*: *secl. Bas.*: καλῶς *Corn.*, *fort. recte*   26–31 ἐπεὶ – ἀπέβη. οὐ – κρίσεως.] οὐ – κρίσεως. ἐπεὶ – ἀπέβη. y: *ordinem sec. Nic. mutavi*   ζ′ y: *numerum plenius praeb. Chart.*   29 ἀπέβην L εἴδεσαν y: *corr. Kühn*   30 ὄψεσθαι ἐσομένην] esse *Nic.*   **31**sq. κατὰ τὴν προτεραίαν *om. Nic.*

sent a man to Sextus' house to wait and bring me back to him after
my examination. So, having seen Sextus, I came to him. "Will 11
you deny what you said yesterday?", he said, "Or do you still stay
by the same opinion?" I told him that I held even more firmly to
my opinion than on the previous day. Then, after breakfast, he sum-
moned me again and asked once more if I was entirely certain that
Sextus would have a crisis. I told him that I could be even more 12
definite than the previous day. +When again on the second day
he asked me+[1] whether I still adhered to my earlier statements
or wished to change anything, he was told that I retracted nothing
and could even add to what I had said. He asked again, "What is 13
this?" and heard that when the seventeenth day was over the
sweating would commence at the second hour of the night. "Well 14
then", he said, "I suppose you have told Peitholaus?" I replied
that I had indeed told him and that he was convinced that I would not
fail in my prediction and treatment. He replied that Peitholaus had 15
assuredly passed this on to the emperor. "Possibly", I said, "he has
told him: but, personally, I am not bothered about my reputation
with such people. I don't go around broadcasting my prognoses and
cures so as to incur greater enmity from doctors and philosophers
and have them calling me wizard and prophet and other such names.
But to you, my friends, who have condemned medicine because of 16
the ignorance of men like that, I declare that this art is worthy of
Apollo and Asclepius, and that these doctors have abused it; just
as those philosophers have abused philosophy who honour themselves
with the august name of philosophy although their way of life is no
better than that of the ordinary man."

That was the gist of my conversation with Severus; and you 17
are well aware, Epigenes, of the maliciousness of almost all the
doctors, who openly prayed for my failure and all day long sent men
to find out and tell them what was going to happen. When they learn- 18
ed that Sextus had had an increase of fever about the seventh
hour, with derisive laughter and obvious delight they sneeringly told
everyone they met that Galen's wonderful prophecy had misfired.
For they did not know that I had predicted to Severus and Peitho-
laus that they would see the crisis beginning that afternoon. When the 19
crisis took place as I had forecast the previous day, they were all put to

[1] +When – me+: see Niccolò's version in the app. crit.

τὴν προτεραίαν [ἔφασαν ἑπομένην ἐναλλὰξ] ἐτρέποντο πάντες αἰσχυνό-
μενοι, καὶ ταῦτα τῆς προγνώσεως οὐδὲν ἐχούσης θαυμαστόν, ὡς ἔδειξά
657 σοι | διά τε τῶν Εἰς ⟨τὸ⟩ πρῶτον ⟨τῶν⟩ Ἐπιδημιῶν ὑπομνημάτων ἔτι
20 τε τὴν Περὶ τῶν κρίσεων πραγματείαν. τούτοις μέντοι τοῖς ἰατροῖς οὐ μόνον
ἀγνοεῖν ὑπάρχει τὰ γεγραμμένα τοῖς παλαιοῖς ἀλλὰ μηδὲ τὰς ἡμέρας
ἀριθμεῖν ἔτι μετὰ τὴν ἑβδόμην, καὶ μάλιστ' ἐὰν ἀπύρετος γενόμενος ὁ
21 κάμνων αὖθις ἐξ ὑποστροφῆς πυρέττῃ· καίτοι παρ' Ἱπποκράτους
κατὰ ⟨τὰ⟩ τῶν Ἐπιδημιῶν βιβλία γεγραμμένων ἁπασῶν τῶν ἡμερῶν
ἐφ' ἑκάστῳ τῶν ἀρρώστων ἄχρι τῆς ἐσχάτης λύσεως οὐ μόνον εἰ κατὰ
τὴν τετταρεσκαιδεκάτην ἡμέραν ἀλλὰ καὶ κατὰ τὴν ἑξηκοστὴν ἢ ὀγ-
22 δοηκοστὴν τύχοι γεγενημένη. αὕτη μὲν οὖν ἡ πρόρρησις, ὡς ἔφην, [ὡς]
εἰ καὶ θαυμαστὴ τοῖς πολλοῖς τούτοις ἰατροῖς ἔδοξεν, ἀλλ' οὐ τοιαύτη
γε κατ' ἀλήθειαν ἦν, ὥσπερ οὐδ' ἡ μετὰ γνώσεως τῶν ἐνεστώτων θερα-
πεία τοῦ παιδὸς αὐτοῦ Κομ⟨μ⟩όδου κατὰ τὴν ἐπιδημίαν ἐκείνου γε-
νομένη.

11. Θαυμαστὴ δ' ὄντως ἡ νῦν ἐπ' αὐτοῦ τοῦ βασιλέως συμβᾶσα,
658 δόξαντος μὲν καὶ | αὐτοῦ καὶ τῶν ἀμφ' αὐτὸν ἰατρῶν ὅσοι συναπεδήμησαν
αὐτῷ παροξυσμόν τινα πυρεκτικὸν ἄρξασθαι, σφαλέντων δὲ πάντων
καὶ τῆς δευτέρας καὶ τρίτης ἡμέρας ἕωθεν καὶ περὶ τὴν ὀγδόην ὥραν.
2 εἰλήφει δὲ τῆς προτεραίας τοῦ διὰ τῆς ἀλόης πικροῦ φαρμάκου πρώτης
ὥρας, εἶτα τῆς θηριακῆς, ὡς ἔθος ἦν αὐτῷ καθ' ἑκάστην ἡμέραν προσφέ-
ρεσθαι, καὶ τότε προσενεγκαμένου περὶ ὥραν ὡς ἕκτην, εἶτα λουσαμένου
περὶ δυσμὰς ἡλίου καὶ βραχὺ τραφέντος, ἐπιγενομένων ὅλης τῆς νυκτὸς
στρόφων ἅμα τῇ διὰ τῆς κάτω γαστρὸς κενώσει, καὶ διὰ τοῦτο πυρέξαντος
αὐτοῦ, καὶ τῶν ἀμφ' αὐτὸν ἰατρῶν ἕωθεν θεασαμένων ἡσυχάσαι τε κε-
λευσάντων, εἶτα ῥοφήματι θρεψαμένων ὥρας ἐνάτης, ἐμοῦ δὲ μετὰ ταῦτα
κληθέντος ὅπως καὶ αὐτὸς ἐν τῷ Παλατίῳ κοιμηθείην, ἧκέ τις καλῶν
3 ἡμᾶς ἄρτι λύχνων ἡμμένων ὑπὸ τοῦ αὐτοκράτορος στελλόμενος. ὡς

3 τῶν^{I} – ὑπομνημάτων] Gal. In Hipp. Epid. I comm. I–III: CMG V 10,1 p. 3–151, *in primis* comm. II: p. 45,14–102,4 4 τὴν – πραγματείαν] *in primis* De crisib. I 14–16: p. 107,11–114,15 Alex. = IX p. 610,15–622,6 K.; III 6–11: p. 185,3–212 Alex. = IX 730,1–738 K. 11 ἔφην] *v. supra* l. 2sq. 13 ἡ–15] *v. infra* p. 130,11 – 134,8 16] *cf.* Gal. De libr. propr. 5: Scr. min. II p. 110,16–111,3 Müller = XIX p. 32,13–33,8 K.

1 ἔφασαν – ἐναλλὰξ *om. Nic.*: *seclusi* 2 ταύτης L ἐδείξατο L 3 τὸ *add. Schöne* τῶν *add. Schöne, Bardong, Nachrichten d. Akad. Göttingen 1942, 6, p. 614* 7 πυρέττει y: *corr. Morel Chart.* 8 τὰ *addidi* 9/11 ἡ . . . τύχῃ y: *sec. Nic.* (si . . . fiat) εἰ . . . τύχῃ *Bas.*: *correxi* 10 ιδ' . . . ξ' . . . π' y: *numeros plenius scripsi* 11 γεγενημένην L ὡς^{I} – 13 ἀλήθειαν *om. Nic.* ὡς^{II} *secl. Bas.* 13 ἡ] εἰ y: *om. Nic.*: *corr. Bas.* 14 τοῦ – Κομμόδου] Commodus filii Pitholai *Nic.* αὐτοῦ] αὐτοκράτορος *coniecerim* Κομόδου y: *corr. Chart.* ἐπιδημίαν] *sec. Nic.* (in peregrinatione) ἀποδημίαν *coni. Bas., fort. recte, sed v. infra comm. ad loc.* 17 αὐτὸν] αὐτῶν L 19 ἢ τρίτης y: *sec. Nic.* (et tercio) *corr. Bas.*: *secl. Corn.* ἕωθεν – ὥραν *om. Nic.* 23 βραχὺ] τράχυ L: τράων M: *sec. Nic.* (modicum) *corr. Ald.* *post* τραφέντος *sec. Nic.* (et) *add.* καὶ *Bas.* ἐπιγενομένου L 25 ἕωθεν *om.* M 26 θ' y: *numerum plenius praeb. Chart.* 28 ὡς τὸν αὐτοκράτορα στελλόμενον y: *sec. Nic.* (a rege missus) *corr. Bas.*

shame and confusion – and this, when my prognosis contained nothing
remarkable, as I have shown you in my 'Commentaries on the first
book of the Epidemics' and also in my treatise 'On crises'. But these 20
doctors are not only incapable of understanding the works of the an-
cients; they cannot yet even count the days beyond seven, especially
if the patient has once become free of fever and then has a relapse. Yet 21
Hippocrates in his 'Epidemics' has described all the days in each
illness to its final conclusion, not only if it should occur on the four-
teenth day, but also if it lasts until the sixtieth or eightieth. This 22
prognosis, therefore, as I have said, even if it appeared remarkable
to the generality of doctors, certainly was not so in fact, any more
than the cure I made of the young Commodus when he was in Rome,
which involved taking into account all the attendant circumstances.

11. Now the cure that I performed on the emperor himself was
really remarkable. He and the medical advisers who had accompanied
him on campaign believed a paroxysm of fever had begun, but they
were all proved wrong on the second and third day, both in the morn-
ing and at about the eighth hour. On the previous day he had taken a 2
draught of bitter aloes at the first hour and then some theriac at
about the sixth, as was his daily custom. He had a bath at sunset
and a light meal. All night long there followed colicky pains and
evacuations through the lower belly, which made him feverish, and
when his court doctors saw him in the morning, they advised him to
rest and fed him some thick gruel at the ninth hour. Although I was
then called in to sleep at the Palace, it was just when the lamps
had been lit that an emissary from the emperor came to summon me.

δὲ τριῶν ὄντων τῶν ἕωθέν τε καὶ περὶ τὴν ὀγδόην ὥραν ἑωρακότων
αὐτόν, ἁψαμένων τε τῶν σφυγμῶν, ἐπισημασίας ἀρχή τις εἶναι πᾶσιν
ἐφαίνετο, σιωπῶν ⟨δ'⟩ εἱστήκειν ἐγώ, προσβλέψας με πρῶτον ἐπύθετο |
659 4 διὰ τί τῶν ἄλλων ἁψαμένων ἐγὼ μόνος οὐχ ἡψάμην. εἶπον οὖν αὐτῷ
ὅτι δὶς ἤδη τούτων ἡμμένων, ἤδη δ' ἴσως καὶ κατὰ τὴν μετά σου γε-
γενημένην αὐτοῖς ἀποδημίαν ἐγνωσμένης τῇ πείρᾳ τῆς ἰδιότητος τῶν
σφυγμῶν σοῦ, μᾶλλον αὐτοὺς ἐλπίζω διαγινώσκεσθαι τὴν ἐνεστῶσαν
5 ἄρτι διάθεσιν. ὡς δ' εἰπόντος μου ταῦτα καὶ αὐτοῦ με κελεύσαντος
ἅψασθαι, φανέντος μοι τοῦ σφυγμοῦ παρὰ τὸ κοινὸν μέτρον ἁπάσης
ἡλικίας τε καὶ φύσεως ἀφεστηκέναι τοῦ δηλοῦντος ἀρχὴν ἐπισημασίας,
ἀπεφηνάμην εἰσβολὴν μὲν οὐδεμίαν εἶναι πυρετοῦ, θλίβεσθαι δ' αὐτοῦ
τὸν στόμαχον ὑπὸ τῆς εἰλημμένης τροφῆς, φλεγματωθείσης μὲν πρὸ
ἐκκρίσεως, ἐμφαινούσης δέ, ἔπαινόν τινα τῆς διαγνώσεως αὐτῇ
λέξει τῇδε τρὶς ἐφεξῆς εἰπών, «αὐτό ἐστιν, αὐτὸ τοῦτο ὃ εἶπές ἐστιν·
αἰσθάνομαι γὰρ ὑπὸ ψυχροτέρας τῆς τροφῆς βαρυνόμενος», ἤρετο τί
6 ποιεῖν χρή. ἐγὼ δ' ἀπεκρινάμην ἅπερ ἔγνων καὶ ἐλέχθη μοι πρὸς αὐτὸν
ὡς εἰ ἄλλος τις ἦν ὁ διακείμενος οὕτως ἔδωκα ἂν αὐτῷ, καθάπερ εἴωθα,
πιεῖν οἶνον πεπέρεως ἐπιπάσας. ἐφ' ὑμῶν δὲ τῶν βασιλέων, ἀσφαλεστά-
660 τοις βοη|θήμασιν εἰωθότων χρῆσθαι τῶν ἰατρῶν, ἀρκεῖ ναρδίνῳ μύρῳ
θερμῷ δεύσαντα μαλλὸν ἐρίου θεῖναι κατὰ τοῦ στόματος τῆς κοιλίας.
7 ὁ δὲ καὶ ἄλλως εἰπὼν ἔθος ἐκείνῳ ὅταν ποτὲ μέμψηται τὸν στόμαχον,
ἀνειλημμένον πορφυρέῳ [τε] ἐρίῳ τὸ νάρδινον μύρον ἐπιτιθέναι θερμὸν
κελεύσας τε Πειθολάῳ πρᾶξαι τοῦτο καὶ ἡμᾶς ἀπολῦσαι, ἐπιθέντος δ'
αὐτοῦ καὶ τῶν ποδῶν ἐκθερμανθέντων ὑπὸ τῶν ἀνατριβόντων θερμαῖς
8 ταῖς χερσίν, ᾔτησεν οἴνου Σαβίνου καὶ πεπέρεως ἐπιβαλὼν ἔπιε. καὶ
τῷ Πειθολάῳ μετὰ τὸ πιεῖν ⟨εἰπὼν⟩ ὡς ἰατρὸν ἔχομεν ἕνα καὶ τοῦτον
ἐλεύθερον πάνυ διετέλει [τε] περὶ ἐμοῦ λέγων ἀεί, καθάπερ οἶσθα καὶ
σύ, τῶν μὲν ἰατρῶν πρῶτον εἶναι, τῶν δὲ φιλοσόφων μόνον· ἐπεπειρᾶτο
γὰρ ἤδη πολλῶν οὐ μόνον φιλοχρημάτων ἀλλὰ καὶ φιλονείκων καὶ φι-
λοδόξων καὶ φθονερῶν καὶ κακοήθων.
9 Ὅπερ οὖν ἔφην ἐγώ, ταύτης τῆς ἐπισκέψεως οὐδεμίαν ἄλλην ἡγοῦ-
μαί μοι γεγονέναι θαυμαστοτέραν. ἐζητημένου γὰρ ἅπασι τοῖς ἄριστα
τὴν περὶ τοὺς σφυγμοὺς τέχνην ἀσκήσασιν, ὧν εἷς καὶ Ἀρχιγένης

8–10 ἐπισημασίας] *exc.* Razes *Kitāb al-ḥāwī* XIV 14,8; XVII 39,10; 42,13
11 sq. ἀπεφηνάμην – μὲν] *exc.* Razes *Kitāb al-ḥāwī* V 80,9; 111,6

1 τε – ὥραν *om. Nic.* ὀγδόην ὥραν *scripsi*: ἕω y 2 *post* τε *sec. Nic.* (duobus) *add.* δυοῖν *Bas.* 3 δ' *sec. Nic.* (uero) *add. Bas.* 5 τότε δὶς y: quoniam hii duo *Nic., sec. quem* ὅτι δύο *coni. Bas.* ἤδη[I] *om. Nic.* 8 *post* διάθεσιν *add.* αὐτῶν *Schöne* αὐτόν ἐμε κελεύσαντα y: αὐτόν ἐμε κελεύσαντος *Bas.*: *correxi* 9 μοι] μοῦ y: *corr. Corn.* 9 sq. παρὰ – φύσεως] multum *Nic.* 12 εἰλημένης L *post* πρὸ *add.* τῆς *Bas., fort. recte* 13 ἐμφαινούσης – 14 τῇδε] ipse autem laudans dignotionem *Nic.* ἐμφαίνων *Corn.* 14 αὐτό ἐστιν *om. Nic.* 16 ἅπερ – 17 ὡς] sic *Nic.* οὐλελέχθη L 18 ποιεῖν L: facere *Nic.* 20 μαλλὸν *om. Nic.* 22 πόρθυρά τε ἔρια y: infusa in eo porfira (porrifira *Nic.*[b]) *Nic.*: *corr. Corn. Chart.* 23 Πιθολάω L 26 εἰπὼν *sec. Nic.* (dicente) *post* καὶ *add. Bas.*: *transposui* ἔχων M 27 τε *secl. Müri, p. 58* 29 ἤδη *om. Nic.* 31 Ὅπερ] sicut *Nic.* 32 ἐζητουμένου L

Three doctors had already examined him at dawn and at the eighth 3
hour; they had taken his pulse; and they agreed that this was ap-
parently the opening of an attack of an illness. When I stood by in si-
lence, the emperor looked at me and asked why, when the others had
taken his pulse, I alone had not done so. I replied that since they 4
had already done so twice and the peculiarities of his pulse were pro-
bably known to them through their experiences on their travels
abroad with him, I expected that they could obtain a better diagnosis
of his present condition than I. On hearing this, he commanded me to 5
take his pulse. It seemed to me that his pulse, compared with the
general norm for each age and constitution, was far from show-
ing the onset of an attack of an illness, and so I said that there was
no attack of fever, but his stomach was overloaded with the food he
had taken, which had turned to phlegm before excretion, and that
this was now quite clear. After praising my diagnosis three times
in these words: "That's it, what you have said is just it: I feel that
some rather cold food is upsetting me", he asked what was to be
done. I told him what I knew and said that, had it been anybody 6
else in that condition, I should have prescribed my usual dose of wine
with pepper on top: but in the case of kings like him, when doctors
should employ the safest remedies, it was enough to place over the
mouth of the stomach a pad of wool impregnated with warm nard
ointment. He replied that in any case, when he had a stomach com- 7
plaint, he used to apply warm nard ointment smeared on scarlet
wool, and he ordered Peitholaus to do that and then dismiss me.
After the ointment had been applied and his feet warmed by the warm
hands of the masseurs, he called for Sabine wine, sprinkled pepper
on it, and drank it. After he had drunk it, he remarked to Peitho- 8
laus, "We have one doctor, and he is a very enlightened gentleman."
As you well know, he was continually speaking of me as the first
among physicians and unique among philosophers: for he had al-
ready met many who were avaricious, quarrelsome, proud, jealous and
spiteful.

As I said, I think that this was the most remarkable of my 9
investigations. For there had been attempts by all the doctors who
were very well trained in the theory of pulses – of whom in fact Ar-

661 ἐγένετο, τί σημεῖον ἴδιον ἐπι|σημασίας, ἐπεί τινων μὲν ἐν ἀρχῇ τῆς κατὰ
τὴν ἀρτηρίαν συστολῆς εὑρίσκεσθαι φάντων [αὐτῶν], τινὼν δὲ μηδ' ὅλως
αἰσθητὴν εἶναι τὴν συστολήν, εὐτυχήσας ἐγώ – τί γὰρ ⟨ἂν⟩ ἄλλο φαίη
τις αἰσθητικωτάτην ἀφὴν τῆς παρὰ μικρὸν ἐν τοῖς σφυγμοῖς διαφορᾶς –
ἁμαρτανόντων εἰς τοσοῦτον ἐνίων ἰατρῶν ἐπειράθην ὡς ἀρχομένους
ἐπισημαίνεσθαί τινας εἰς τὸ βαλανεῖον ἐκπέμπειν ἢ τραφῆναι κελεύειν, ἐκώ-
10 λυσα. διὰ παντὸς οὖν ἀκριβῶς ἐμαυτοῦ πεπειραμένος διαγνόντος ἀρχὴν
παροξυσμοῦ προπετέστερον μὲν ἴσως, ὅμως δ' ἐτόλμησα βασιλεῖ δια-
τεινάμενος εἰπεῖν, ὅτε πρῶτον ἡψάμην, ἐναντίαν ἀπόφασιν ἧς αὐτός τε
καθ' ἑαυτὸν ἐδόξαζε καὶ τῶν ἰατρῶν ἤκουεν.
12. Τὸ μέντοι κατὰ Κόμ⟨μ⟩οδον ἔχειν μέν φασί ⟨τι⟩ μέγιστον, τῇ
δ' ἀληθείᾳ πάμπολυ λείπεται τοῦδε. τῆς παλαίστρας γὰρ ἀπαλλαγέντος
αὐτοῦ πρὶν σιτίων ὥρας ὀγδόης εἰσέβαλε θερμὸς ἱκανῶς πυρετός· ἁψα-
μένῳ δέ μοι τῶν σφυγμῶν φλεγμαίνειν τι μόριον ἐφαίνετο· καὶ ταῦτ' ἀκού-
662 σας ὁ Πειθόλαος θαυ|μάζειν ἔφησεν εἰ τῶν παρισθμίων ἡ φλεγμονὴ
2 τὸν σφυγμὸν ἠλλοίωσε τοῦ παιδός· οὐδὲν γὰρ ἄλλο μέρος αὐτοῦ φλεγ-
μαίνει. κἀν τούτῳ διανοίξας αὐτῷ τὸ στόμα κελεύει μοι θεάσασθαι. φα-
νέντων δὲ τραχέων καὶ λίαν ἐρυθρῶν, οὐ μέντοι μέγαν ὄγκον ἐχούσης
τῆς φλεγμονῆς, ἠρόμην τίς ὁ ἀνατρίψας εἴη στοματικῷ φαρμάκῳ σφο-
3 δροτέραν τῆς ἁρμοττούσης τῷ παιδὶ στῦψιν ἔχοντι. τοῦ δὲ φάντος ἑαυτὸν
εἶναι τὸν ἀνατρίψαντα τῷ διὰ μέλιτος καὶ ῥοῦ φαρμάκῳ, μεταβῆναι μὲν
ἐπὶ μελίκρατον ἐναφεψημένων ῥόδων ἐκέλευσα καὶ τούτῳ μόνῳ χρῆσθαι
διά τε τῆς νυκτὸς καὶ τῆς ἐχομένης ἡμέρας ὅλης πολλάκις ἅμα τῇ μετ' αὐτὴν
4 νυκτί. τῇ δὲ τρίτῃ τῶν ἡμερῶν ἕωθεν, ἐπειδὴ τά τε τῆς φλεγμονῆς ἐπέπαυτο
τελέως ἀπύρετός τε μικροῦ δ⟨εῖν⟩ ἦν ὁ παῖς, ἔπεισα δ' οὖν τὸν Πειθόλαον
εἰς βαλανεῖον ἐγγὺς ὂν τοῦ κοιτῶνος εἰσαγαγόντα, μετ' οὐ πολὺ τῷ
κατὰ τὴν π[τ]ύελον ὕδατι χρήσασθαι, διαβρεχομένων μὲν ἁπάντων τῶν
ἄλλων μορίων, μόνης δὲ τῆς κεφαλῆς καταντλουμένης δαψιλῶς τραφέντι
663 5 αὐτῷ. περὶ τρίτην ὥραν ἧκεν Ἀννία Φαυστῖνα, | συγγενὴς οὖσα τῷ
αὐτοκράτορι ἔγγιστα, παραιτουμένη διότι δευτεραῖον αὐτὸ⟨ν⟩ οὐκ εἶδε·

1–3 εὐτυχήσας] *cf.* Gal. De dign. puls. I 3: VIII p. 788,18–790,10 K. τινων – 3 συστολήν] *cf.* Gal. De dign. puls. I 1: VIII p. 771,2–772,7 K.; I 3: VIII p. 786, 13–790,10 K. Syn. de puls. 5: IX p. 443,11–444,8 K. M. Wellmann, Die pneumatische Schule (Berlin 1895), p. 169sq.

1 ἐπεί *om. Nic.*: καὶ *coni. Bas.* ἐν ἀρχῇ *om. Nic.* 2 αὐτῶν *om. Nic.*: *secl. Corn.*: τὸ αὐτὸ *sscr.* L^{2} 3 ἂν *add. Kühn* 4 αἰσθητικωτάτην ἀφὴν] cum ... cognouerim *Nic.* αἰσθηκωτάτην L 5 ὧν y: *sec. Nic.* (ceu [seu *Nic.*^{z}]) *corr. Bas.* 6 ἐπισημαίνεσθαί *ex* ἐπισημθαιν- *corr.* L 7 διαγνῶντος L 9 ὅτε] οὗ y: *sec. Nic.* (cum) *corr. Corn. Kühn* 11 κατὰ *postea add.* L *ante* Κόμμοδον *add.* τὸν L Κόμοδον y: *corr. Chart.* τι *sec. Nic.* (quid magnum) *add. Bas.* μεγίστην y: *corr. Bas.* 13 πρὶν – ὀγδόης] ante horam sextam *Nic.* 15 παρισθμίων M 16 φλεγμαίνειν *scripserim* 18 *post* δὲ *sec. Nic.* (locis) *add.* τόπων *Bas.* 20 φανέντος M 21 ῥοῦ] κήρου y: *sec. Nic.* (sumac [sumach *Nic.*^{zv}]) *corr. Bas.* 24 ἐπειδὴ] quia iam *Nic.* 25 δ' ἦν y: *sec. Nic.* (paulominus) δεῖν *Bas.*: *correxi* 26 ὢν y: *corr.* N *Ald.* μεθ' οὗ y: *corr. Corn.* 27 πτύελον y: *corr. Ald.* 28sq. τραφέντι αὐτῷ] demum (deinde *Nic.*^{cev}) cibare eum *Nic.* 29 Ἀνία M Φαυστίνη y: *correxi* 30 αὐτὸ y: *sec. Nic.* (eum) *correxi* οἶδε M

chigenes was one – to discover the particular indication of an access of
an illness. Some of them declared that it was to be found at the begin-
ning of an arterial systole, others that the systole was imperceptible. I
was lucky – how else could one describe a very sensitive touch, capable
of detecting the slight differences between pulses? – and I found some
doctors whose errors were so big that I had to stop them sending to the
bath patients who were starting to show signs of an attack or prescrib-
ing them food. Thus having tested my own diagnosis of the beginning 10
of a paroxysm long and carefully, I dared tell the emperor, a little
hastily, perhaps, but nevertheless I insisted upon telling him, as soon
as I had touched his pulse, an opinion contrary to what he had conjec-
tured himself and had been told by his doctors.

12. My treatment of Commodus is said to be extremely remark-
able, but in fact it is far from it. After leaving the palaestra, before
eating, he was seized with quite a hot fever at the eighth hour, and
it became clear to me on taking his pulse that some part was inflamed.
When Peitholaus heard this, he expressed surprise that inflammation
of the tonsils could alter the boy's pulse; for no other part was in-
flamed. At this he opened the boy's mouth and told me to examine 2
it. Since some rough and excessively red patches were visible, al-
though the inflammation had no great swelling, I asked who had rub-
bed him with a mouthwash containing a stronger styptic than was
suitable for a boy. When he replied that he had done so, using a mix- 3
ture of honey and sumac, I instructed him to change to a solution
of honey and rosewater and to apply only this for that night, the whole
of the next day and the following night. In the morning of the third 4
day, when the effects of the inflammation had entirely ceased and the
boy was nearly free of fever, I persuaded Peitholaus to bring him
to the bath, which was near his room, and without delay, using
the water in the trough, to drench all the parts of his body thor-
oughly, except for his head, which was to be sprinkled lightly after
he had been given food. About the third hour, Annia Faustina, 5
a very close relative of the emperor, arrived, complaining that she
had not seen the lad for two days: for she said that she had heard

χθὲς γὰρ ἔφη[ν] μετ' ἄριστον ἐγνωκέναι περὶ τοῦ γενομένου πυρετοῦ·
καὶ τούτοις ἔτι προσετίθει δῆλον εἶναι μέλλοντας ἡμᾶς ὑπερβάλλειν τὴν
6 ὀγδόην ὥραν καθ' ἣν εἰσέβαλεν ὁ παροξυσμός. μειδιάσας οὖν ὁ Πειθό-
λαος, «πῶς δ' οὐ μέλλομεν», ἔφη, «τὴν Θεσσαλείαν ὑπερβάλλειν διά-
τριτον; ἀλλὰ Γαληνὸς οὗτος», ἔφη, «θεασάμενος ἕωθεν ἰσχνόν τε ⟨. . .⟩
πυρέξειν ἔφη· καὶ μέντοι καὶ λούειν αὖθις ἑσπέρας ἐπηγγείλατο καὶ
7 δεῖπνον παρέχειν ὁποῖον ὑγιαίνων δειπνεῖ.» ταῦτ' ἀκούσασα, βραχύ τι
χρόνου αὐτόθι διατρίψασα ἡ Φαυστῖνα, λαβομένη τῆς χειρὸς ἑαυτῇ
συνεξήγαγεν ἰατρόν τινα τῶν συνηκολουθηκότων αὐτῇ μεθοδικῶν, παί-
ζουσα, «Γαληνόν», ἔφη, «τοῦτον ἴσθι μὴ λόγοις ἀλλ' ἔργοις ὑμῖν τοῖς
8 μεθοδικοῖς πολεμεῖν. πολλάκις γὰρ ἤδη πολλοὺς τῶν ἀρχομένων
⟨πυρέττειν⟩ ἔλουσέ τε καὶ ἔδωκεν οἴνου πιεῖν· ἐνίους δὲ καὶ κατὰ τὴν
πρώτην, ἐνίους τῇ τρίτῃ τῶν ἡμερῶν ἀπέλυσεν ἐπὶ τὰς συνήθεις πράξεις·
664 ἐν ᾗ πάντες ὑμεῖς ταῖς πρώταις ἡμέραις δύο προασιτῆσαι κελεύσαν|τες,
9 ὑπερβάλλειν τὰς ὑπόπτους ὥρας κατακειμένους φυλάττεσθε. καὶ νῦν
οὖν», ἔφη, «τὸ τῆς ἐπιστήμης βέβαιον ἐπιδείκνυται, βασιλικοῦ παιδὸς
ἀποδημοῦντος τοῦ πατρὸς ἐν ταῖς πρώταις δύο πυρέξαντος σφοδρῶς,
ὡς καὶ ὑμεῖς χθὲς ἠκούσατε, κατὰ τὴν τρίτην ἡμέραν οὐχ ὑπερβάλλειν,
ὡς ὑμεῖς ἀξιοῦτε, τὴν ὀγδόην ὥραν ἀναμείνας ἀλλ' ἤδη λούσας τε καὶ
θρέψας ⟨ἐθεράπευσεν⟩· ὅ τε τροφεὺς αὐτῷ Πειθόλαος, ἀκριβέστατος
ὢν περὶ τὰ τοιαῦτα ὡς δειλίαν εἶναι τὴν ἀκρίβειαν αὐτοῦ, διὰ τὸ προ-
πειρᾶσθαι τῆς τέχνης τοῦ ἀνδρὸς ἐπείσθη καὶ λοῦσαι καὶ θρέψαι πρὸ τῆς
ὑπόπτου.»
10 Ἡ μὲν τοιαῦτ' ἔλεγε διαβαδίζουσα μέχρι τοῦ ὀχήματος· ἐγὼ δὲ
μελλούσης αὐτῆς ἐπιβαίνειν αὐτοῦ χωριζόμενος εἶπον, «ἐποίησάς με πολὺ
μᾶλλον ἢ πρόσθεν ὑπὸ τῶν ἰατρῶν μισεῖσθαι», χωρισθείς τε τῷ Πειθο-
λάῳ διηγούμην ταῦτα καὶ μέντοι καὶ ὅτι διὰ τοὺς τοιούτους ἰατροὺς
ἔναγχος ἔγραψα τρεῖς πραγματείας, μίαν μὲν τὴν Περὶ τῆς διαφορᾶς τῶν
πυρετῶν, ἑτέραν δὲ τὴν Περὶ τῶν κρισίμων ἡμερῶν καὶ τρίτην τὴν Περὶ τῶν
κρίσεων, ἐπιδεικνὺς ὑφ' Ἱπποκράτους γεγράφθαι τὴν θεωρίαν ἀφ' ἧς
665 11 ἄν τις προγινώσκοι τὰ γενησόμενα περὶ | τοὺς ἀρρώστους. οἱ δ' οὕτως
εἰσὶν ἀφυεῖς ὥστε μηδὲ μετὰ τῆς ἐμῆς ἐξηγήσεως δύνασθαι αὐτὰ μαθεῖν.

28sq. Περὶ τῆς διαφορᾶς τῶν πυρετῶν] VII p. 273–405 K. 29 Περὶ τῶν κρισίμων ἡμερῶν] IX p. 769–941 K. 29sq. Περὶ τῶν κρίσεων] p. 69–212 Alex. = IX p. 550–768 K.

1 ἔφην y: *sec. Nic.* (dixit) *corr. Chart.* πυρετοῦ] in puero *Nic.* 3 ὥραν *om.* M *Nic.*[ce] 4 τὸν Θεσσαλεῖον y: *correxi* 5 ἔφη *om. Nic.*: *secluserim lacunam indicavi*: et aridum (arr- *Nic.*[b]) corpus pueri totum balneauit et cibauit nequaquam *Nic.*: καὶ ξηρὸν μὴ *add. Bas.*: καὶ ξηρὸν τὸ σῶμα τοῦ παιδὸς ἅπαν λούσας τε καὶ θρέψας αὐτὸν μὴ *sec. Nic. addiderim* 6 ἔφη] dicens *Nic.* 7 ἀκουσάσασα M 8 χρόνον y: *corr. Ald.* αὐτῇ y: *correxi* 12 πυρέττειν *sec. Nic.* (febrire) *add. Bas.* 14 ἡμεῖς y: *corr.* N *Bas.* 15 φυλάττεται L 17 *post* πρώταις *add.* diebus *Nic.* 19 ἀξιοῖτε L 20 ἐθεράπευσεν *addidi* 21 δειλίαν] timiditas *Nic.*: δήλην *scripserim* 23 *post* ὑπόπτου *add.* horam *Nic.* 27 ταῦτα *sec. Nic.* (hec) *scripsi*: τε αὐτὸς y: αὐτὸς *Corn. Chart.* 28 τρεῖς] τὰς y: *sec. Nic.*[v] (tres) *corr. Corn.*: *om. Nic.*[x] τῆς] τὰς y: *corr.* NN2 *Corn.* differentiis *Nic.* 30 ἀφ'] ἐφ' *edd.* 31 προγινώσκει y: *corr. Bas.* 32 μετὰ] post *Nic.* δύνασθαι *om. Nic.*

the previous day after breakfast about his fever, and she also added that we were clearly going to let the eighth hour, at which the paroxysm had attacked him originally, go past. With a smile Peitholaus 6
said, "Why should we not go beyond the three day period of Thessalus? For Galen here, who this morning saw that +the boy's body was all thin and dry and who then bathed and fed him, has declared that he will not now be feverish+[1]. Moreover, he has announced that he is going to bath him again this evening and to give him a meal fit for a healthy man." When she heard this, Faustina paused for a 7
moment, then, taking by the hand one of the Methodist doctors who followed her, she led him forward and said sarcastically, "This is Galen, who battles against you Methodists with deeds, not words. For often 8
already he has bathed many of those who were beginning to be feverish and given them wine to drink; and he has returned them to their normal lives, some on the first, others on the third day, while you all tell them to fast for the first two days and you take care that they should pass the suspected hours lying down. And indeed now", 9
she said, "there is clear proof of his learning. Although the son of our emperor has been in a high fever for the last two days – his father is abroad –, as you also heard yesterday, he has not waited to let the eighth hour go by on the third day, as you insist, but he has already treated him by giving him a bath and some food. And his tutor, Peitholaus, a very shrewd man in these matters, whose hesitancy is part of his shrewdness, has been persuaded by his previous experience of this man's skill to wash and feed the boy before the suspected hour."

She said this as she made her way to her chariot, but as she was 10
about to climb in, I turned away, saying, "You have made me even more hated by the physicians." Then I withdrew and told it all to Peitholaus, especially how I had just written three treatises because of these doctors, one 'On the differences between fevers', another 'On critical days', and a third 'On crises', to show that the theory whereby one might predict the future course of an illness had been laid down by Hippocrates. But they are so ignorant that 11
they could not learn this even with the aid of my commentary. You

[1] +the – feverish+: see the addition to the text proposed in the app. crit.

αὐτὸς γὰρ σύ, Ἐπίγενες φίλτατε, τὰ γεγραμμένα μοι περὶ τούτων ἁπάντων ὧν ἐθεάσω με προλέγοντα γινώσκεις ἐπιδεδειγμένα πρὸς Ἱπποκράτους εἰρῆσθαι, μόνην αὐτοῖς προσθέντος τὴν περὶ τοὺς σφυγμοὺς θεωρίαν ἥνπερ καὶ μόνην οὐκ ἐξειργάσατο, καθάπερ οἱ μετ' αὐτὸν ἄλλος ἄλλο τι προσθεὶς αὐτῇ μέχρι ⟨τῶν⟩ καθ' ἡμᾶς χρόνων
12 ἐπεκόσμησαν. καὶ γὰρ ἡ γνῶσις τῶν τοῦ σώματος διαθέσεων ἐκ τῆς θεωρίας ταύτης, ὥσπερ γε πάλιν ἐκ τῆς τῶν διαθέσεων ἀκριβοῦς γνώσεως ἡ τῶν μελλόντων ἔσεσθαι πρόγνωσις.

13. Καὶ τό γε παρόντος γενόμενον ἡνίκα περὶ φλεβοτομίας ἐσκέπτοντο τῶν ἐν Ῥώμῃ πρωτευόντων ἔνιοι διὰ τῶν ὑπομνημάτων ὧν
2 ἐποίησα δείκνυται δεδειγμένον ὑφ' Ἱπποκράτους τελεώτατα. πέμπτην γὰρ ἡμέραν ἦγε τοῦ νοσήματος ὁ νεανίσκος, ἐφαίνετο δὲ παραλελεῖφθαι τὸ
666 τῆς φλεβοτομίας βοήθημα, δεο|μένου τοῦ πάθους ἐν ἀρχῇ γεγονέναι περὶ
3 δευτέραν ἢ τρίτην ἢ πάντως γε τὴν τετάρτην ἡμέραν αὐτήν. εἶτ' ἐπειδὴ μήθ' ἡ ὥρα τοῦ ἔτους μήθ' ἡ ἡλικία τοῦ κάμνοντος ὥσπερ γε μηδ' ἡ κατὰ τὴν ζωτικὴν δύναμιν ἀσθένεια μήθ' ἡ προγεγενημένη δίαιτα τοῦ νοσήματος ἀντεδείκνυτο, πάντα δ' ἀλλήλοις ὡμολόγει τὴν φλεβοτομίαν ἐνδεικνύμενα, συνεβούλευσαν οἱ ἰατροὶ τέμνειν τὴν φλέβα, προσηκόντως
4 φρονοῦντες. ἐγὼ δὲ περινοήσας ἀκριβῶς ἅπαντα τὰ φαινόμενα τὰ πρὸς Ἱπποκράτους εἰρημένα τῶν αἱμορραγήσειν μελλόντων σημεῖα, καλῶς μὲν ἔφην αὐτοὺς ὁρίζειν τὴν ἀφαίρεσιν τοῦ αἵματος, ἔρχεσθαι δ' ἐπὶ τοῦτο καὶ τὴν φύσιν ἐπειγομένην ἀποκρῖναι τὸ βαρῦνον αὐτήν· καὶ τοῦτ'
5 αὐτίκα μάλα γενήσεσθαι κἂν ἡμεῖς μὴ ποιῶμεν. οἱ μὲν ⟨οὖν⟩ ἰατροὶ ταῦτ' ἀκούσαντες ἐθαύμαζον δῆθεν, ἐξαναστάντος δ' ἐπὶ τῆς κλίνης τοῦ νοσοῦντος ὡς ἀναπηδῆσαι θέλοντος, ἐρωτηθέντος δὲ τίνος ἕνεκεν ἀνεπήδησε
667 μηδενὸς ὄντος φόβου, φάντος δὲ τὸν ἐρυθρὸν ὄφιν ἐξέρποντα | τῆς ὀροφῆς θεασάμενον αὐτὸν δεῖσ[θ]αι μή πως ἀποσφαλεὶς ἐπ' αὐτὸν κατενεχθείη, καὶ διὰ τοῦτο φυγεῖν τὸν τόπον ἐν ᾧ κατέκειτο, τοῖς μέντοι οὐδέν τι συντελεῖν ἐδόκει τοῦτο πρὸς τὴν μέλλουσαν αἱμορραγίαν.
6 ἐμοὶ δὲ τά τ' ἄλλα διασκεψαμένῳ πάντα καὶ [τὸ] κατὰ τὸ δεξιὸν μέρος τῆς

4 καθάπερ – 6 ἐπεκόσμησαν] *cf.* Gal. Meth. med. VI 4: X p. 420,9–16 K. 7sq. ὥσπερ – πρόγνωσις] *cf.* Gal. De praes. ex puls. IV 11: IX p. 418,9–16 K. 9–138, 12] *cf.* Gal. De exam. medico: Meyerhof, p. 80,13–17 De caus. procat. 2,16sq.: CMG Suppl. II p. 14,32–15,10 De nominib. medic. p. 20,4–21,5 19–138,4] *exc.* Razes *Kitāb al-ḥāwī* XVIII 46,11

1 σύ] σοί L 3 *ante* μόνην *addiderim* ἐμοῦ 4 οὐκ – καθάπερ *om. Nic.* 5 τῶν *addidi* χρόνον M 6sq. ἐκ – διαθέσεων *om.* M 7 *post* θεωρίας *sec. Nic.* (fit) *add.* γίνεται *Bas., fort. recte* 9 *ante* γε *sec. Nic.* (te presente [in presenti *Nic.*[ce]]) *add.* σοῦ *Bas., fort. recte* *post* γενόμενον *add.* in quodam iuuene *Nic.* 10 *post* ἔνιοι *add.* medicorum *Nic.* 11 δεδειγμένων y: *sec. Nic.* (monstratum) *corr. Guinther Corn.* 12 *post* ἦγε *add.* a principio *Nic.* 15 ἡ[II] *om.* M 16 ἀσθένεια] robur *Nic.* μήθ'] μηδ' y: *corr. Bas.* 17 ἀντενεδείκνυτο *coni. Durling* 18 προσηκότες M 21 τούτῳ L 23 οὖν *sec. Nic.* (igitur) *add. Bas.* 24 ἐπὶ y: de lecto *Nic.*: ἀπὸ *Schöne, fort. recte* 26 ὄντος *ex* ἔντος *corr.* M φόβου *om.* M: *sec. Nic.* (timoroso) φοβεροῦ *Bas.* φανέντος y: *sec. Nic.* (dixit [dissit *Nic.*[c]: dixisset *Nic.*[a]]) *corr. Bas.* 27 δεῖσθαι y: timere *Nic.*: *corr. L. Dindorf, Thesaurus Linguae Graecae II, p. 937* 28 κατενεγχθείη M τοῖς] τούτοις *sec. Nic.* (hiis) *coni. Durling* 30 τὸ[I] *om. Nic.*: *seclusi*

yourself, my dear Epigenes, know that I have said that everything
that I have written about all the predictions you have seen me make
was demonstrated by Hippocrates, and that I only added the
theory of pulses, which was all that he had not worked out, just as
his successors down to our time have made various additions, one
after another. Indeed, a knowledge of the dispositions of the body 12
depends on this theory, just as in turn the prognosis of future events
depends upon an accurate knowledge of these dispositions.

13. Besides, what happened in your presence when some of the
leading men in Rome were considering venesection is discussed in my
commentaries, where I show that Hippocrates gave a full demon-
stration of it. The young man was in the fifth day of his illness: the 2
help of venesection seemed to have been omitted, although, from the
outset, his condition demanded it on the second, third, or, at the la-
test, the fourth day. But since neither the season of the year nor the 3
age of the patient nor any lack of vital power nor the previous regimen
in his illness offered any indication to the contrary, but all agreed to-
gether in pointing to venesection, the doctors reached a fair decision
and determined to cut the vein. But I carefully observed all the ob- 4
vious signs that were said by Hippocrates to portend a haemor-
rhage, and then said that, although they had rightly decided to ex-
tract some blood, the patient's own nature also was fast coming to
this by itself as it strove to expel what was oppressing it: this would
occur soon, even if we did nothing. When the doctors heard this, they 5
were indeed surprised, but then the patient stood up in bed, as if
he wanted to jump out. When asked why he had jumped up when
there was nothing to fear, he said that he saw a red snake crawling
from the roof and was scared that it might lose its hold and fall on him:
he was therefore avoiding the place where he had been lying. They 6
still thought that this had nothing to do with the impending haemor-
rhage, but I examined everything closely, including the right side

ῥινὸς ἄχρι τοῦ μήλου θεασαμένῳ τὴν τέως ἀμυδρὰν ἐρυθρότητα πολὺ δή
τι νῦν ἐμφανέστερον γενομένην, ἐπίδοξον ὅσον οὔπω κατὰ τὸν δεξιὸν
7 μυκτῆρα τὸ τὴν αἱμορραγίαν ἔσεσθαι σαφῶς ἐφαίνετο. καί τινι τῶν
παρόντων οἰκετῶν τοῦ κάμνοντος ἠρέμα διαλεχθεὶς ἀγγεῖον ἔχειν
ἕτοιμον ὑπὸ τὴν ἐφεστρίδα τῶν ἐπιτηδείων δέξασθαι τὸ αἷμα, κἄπειτα
φθεγξάμενος εἰς ἐπήκοον πάντων ἰατρῶν, ἐὰν βραχύτατον προσμείνωσι,
θεάσασθαι τὸν ἄνθρωπον ἐκ δεξιοῦ μυκτῆρος αἱμορραγοῦντα, τῶν δὲ
γελασάντων ἐν τῷ προειρῆσθαι προ[σ]κεῖσθαι κατὰ τὸν λόγον τὸν δεξιὸν
μυκτῆρα, «καὶ μήν», ἔφην, «ἢ ἀμφότερα δεῖ γενέσθαι ἢ περὶ θάτερά με
8 σφαλῆναι. ἀπὸ γὰρ τῆς θεωρίας ἀμφότερα τὴν πρόγνωσιν ἔχει, τό θ᾽
668 αἱμορραγῆσαι τὸν νοσοῦντα τό τ᾽ ἐκ δεξιοῦ μυκτῆ|ρος, ἐφ᾽ ᾧ τεκμήρα-
σθαι ⟨. . .»⟩
9 ⟨. . .⟩ προσέχειν ἠξίωσα τῷ γινομένῳ τὸν κρύπτοντα τὸ ἀγγεῖον
ὅπως, ἐπειδὰν ἴδῃ τὸ αἷμα τοῦ μυκτῆρος ἐκχεόμενον, προσδραμὼν
10 ὑποθῇ τὸ σκεῦος. ἅμα τ᾽ οὖν ἔλεγον ταῦτα καὶ τὸν δάκτυλον ᾑμαγμένον
ὁ κάμνων ἐξείλκυσεν ὅ τ᾽ οἰκέτης προσδραμὼν ὑπέθηκεν αὐτῷ τὸ ἀγγεῖον,
ἐφ᾽ ᾧ μεγίστης κραυγῆς, ὡς οἶσθα, γενομένης οἱ μὲν ἰατροὶ πάντες
ἔφυγον, ἐγὼ δ᾽ ἐρομένῳ σοι τὴν θεωρίαν τῆς προγνώσεως ἐδήλωσα πᾶσαν
ἐκ τῶν ὑφ᾽ Ἱπποκράτους εἰρημένων δεδιδαγμένος, ἔτι δὲ καὶ τοῦτο
11 προσέθηκα σφοδρὰν ἔσεσθαι προσδοκᾶν τὴν αἱμορραγίαν. ἥ τε γὰρ
ὁρμὴ τῆς φύσεώς ἐστιν ἰσχυρὰ καὶ ἡ νόσος ἄπεπτος· εἰώθασι δὲ τοῖς
12 τοιούτοις αἰτίοις ἄμετροι κενώσεις γίγνεσθαι. διὸ καὶ παραμεῖναι χρόνον
τῷ κάμνοντι κάλλιον εἶναι νομίσας ἔπεμψα τὸν ἀκόλουθόν μου παῖδα
κομίσαντα σικύαν μεγάλην ἀφανῶς τοῖς πολλοῖς· ἐν τάχει δ᾽ αἵματος
πολλοῦ κατὰ τὸ ἀγγεῖον ἀθροισθέντος ἕτερον αἰτήσας, δεξάμενος τὸ
669 αἷμα καὶ τὸν σταθμὸν | ἰδὼν τοῦ κενουμένου λιτρῶν ὄντα τεττάρων καὶ
ἡμισείας ἀνάρροπόν τε τὸν κάμνοντα σχηματίσας καὶ ψυχρὸν ὀξύκρατον

6 ἐὰν – 13 ⟨κνίζοντι⟩ *(v. app. crit.)*] *cf.* Gal. De diff. puls. III 3: VIII p. 656,9sq. K. De crisib. III 3: p. 170,15sq. Alex. = IX p. 708,3sq. K.; III 11: p. 210,18–211,5 Alex. = IX p. 766,4–17 K. Meth. med. ad Glauc. I 16: XI p. 68,12–18 K. In Hipp. Prorrhet. I comm. III 32: CMG V 9,2 p. 144,19–146,6 19 Ἱπποκράτους] *cf. exempli gratia* Hipp. Epid. IV 25: V p. 170,1 L.; VI 12: V p. 272,12 L. Prorrhet. I 125: V p. 554,3–5 L. Progn. 7: I p. 84,10–16 Kw. = II p. 126,12–128,4 L. 26 ἰδὼν – 138,4] *exc.* Razes *Kitāb al-ḥāwī* III 76,20

2 ἐπίδοξον . . . οὔπω] quam cito *Nic.* 3 τῆς αἱμορραγίας y: *correxi* σαφῶς ἐφαίνετο] putaui *Nic.* 4 ἠρέμα *om. Nic.* 7 θεάσεσθαι *Chart., fort. recte* τῶν – 9 μυκτῆρα *om. Nic.* 8 *post* προειρῆσθαι *iter.* ἐν τῷ L προσκεῖσθαι y: *correxi* 9 ἔφην] dixerunt *Nic.* 12sq. *lacunas indicavi*: illi quidem riserunt sicut nosti. ego autem uidens egrum ponentem digitum indicem intra narem quasi habens ibi pruritum *Nic.*: *sec. Nic.* προσέχειν *(non hab. Bas.)* ἠξίωσα (ἐξίωσα *Bas.*). θεασάμενος οὖν *(non hab. Bas.)* τὸν *(om. Chart.)* νοσοῦντα δάκτυλον *(ante* δάκτ. *add.* τὸν *Chart.)* ὡς κνίζοντι τῷ μυκτῆρι ἐνερείδοντα (ἐνεραί- *Bas.*) *post* μυκτῆρος *add. Bas., post* τεκμήρασθαι *Chart.*: ἠξίωσα.» Οἱ μὲν οὖν ἐγέλασαν, ὡς οἶσθα, ἐγὼ δὲ θεασάμενος τὸν νοσοῦντα δάκτυλον ὡς κνίζοντι τῷ μυκτῆρι ἐνερείδοντα *addiderim* 14 ἤδη y: *corr.* N *Corn. Chart.* 16 ὁ κάμνων *om.* M 18 ἐρωμένῳ L 19 καὶ τοῦτο *om. Nic.* 22 *ante* χρόνον *add.* ὀλίγον *sec. Nic.* (modico tempore) *Bas., sed cf. L-S-J, p. 2008; si adiectivum addere velis,* βραχὺν *scribendum* 24 σηκυίαν y: *correxi* δὲ *in* τε *mut.* L²: τε M: autem *Nic.* 24sq. αἷμα τὲ πολοῦ L 26 δ´ y: *numerum plenius scripsi*

of his nose, extending to the cheek bone, where I saw a redness, hi-
therto faint, had now begun to be much more prominent. It then be-
came clearer than ever that the haemorrhage would come from his
right nostril. So I spoke quietly to one of the invalid's slaves there, 7
and told him to have ready under his cloak a bowl suitable for re-
ceiving blood, and then I announced in the hearing of all the doctors
that, if they would only wait a moment, they would see the man bleed-
ing from the right nostril. They laughed at me for proposing to
include the right nostril in my prognosis. "Well then", I said, "either
both must happen or I must be wrong on both counts: for both de- 8
rive their prognosis from the same theory. The patient will suffer a
haemorrhage and this will come from the right nostril, which +I have
asked+[1] you to observe."

+They broke into laughter, as you recall; but as soon as I saw the 9
invalid scratching his nostril as if it was itching,+[2] I told the servant
hiding the bowl to pay attention to what was happening and, when he
saw blood pouring from the nostril, to run and put the vessel under
it. Just as I was saying this, the patient drew out his bloodstained 10
finger, at which the servant rushed forward and held the bowl under-
neath. As you know, there was a great shout and all the doctors fled.
In response to your query, I showed that I had learned the whole theory
from the pronouncements of Hippocrates, adding that we should
expect the haemorrhage to be severe; for the impulse of his nature 11
was strong and the disease unconcocted, which together usually pro-
duce excessive evacuations. So, thinking it best to stay a little while 12
with the invalid, I sent my accompanying slave to fetch a large cup-
ping glass without attracting most people's attention. Quickly col-
lecting a large amount of blood in the bowl, I asked for another, and
on receiving the blood I calculated the weight of the evacuated blood
at four and a half pounds. I kept the patient elevated, ordered him

[1] +I – asked+: see the addition to the text proposed in the app. crit.

[2] +They – itching,+: see the addition to the text proposed in the app. crit.

ἀναρροφεῖν τῷ μυκτῆρι κελεύσας ἐπιθείς τε τῷ μετώπῳ σπόγγον ἐκ ψυχροῦ βεβρεγμένον μελικράτου καὶ τὰ κῶλα διαδήσας, ὡς οὐδὲν ὅλως ἤνυσε ταῦτα, τὴν σικύαν κατὰ τὸ δεξιὸν ὑποχόνδριον ὑποβαλὼν εὐθέως ἔστησα τὴν αἱμορραγίαν· ὅπερ ὅτι καὶ αὐτὸ τῆς Ἱπποκράτους
13 ἐστὶ τέχνης ἐδήλωσά σοι. καί μοι διὰ τοῦτο καὶ ταῦτα καὶ τἆλλα πάνθ' ὅσα διὰ τῶν ἔργων ἐπεδειξάμην ἐγράφη. καὶ γὰρ ῥῖγος ἐσόμενον ὅπως χρὴ προγινώσκειν ἔγραψα καὶ διάρροιαν γαστρὸς ἔμετόν τε καὶ πλῆθος οὔρων ἄμετρον ἢ ἐπίσχεσιν ἱδρῶτάς τε καὶ παρωτίδας ἐσομένας ἀποστήματά τε παραφροσύνην τε καὶ καταφορὰς ἅπαντά τ' ἄλλα συμπτώ-
14 ματα. τινὰ δέ, ὡς ἔφην καὶ πρόσθεν, ὁ προμαθὴς ταῦτα προσεπιλογίζεται πρὸς ἑαυτοῦ, καθάπερ ἐπὶ τοῦ Βοηθοῦ παιδὸς προσεπελογισάμην ἐγὼ ἐπί τε τῆς ἐρώσης καὶ τοῦ διὰ φόβον ἀθυμοῦντος.
670 14. Ἔναγχος ⟨δέ⟩, ὡς οἶσθα, καὶ τοιόνδε τι | προειπόντος μου τοὺς πολλοὺς ἐξέπλησσεν ἡ πρόγνωσις. οἰκονόμος γάρ τις ἅπαντα διοικῶν ὀρθῶς τὰ τοῦ δεσπότου καὶ διὰ τοῦτο τιμώμενος, ἑτέρων αὐτὸν ἰατρῶν ἰωμένων, ἐκρίθη μὲν ἑβδομαῖος ἱδρῶτι, τῇ δ' ὑστεραίᾳ διαλείποντα τὸν σφυγμὸν εὑρόντες αὐτοῦ κακοήθη διάθεσιν ἐν τῷ σώματι φωλεύειν
2 ἔδοξαν, σφαλέντες μεγάλως. εἶτα τῆς οἰκίας ἐξελθόντες ἅμα τῷ δεσπότῃ τοῦ νεανίσκου κατὰ τύχην ἀπήντησάν μοι διηγησάμενοί τε τὰ προγεγονότα καὶ τὰ παρόντα συμπτώματα, τί ποτε σημαίνει τὸ κατὰ τὸν
3 σφυγμὸν ἀλόγως γεγονὸς ἐδέοντο μαθεῖν. κἀγὼ πυθόμενος πλησίον εἶναι τὴν οἰκίαν ἐν ᾗ κατέκειτο συνῆλθον αὐτοῖς ἀψάμενος τῶν σφυγμῶν τοῦ νεανίσκου. κατὰ γὰρ αὐτὴν τὴν αἰσθητικὴν διάθεσιν, ⟨ὡς⟩ εἶπόν σοι, πολλάκις οὐκ ὀλίγα σφάλλονται καὶ τῶν ἀξιολόγων ἰατρῶν ἔνιοι, μέγα⟨ν⟩ ἡγούμενοι τὸν οὐ μέγα⟨ν⟩ σφυγμόν, ὥσπερ γ' ἐνίοτε καὶ ταχὺν
4 τὸν οὐ ταχὺν ἢ τὸν βραδὺν οὐ βραδύν. ὡσαύτως δὲ περὶ ⟨τὴν⟩ τῶν ἀμυδρῶν τε καὶ σφοδρῶν καὶ σκληρῶν καὶ μαλακῶν σφυγμῶν διάγνωσιν
671 σφάλλονται, καὶ μᾶλλον ἔτι περὶ τὴν τῶν | ἀτάκτων τε καὶ τεταγμένων, ὁμαλῶν τε καὶ ἀνωμάλων, ἐν ἀθροίσματί τε καὶ κατὰ μίαν διαστολήν, δι' οὓς κἀγὼ τέτταρα Περὶ τῆς διαγνώσεως τῶν σφυγμῶν ἔγραψα βιβλία, προηγούμενα τεττάρων ἑτέρων ἃ Περὶ τῶν ἐν σφυγμοῖς αἰτιῶν

3 τὴν – 4] *cf.* Gal. De hirudin. 2: XI p. 319,15–17 K.; 3: XI p. 321,4–6 K. 6–10] *cf. supra* p. 70,2–5. Gal. Meth. med. ad Glauc. I 16: XI p. 69,1–8 K. 10 πρόσθεν] *v. supra* p. 120,8–12 11 καθάπερ – 12] *v. supra* p. 100,21–110,12 14–140,24] *cf.* Gal. In Hipp. Progn. comm. III 42: CMG V 9,2 p. 369,18–20 30 Περὶ τῆς διαγνώσεως τῶν σφυγμῶν] VIII p. 766–961 K. 31 Περὶ τῶν ἐν σφυγμοῖς αἰτιῶν] IX p. 205–430 K.

2 ψυχροῦ *ex* χυχροῦ *corr.* L μελικράτου] oxicrato *Nic.* 3 σηκυίαν y: *corr. Chart.* ὑπολαβὼν L 8 ἄμετρον N: ἀμέτρων L *(ex* ἄμετρον *mut.)* M ἀποσκήμματά L *Bas.*: ἀποσκήμματός M: *sec. Nic.* (apostases) *correxi* 9 παραφορὰν y: *sec. Nic.* (cataforas [cathaforas *Nic.*[ba]: catoforas *Nic.*[ev]]) *correxi* 11 ἑαυτῷ L: ἑαυτῆς M: *sec. Nic.* (seipso) *corr. Chart.* προσεπιλογισάμην y: *corr. Kühn* 12 φόβου *edd.* 13 δέ *sec. Nic.* (autem) *add. Corn.* 17 κακοήθη] aliquam *Nic.* (malignam *coni. Durling*) 18 σφαλέντες μεγάλως *om. Nic.* ἐξελθόντος y: *sec. Nic.* (egressi) *et Rotam* (exeuntes) *correxi* 19 διηγησάμενοί – 20 συμπτώματα *om. Nic.* τε] με y: *corr. Corn.* 22 τῶν σφυγμῶν] τε σφυγμῶν y: τὸν σφυγμὸν *Kühn*: pulsum *Nic.*: *correxi* 23 ὡς *sec. Nic.* (ut) *addidi* 24 ὀλίγα] pauci *Nic.* καὶ – ἔνιοι *om. Nic.* 25 μέγα *(bis)* y: *corr. Ald.* 26 τὴν *add. Bas.*

to sniff cold sour wine and water, then applied a sponge soaked in
cold honey and water to his forehead and bandaged his limbs. When
none of these proved efficacious, I applied the cupping glass to his
right hypochondrium and stopped the bleeding immediately. I have
shown you that this treatment also belongs to the art of Hippocrates.
It was for this reason that I wrote down this and everything else that 13
I demonstrated in my actions; for I also described how one should
predict an impending rigor, diarrhoea, vomiting, an excessive emission
or retention of urine, sweats, abscesses of the ear and elsewhere,
attacks of delirium or lethargy and all other symptoms. Some of them, 14
as I said earlier, the man who is equipped with such foreknowledge can
calculate for himself, as I did in the cases of the son of Boethus, of
the woman in love, and of the man who was depressed through fear.

14. Recently, as you know, when I made a particular forecast,
my prognostication startled many people. A steward who was a sound
administrator of his master's property and respected for that came
to a sweating crisis on the seventh day, despite the attentions of other
doctors. On the next day, finding his pulse missing a beat, they
concluded that some noxious condition was lurking in his body; but
they were wildly wrong. On their way from the house with the young 2
man's master they met me by chance, and after describing his past
and present symptoms, they demanded to know what this strange
phenomenon in his pulse rate signified. Learning that the house in 3
which he was lying was close by, I went with them and took the young
man's pulse. For in this particular sensory condition, as I have told
you, even some reputable doctors often make big mistakes, for example
when they consider a pulse that is not large to be large, or sometimes
one that is not swift to be swift, or one that is not slow to be slow.
Similarly they are at fault in their diagnosis of weak and strong, hard 4
and soft pulses, and even more so when they come to diagnose those
that are regular and irregular, equal and unequal, or exist in a group
of beats or merely in a single diastole. For them I wrote four books
'On the diagnosis of pulses', which precede four more entitled 'On the

ἐπιγέγραπται. δεῖται γὰρ ἀμφοτέρων τῶν πραγματειῶν ἡ Περὶ τῆς διὰ
τῶν σφυγμῶν προγνώσεως, ἐν τέτρασι [τε] καὶ αὐτὴ γεγραμμένη βι-
βλίοις, δι' ἣν καὶ αἱ προειρημέναι δύο τυγχάνουσιν οὖσαι χρησιμώταται·
5 τῆς δὲ καθ' ἕνα σφυγμὸν ἀνωμαλίας οὔσης, ὡς ἐπιδέδεικται, γυμνασίας
ἰσχυροτέρας [αἰσθανομένους, ὡς μηδὲ πράττειν ἢ ὑπομένειν ἃ πρότερον
ἀμέμπτως ἔπραττον ἀλλὰ κατακλιθῆναί τε καὶ δεῖσθαι σκεμμάτων καὶ
τοῦτο παθόντας ἐνίους μὲν ὥραις τρισὶ τοῦ φυγεῖν αὐτὴν τὴν γλωσ-
σολαλίαν· οὐδὲ γὰρ οὐδὲ βλάβη ἕως ὧδε πολλῆς] δεομένης εἰς διάγνωσιν
ὡς ἂν πολλὰς ἐχούσης διαφοράς, ὅταν ὁ σφυγμὸς ὅ τε κατὰ μίαν ἐνέρ-
γειαν ὅ τε κατὰ πλείους ἐφεξῆς ἀλλήλων μηδὲν ἔχῃ παρὰ φύσιν ἄλλο
πλὴν τοῦτο μόνον ὃ κατὰ διάλειψιν γίνεται, γινώσκειν οὖν χρὴ τὸ
τοιοῦτον ἐκ γενετῆς εἶναι σύμπτωμα. διαγινώσκεσθαι δὲ χαλεπώτατόν
ἐστιν, μᾶλλον δ' ἀδύνατον ἄνευ τοῦ πασῶν τῶν κατὰ τοὺς σφυγμοὺς
διαφορῶν ἀκριβῶς αἰσθάνεσθαι.
672 6 Θεασάμενος οὖν τὸν ἄνθρωπον οὕτως ἔχοντα συνε|βούλευσά τε
τοῖς ἰατροῖς ἀναληπτικῶς ἄγειν αὐτὸν ἀσφαλῶς κεκριμ[μ]ένον, εἶθ' ὅταν
προέρχηται ἤδη καὶ τὰ συνήθη πράττῃ, τότε τῶν σφυγμῶν ἁψαμένους
αὐτοῦ, διαλιπόντας εὑρήσειν ἔφην ὡς καὶ νῦν. τοῦτο γὰρ αὐτῷ φύσει
7 συμβεβηκέναι, οὐκ ἐξ ὑποπιπτούσης αἰτίας τινὸς νοσώδους. ἐκ μὲν οὖν
τοῦ παραχρῆμα τὸ ῥηθὲν αὐτοῖς ἄπιστον ἐφαίνετο· κατὰ δὲ τὸν ἑξῆς
χρόνον ἅπαντα διαλιπόντα μίαν πληγὴν τὸν σφυγμὸν εὑρίσκοντες
ἄλλοτε κατ' ἄλλον ἀριθμόν, ὕστερον δέ ποτε προσελθόντες μοι παρεκά-
λουν ἀκοῦσαί μου διὰ τίνος σημείου τὴν φύσιν ἐγνώρισα τοῦ νεανίσκου
8 τοιαύτην οὖσαν. ἀπεκρινάμην οὖν αὐτοῖς ὅπερ ἤκουσά ποτε εἰπεῖν
Ἰσοκράτην τὸν ῥήτορα τῶν ἑταίρων τινὶ πυνθανομένῳ περὶ τριῶν
ἐτῶν ἀσκήσεως εἰ δυνήσεται καὶ ⟨αὐτὸς⟩ ἀσκήσας ἐν τοσούτῳ χρόνῳ
⟨πρὸς⟩ ἕκαστον τῶν προβαλλομένων εἰπεῖν ὡς ἑώρα λέγοντα τὸν
9 Ἰσοκράτην· φασὶ γὰρ ἀποκρίνασθαι τῷ μειρακίῳ τὸν ἄνδρα, «σοὶ μὲν

1sq. Περὶ τῆς διὰ τῶν σφυγμῶν προγνώσεως] IX p. 205–430 K. 4 ὡς ἐπιδέδεικται] Gal. De diff. puls. I 21–28: VIII p. 547,9–556,16 K.; 30: VIII p. 558,3–565,12 K. 5 αἰσθανομένους – 7 τρισὶ] Gal. De morb. temp. 2: VII p. 411,3–6 K. 26 εἰ – 142,3] *cf.* Gal. De dign. puls. I 1: VIII p. 770,10–15 K.

1 ἀμφότερα y: ἀμφοτέρᾳ *Bas.*: *sec. Nic.* (ambabus operis) *corr. Corn.* 2 πρόγνωσις y: *sec. Nic.* (de pronosticatione) *corr. Bas.* τε *seclusi* 3sq. οὖσαι· χρησιμωτάτης δὲ τῆς y: *sec. Nic.* (sunt ualde utiles. ea uero) *corr. Corn.* 4 ὡς ἐπιδέδεικται *post* διάγνωσιν *(l. 8) trsp. edd.* 5 αἰσθανομένους – 8 πολλῆς *om. Nic. Guinther Rota Iacchinus Chart., secl. I. Caius, Cl. Galeni Pergameni libri aliquot Graeci, Basileae 1544, p. 322* ὡς – 8 ὧδε *secl. Corn.* 9 ὅ τε] ὅτε L: ὅταν M: *corr. Corn. Chart.* 11 *ante* διάλειψιν *add.* τὴν L 12 συμπτώματα y: *corr.* N *Corn. Chart.* 15 τὸν ἄνθρωπον] illum *Nic.* 16 κεκριμμένον L: κεκρυμμένον M: *corr. Bas.* 17 πράττει y: πράττοι *Bas.*: *corr. Morel Chart.* ἁψάμενος y: *sec. Nic.* (si ... tetigeritis) *correxi* 21 χρόνον] λόγον y: *sec. Nic.* (tempore) *et Guinther* (tempus) *corr. Corn.* εὑρίσκεσθαι y: *sec. Nic.* (inuenientes) *corr. Corn.* 22 ἀριθμόν] modum rithimi *Nic.*[ba]: modum rythmi *Nic.*[d]: modum richimum *Nic.*[ce]: rithimi *Nic.*[v] 25 Ἰσοκράτην] Socrates *Nic.*: Ysocrates *Nic.*[c3e2] τῶν ἑταίρων *om. Nic.* ἑτέρων L 26 αὐτὸς *sec. Nic.* (ipse [uxor *Nic.*[ce]]) *addidi*: οὗτος *Schöne* 27 πρὸς *add. Schöne, qui et* εἰς *coni., Rheinisches Museum 73, 1924, p. 158* 28 Ἰσοκράτην] Socratem *Nic.*: Ysocratem *Nic.*[e2] συ y: σε *Chart.*: *corr. Corn.*

causes of pulses'. Both these works are essential to the understanding
of 'On prognosis through the pulse' – also in four books –, which makes
the first two treatises of great practical value. An irregularity in a 5
single pulsation, as has been shown, requires more training before it
can be diagnosed, since there are many different possible causes. So
when a pulse in one action or in several, one after the other, displays
no other unnatural feature except that it misses a beat, one should
realise that this condition has existed from birth. It is extremely hard
to diagnose, in fact impossible, without a sound appreciation of all the
differences between pulses.

When I saw that the man was in this condition, I advised the 6
doctors that he was recovering after a safe crisis, and that, if they took
his pulse when he was out and about again at his normal work, they
would find it still missing a beat, just as now. This happened to him
naturally, not through some underlying harmful cause. At first my 7
statement seemed implausible, but when, from then on, they found
that his pulse missed a beat occasionally and in a different ratio, they
later came to me and asked to hear by what indication I had realised
that the youth's natural condition was like that. My reply was similar 8
to that attributed to Isocrates the orator. When one of his students,
concerned about his three year course, asked him if he himself, after
studying so long, would then be able to speak on any given topic with
the same fluency as he saw Isocrates display, the man is said to 9

ἄν, ὦ παῖ, συνηυξάμην μὲν κἂν ἐν ἡμέρᾳ μιᾷ δύνασθαι μαθεῖν ὅπερ πυνθάνῃ· αὐτὸς δ᾽ ἂν ἐμαυτοῦ καταγνοίην ἀφυίαν, ἔτεσι πολλοῖς ἀσκήσας αὐτό[ν].» |

673 10 «Γνώσεσθε δέ», ἔφην, «ὅσαι παρὰ φύσιν εἰσὶν ἐν τοῖς σφυγμοῖς διαφοραί, τουτὶ τὸ βιβλίον ἀναγνόντες.» [ἦν δὲ τὸ πρῶτον Περὶ τοῦ τὰς τῶν σφυγμῶν διαφορὰς ἁπάσας διαγινώσκειν, ἁπτόμενον ἀσκήσεως τὴν ὁδὸν ἐν τέταρσι γεγράφθαι βιβλίοις ἃ λαβεῖν ἔξεστιν ὑμῖν ὅταν ἀπὸ στόματός μου τὰς γεγραμμένας ἐν τῷδε τῷ βιβλίῳ διαφορὰς εἴπητε.]

11 τοῦτ᾽ οὖν, ὦ Ἐπίγενες, ἀξιόλογον ἔργον ἰατρικῆς προγνώσεώς ἐστιν, ὥσπερ καὶ τὸ κατὰ τὸν αὐτοκράτορα τῆς δοκούσης αὐτῷ εἰσβολῆς

12 γεγενῆσθαι τοῦ παροξυσμοῦ. τῶν δ᾽ ἄλλων ὅσα θαυμάζουσιν οἱ πολλοὶ τῶν ἰατρῶν οὐδὲν οὐδ᾽ ἐγγὺς ὅμοιόν ἐστι τοῖσδε· θαυμαστὸν γὰρ εἶναι φαίνεται διὰ τὴν τῶν πολλῶν ἄγνοιαν, οὐ δι᾽ ἑαυτά, τοῖς νομίμως ἠσκηκόσι τὰ κατὰ τὴν τέχνην οὐκ ἔχοντα δύσκολον τὴν πρόγνωσιν.

10 ὥσπερ – 11] *v. supra* p. 126,16–128,30

1 μὲν *secl. Bas.* ἐν *secluserim* ὅπερ – 3 αὐτό] quod ego didici (didixi *Nic.*[a]: didisci *Nic.*[d]) (in *add. Nic.*[c]) tribus annis. sed secundum ineptitudines discentium anni multiplicantur *Nic.* 2 ἐμοι τοῦ κατὰ γνώμην y: *corr. Schöne* 3 αὐτόν y: *corr. Schöne* 4 γνώσεσθαι y: *sec. Nic.* (scietis) *corr. Schöne* 5 ἦν – 8 εἴπητε *om. Nic., seclusi* *post* Περὶ *lacunam indic. Schöne* 6 ἁπαγομένων M: ἐπαγομένων *Bas.*: ἐπαγόμενον *Schöne* 8 μοι *Schöne* αἴτητε *Corn.* 12 θαυμαστὰ *sec. Nic.* (miranda) *coni. Schöne, fort. recte* 14 οὐκ *om. Nic.* τέλος Γαληνοῦ περὶ τοῦ προγινώσκειν *subscr.* L

have replied to the youth, "I should like you to be able to learn in one
day all you ask, my child; but I would then condemn myself for ignor-
ance because I have studied it for many, many years."
"You will be aware", I said, "of the natural differences between 10
pulses if you read this book." This then, Epigenes, is an important 11
practical demonstration of medical prognosis, as in the case of the
emperor who believed that he had suffered the onset of a feverish
paroxysm. None of my other cases which surprise most doctors is in 12
any way like that: they appear surprising because of the ignorance of
the crowd, not because they are so intrinsically, since they present
no great difficulty of prognosis to those who have made a proper study
of all aspects of the medical art.

COMMENTARY

A decision to write a literary and historical commentary upon 'On prognosis', allegedly a work of medicine, requires little apology, for, together with De libris propriis, De ordine librorum suorum and De animi erroribus, it forms the basis for any biographical study of Galen and it offers important insights into the cultural environment in which he lived. The second century was an age in which culture mattered, in which emperors and senators were expected to show a sensitive acquaintance with the literature of the past and in which possession of the necessary linguistic, rhetorical and even philosophical skills could bring a man quickly to positions of power, not only in his local city but in the Roman Empire. The Greek renaissance that is associated with the so-called Second Sophistic is as much a social as an intellectual movement, and the patronage of men of letters from the provinces by political leaders at Rome helped in bringing a cultural unity to a scattered Empire. Philostratus' 'Lives of the Sophists' is a panegyric on the great orators and teachers of the second century and recreates in its optimism the excitement and vitality of the great age of the sophists which coincided with the lifetime of Galen. 'On prognosis', which describes incidentally Galen's rise to imperial favour, is thus extremely important for the understanding of the intellectual and social history of the second century. It introduces us to sophists and senators, to the Aristotelians in Rome and to the emperor himself; it offers glimpses of the workings of patronage; it provides unique information about conditions in Rome and Asia Minor. It is also the most detailed single source for a doctor's career – and indeed for the social position of doctors in general – in classical antiquity, and has been often used as such by historians of medicine. But when such richness is found in a single treatise it is only too easy to overvalue it, credulously to consider all its statements true, and to make sweeping generalisations from its evidence alone. In an attempt to avoid this natural prejudice in favour of Galen – a difficult task since his rhetoric is so persuasive – I have tried to put his statements into the context of the second century as a whole, so that a fairer impression of his veracity may be obtained. If this has led me to cite inscriptions and parallels from non-medical sources at what may seem to be undue length, I can claim in justification that the absence of any satisfactory biography of Galen or of any history of the medical profession in antiquity prevents me from taking the easy way out of the difficulties of the evidence and referring to an accessible and accurate secondary source.

'On prognosis' also gives us important information about Galen's thought-world, about his own attitudes and the intellectual heritage and attainments that go to make them up. More than in any other treatise, we can see the effects of his rhetorical and sophistical training, which are clear in his thought as well as in his language (above, pp. 59–63). Like many of his contemporaries he was well acquainted with, if not expert in, the art of rhetorical mimesis, the imitation, transformation and adornment of common themes, and it is essential to distinguish, if possible, between these common places, other literary influences on him, and his individual inventions, however few they may be. Thus I have referred the reader to parallel passages in other authors and I have identified many allusions in an attempt to delineate Galen's own ideas, for, even if he proves to be entirely derivative in his style and content, the sources on which he drew contribute to his intellectual biography. The preconceptions and the modes of thought that he took from his literary and philosophical studies, both of which appear in 'On prognosis', play an important part in the growth of his medical ideas, but one that is rarely recognised. I have also thought it useful to collect and discuss examples of Galen's non-Attic and colloquial usages to illustrate his technical and literary prose style.

It has been my aim throughout this commentary to emphasise the value of this treatise as a contribution both to the history of the Antonine period and to the biography of Galen himself. Even if, in the end, he appears more flawed and more prejudiced than his admirers might wish, by placing him in the context of the intellectual movements of his time I hope to have laid a firmer foundation on which to base any estimate of his medical, philosophical and cultural achievements.

P. 68,2: Chartier's insertion of πρὸς Ἐπιγένην before βιβλίον rests on very slight Ms. evidence, that of N Nic. ad and c^3. Since neither Galen himself (above, pp. 48f.) nor the Arabic authors (above, p. 53, n. 4) mention Epigenes, the words may be regarded as the invention of a scribe who wished to distinguish this from the other treatises on prognosis ascribed to Galen (XIX, pp. 497–511 K.; ib., pp. 512–518 K.; and ib., pp. 529–573 K.). There is little reason why Galen should single out Epigenes for such prominence when other friends such as Hieron, Bassus, Boethus and Teuthras are not mentioned at the head of treatises directed to them.

P. 68,3–74,12: J. Ilberg (NJ, p. 285) rightly noted that this prologue is a masterpiece of rhetoric, highly pessimistic and dubiously true. Galen's complaints about the decline of medicine, the maltreatment of worthy doctors and philosophers, and the evils of modern life may be fitly compared with those of Lucian, which stylistically derive from the well known type of diatribe against wealthy philistines. But

B. P. Reardon (pp. 178–180) warns us that Lucian's treatment owes more to the lucubrations of the study than to the realities of the street: "là où à première vue l'œuvre de Lucien semble le plus actuelle, elle est en fait imprégnée, et même construite, de souvenirs littéraires. De mensonges, en fait, si l'on veut." I would not go as far as this in my analysis of this passage, for it is quite clear from other anecdotes that Galen met with opposition, but the reasons that he gives for the poor state of medicine and philosophy are entirely traditional. The opening sentences owe a great deal to Plato, especially to such well known sections as Gorgias 502E and 517A, and Republic 491A–494D, which lie behind the similar polemic at Meth. med. I 1: X, pp. 1,11–4, 15 K.; cf. also the commentary on 68,7; 72,1; 72,17; 72,23; and 74,9. Although it is possible that Galen is here reciting philosophical commonplaces – "the pursuit of virtue for itself, not for its externals", was especially beloved of the Stoics –, it is more likely, given his respect for Plato, that he took the ideas and the language directly from him.[1]

P. 68,3f.: An ugly opening sentence, mainly because the dative τοῖς πολλοῖς, dependent upon ἐπί, is also logically required as the dative associated with the verb ἀδύνατόν ἐστι. On the inceptive use of μέν see Denniston, pp. 382f.: "The budding speaker at the turn of the fourth and fifth centuries was recommended, as a kind of stylistic convention, to start off with a μέν and to trust more or less to luck that he would find an answer to it, and not to care greatly if he did not." The convention was evidently still alive in the time of Galen.

P. 68,3: Although Epigenes has been considered the private doctor of Eudemus[2], this is not immediately certain. From this treatise it is clear that he was a man of wealth and education, p. 120,11f., a fellow countryman of Galen and Eudemus, and well acquainted with medical learning, pp. 74,29–76,2. If he is the addressee of Galen's treatise De parvae pilae exercitio, which is open to doubt,[3] he may have practised medicine: τοῦ πάντων ἠσκηκότος ἄριστα τὴν ἐν αὐτοῖς τέχνην (De parv. pil. exerc. 1: Scr. min. I, p. 93,7f. Marquardt = V, p. 899,10 K.). But in an age when it was intellectually

1 Much evidence for Galen as a Platonist was assembled by K. Deichgräber, Galen als Erforscher des menschlichen Pulses, Sitzungsber. d. Deutsch. Akademie d. Wiss., Kl. f. Spr., Lit. u. Kunst 1956, 3, Berlin 1957, App. II, pp. 33–36, and by P. De Lacy, Galen's Platonism, American Journ. of Philology 93, 1972, pp. 27–39, but neither considers the evidence of Galen's philosophical and literary vocabulary.

2 J. Walsh, Galen's clashes with the medical sects at Rome, Medical Life 35, 1928, p. 423.

3 The words ὦ 'Επίγενες (De parv. pil. exerc. 1: Scr. min. I, p. 93,3 Marquardt = V, p. 899,4 K. = E. Węnkebach, Sudhoffs Archiv f. Gesch. d. Med. 31, 1938, p. 258,1) are missing from the Greek Mss. and are derived from the Latin version ascribed to Niccolò. But of the Latin Mss. I have seen, two, Vatican, Pal. Lat. 1098, fol. 5^{v}, and Munich, CLM 490, fol. 78^{r}, name Epigenes both in the title and the text; two more, Vatican, Lat. 2384, fol. 28^{v}, and London, Wellcome 286, fol. 116^{v}, only in the text; and another, Cesena, S. V 4, fol. 36rb, in neither.

respectable to be interested in medicine (cf. Aulus Gellius, Noctes Atticae, XVIII 10,8; Athenaeus, cited by Oribasius, Coll. med. rel., lib. inc. 39,21: CMG VI 2,2, p. 141,5–9; and G. W. Bowersock, pp. 59–75) this may not be enough to distinguish Epigenes from the ἰδιῶται and from those who turned to politics after dabbling in medicine (Gal., De ord. lib. suor. 4: Scr. min. II, p. 89,3f. Müller = XIX, p. 60,1f. K.). Despite Wenkebach's arguments to the contrary[1], it is still possible to believe that Epigenes was an imperial official, a friend or client of Eudemus, who attended the medical debates and consultations in which Galen took part out of a keen amateur interest in medicine. Alternatively, he is a colleague and pupil of Galen.

P. 68,7: εὐδοκιμεῖν παρὰ τοῖς πολλοῖς is another Platonic allusion, repeated at p. 72,21, either of Theages 127A or, more likely, of Republic 605A, εἰ μέλλει εὐδοκιμήσειν ἐν τοῖς πολλοῖς. Although εὐδοκιμεῖν had been used as a term of abuse in an earlier academic debate[2], it is occasionally found on the honorific inscriptions of doctors from Hellenistic times onwards, see L. Robert, OMS I, pp. 256–259 and Bulletin Epigraphique 1958, n. 336, who cites examples from Delphi, the Tauric Chersonnese, Andros and Istria.

P. 68,8–11 : The morning salutation and the constant attendance demanded of clients were among the common complaints of the satirists, cf. the examples given by J. E. B. Mayor in the notes to his edition of Juvenal, London 1880, at Sat. I 127ff., Lucian, Nigrinus 56, 59f. and De mercede conductis 664f., but, as far as I know, only Galen refers to the 'salutatio', a Roman custom, as existing in the cities of the East, although probably only in the great coastal cities of Asia Minor.

P. 68,11: For the accusative ταῦτα used for variation with the following causal datives, see W. Schmid, I, p. 428; II, p. 309; III, p. 344; and IV, p. 50.

P. 68,12: Galen has a sound Hippocratic precedent for his dislike of showy clothes and rings in De decent. habitu 2f.: CMG I 1, p. 25,17–19 and 21f., and he defines the clothing of his ideal doctor in Hippocratic terms (In Hipp. Epid. VI comment. IV 10: CMG V 10,2,2, p. 205, 21ff., cf. K. Deichgräber, Medicus gratiosus, pp. 41f.). Rings are displayed prominently on statues of local worthies[3], and might be beautifully engraved with exquisite mythological scenes (cf. Gal., De usu part. XVII 1: II, p. 448,14–20 Helmr. = IV, p. 361,13–17 K.). Lucian often expresses similar suspicions of those who appear in glorious clothing, Nigrinus 52 and 59, with much silver and gold, De mer-

[1] E. Wenkebach, ibid., pp. 286f.

[2] H. Raeder, Alkidamas und Platon, Rheinisches Museum 63, 1908, pp. 508f.

[3] E. g. the statue of the doctor, Oulis Euxinou, from Velia in S. Italy, La Parola del Passato 25, 1970, pp. 267–284 and fig. 1; and on a statue from Ephesus, Jahreshefte d. Österreich. Archäolog. Instituts 27, 1932, Beibl. pp. 39–41. A gold ring was a sign of equestrian rank, cf. the gold ring given by Augustus to his physician, Antonius Musa (Suetonius, Aug. 59; Cassius Dio, Hist. LIII 30).

cede conductis 661, displaying ivory instrument cases, silver cupping glasses and gold plated knives, Adv. indoct. 124, although their knowledge and experience is limited. He also warns against placing excessive trust in the number of clients and companions about a man, although he recognises that such a following is essential for success, De mercede conductis 682, Nigrinus 34.

P. 68,16: As Galen says elsewhere (De pecc. dign. 4,1: CMG V 4, 1,1, p. 53,9), a false supposition about ends is often the source of moral error. Such 'Socratic' ideas on right aims are also transferred to a Roman context by Dio Chrysostom (Or. XIII 13; 29; 34–36).

P. 68,19f.: This is a reference to Thessalus and his followers, who are mercilessly pilloried by Galen, especially at Meth. med. I 1: X, pp. 5,1–7,9 K. He not only flattered the rich at Rome but also claimed to teach the whole of medicine in six months, thus attracting many pupils, especially young household slaves. An edict of Trajan (Fontes Iuris Romani Anteiustiniani I 77, cf. PIR² G. 107) withdrew the privileges of tax immunity granted by Vespasian to doctors and teachers who, "eager for gain rather than for the benefit of humanity", taught medicine to slaves and who thereby released a flood of half-trained servile practitioners. C. A. Forbes believed that this edict succeeded in raising standards [1], but this is too simple an explanation of the decline in the number of slave and freedman doctors recorded on inscriptions. In the later second century the lawyer Julian (Dig. 38, 1,25,2) mentions doctors who train slaves to profit by them, and such instruction is also noted by Galen at Protrept. 6: Scr. min. I, p. 108, 27f. Marquardt = I, p. 9,13–15 K.

P. 68,20f.: The evidence to substantiate this statement is hard to come by, unless it alludes to the growing interest in medical theory among men of wealth in the Eastern provinces, for which G. W. Bowersock, pp. 30–35, 59–75, provides a preliminary orientation. This is only to be expected, for backstairs intrigue is unlikely to figure prominently in the sources of our information, although cf. the reputed influence of C. Stertinius Xenophon over the emperor Claudius [2]. Doctors occasionally belonged to important political families in the East: the Statilii played an important part in the administration of Heraclea under Salbace (J. and L. Robert, Carie, pp. 179 and 220); the Philalethae, priest kings at Men Karou in the Maeander valley, numbered doctors among them [3]; and other examples come from Aperlae (IGR III 693), Saribeiler in Phrygia (IGR IV 520), Thyateira (IGR IV 1278) and Thessalonica (IG X ii, 1, 163).

[1] C. A. Forbes, The education and training of slaves, Trans. Amer. Philolog. Assoc. 86, 1955, pp. 345f.

[2] Tacitus, Annals XII 61 and 67; R. Herzog, Nikias u. Xenophon von Kos, Hist. Zeitschr. 125, 1922, pp. 189–247.

[3] Strabo, Geogr. XII 8,20, with the discussions of W. M. Ramsay, Cities and Bishoprics of Phrygia, Oxford, 1895, p. 52, and L. Robert, in J. Des Gagniers (ed.), Laodicée du Lycos: Le Nymphée, Quebec and Paris 1969, pp. 290–292.

P. 68,22: The unworthiness of contemporary τεχνῖται is a commonplace (cf. Cassius Dio, Hist. LXXI 35,2; Libanius, Or. II: p. 215, 11, ed. Förster) and was used by Herodian (Hist. I 1) likewise as a justification for the writing of his History.

P. 70,2: This passage cannot be used to imply that the teaching of medicine was prescribed either by civil law or by the Law of Hippocrates (CMG I 1, pp. 7f.), for although Galen claims to follow the Hippocratic tradition, whether in the Law, the Oath or the Testament (ed. K. Deichgräber, Medicus gratiosus, pp. 88–103), there is little evidence that these writings were widely accepted. Only Erotian (p. 116, ed. Nachmanson) refers for certain to the Law, and the Oath had far less effect in antiquity than in the Middle Ages.[1] No course of instruction was ever laid down for doctors by the imperial government, and experience, rather than learning, seems to have been the main legal criterion for a doctor.

P. 70,3f.: In Galen and Hippocrates, αἱμορραγία, when found alone, means bleeding from the nose (cf. Gal., In Hipp. Epid. I comment. I 10: CMG V 10,1, p. 29,30–32). A flow of morbid humours from the main area of damage was often regarded as beneficial, for it would strike a stronger or a less important part of the body and might even be drained away by the physician if it appeared as pus or as a swelling. In all Hippocratic medicine, such a flow is called ἀπόστασις, which is customarily translated into English as 'abscession'. When this flow is to the ears (Hipp., Progn. 18: p. 97,17f. Kw. = II, p. 158,3 L.) or to the glands behind the ears (Gal., In Hipp. Progn. comment. II 65: CMG V 9,2, p. 316,5f.) the affliction or swelling that results is termed παρωτίς.

P. 70,8: Magic, γοητεία, was a crime when it was performed with an evil intention to harm or defraud another, and was punishable by death (Apuleius, Apol. 26; Institutes IV 18,5) even when no murder had been committed (Paul, Sentent. V 23; Dig. 48,8,13). White magic, which Augustine (Civ. Dei X 9) carefully distinguishes from black, the art of the γόης, was tolerated rather than harassed. The doctor who was skilled in prognosis would easily fall under the suspicion of being a magician or a diviner, against whose predictions, especially when they related to the emperor, the law laid down strong prohibitions (cf. Tacitus, Annals II 32; XII 52; Paul, Sentent. V 21,1; Ulpian, Coll. leg. Mos. 15,2,2,3). The problems of the relationship between white magic and the Roman law have never received a satisfactory treatment from modern scholars.[2]

[1] In addition to the standard accounts of W. H. S. Jones, The Doctor's Oath, Cambridge 1924, and L. Edelstein, pp. 3–63, see F. Rosenthal, An ancient commentary on the Hippocratic Oath, Bull. of the History of Med. 30, 1956, pp. 52–87, and two papyri, Pap. Oxy. 437 (with the notes of H. Schöne and K. Deichgräber, Quellen u. Studien z. Gesch. d. Med. 3,2, 1932, p. 47) and Pap. Oxy. 2547.

[2] The best account is still that of Th. Mommsen, Le droit pénal romain, Paris 1907, II, pp. 356–361; III, pp. 190–194. Cf. also the collections of texts made

P. 70,12: Schöne's suspicions of σφετέραν, a literary flosculus common among second century authors, are unfounded (cf. W. Schmid, II, p. 21 and III, p. 67; Gal., De diff. puls. II 10: VIII, p. 630,6f. K.; IV 6: VIII, p. 732,11 K.; De dign. puls. I 2: VIII, p. 781,17f. K.; CMG V 10,2,3, p. 219), but the phrase is still difficult. Since this request is made by persons who are favourably inclined towards prognosis and do not reject it immediately, there would be no reason, apart from personal spite, for a doctor who knew all the facts not to declare that prognosis had been used and described earlier. Given that ἴσως – ἀγνοοῦντας is correct, the first phrase should mean either that the doctors concealed their knowledge, or that they pretended ignorance, or that they knew something of prognosis but not enough to benefit from it, and that it was through fear of having their poor learning shown up that they resorted to outright denial. The last explanation, which distinguishes between ἄγνοια and ἀμαθία, demands no emendation and is supported by a similar use of ἀμαθία at Gal., De dign. puls. IV 3: VIII, p. 956,8–12 K. and possibly by a Platonic parallel, Gorgias 492A: ἀποκρυπτόμενοι τὴν αὑτῶν ἀδυναμίαν.

P. 70,16: Galen's respect for Hippocrates, who hymned the justice and foresight of Nature (De usu part. III 10: I, p. 172,15–17 Helmr. = III, p. 235,7 K.) is well known. As he stated at Meth. med. VI 4: X, p. 420,9–16 K. (cf. above, p. 134,1–6), he intended his medical writings, not to supersede the works of Hippocrates, but to provide an explanatory commentary upon them and to supplement their deficiencies. L. Garcia Ballester has sought to define four different periods in Galen's attitude to his predecessor[1], but this is much too schematic and it may be better to accept the verdict of Palladios (II, p. 157,18f., ed. Dietz): Ἱπποκράτης μὲν ἔσπειρεν, ἐγεώργησε δὲ ὁ Γαληνός.

P. 70,22: The examples of Quintus and of the young man murdered because of his success (above, p. 92,23–26) may indicate that the envy of Galen's opponents was as malignant as he implies. But φθόνος was a favourite theme, either within a diatribe, as with Lucian (De mercede conductis 698ff.), or forming the subject of an entire sophistic oration (cf. Dio Chrysostom, Or. 77 and 78) or of political moralising (cf. C. P. Jones, p. 112), and Galen may again be elaborating a common theme. He will also have dealt with this in his autobiography, entitled 'On slander' (De lib. propr. 12: Scr. min. II, p. 122,2 Müller = XIX, p. 46,5 K.), although the date of its composition cannot be determined with certainty.

by C. Pharr, The interdiction of magic in Roman Law, Trans. Amer. Philolog. Assoc. 63, 1932, pp. 269–295; and by F. H. Cramer, Astrology in Roman Law and Politics, Philadelphia 1954, pp. 276–281.

[1] L. Garcia Ballester, Galeno, Madrid 1972, pp. 59–68. A better account, stressing the general Hippocratic basis of second century medicine, is given by O. Temkin, Geschichte des Hippokratismus im ausgehenden Altertum, Kyklos 4, 1932, pp. 10–18, and by K. Deichgräber, Medicus gratiosus, pp. 45–48.

P. 70,23: Quintus, the master of Satyrus and Pelops, is regarded by Galen as the greatest doctor of his generation, "a man eminent at Rome during the reign of Hadrian" (Anat. admin. XIV 1: p. 183 Dkw.), although the two never met. He was a great anatomist and commentator upon Hippocrates but, as can be gathered from the anecdotes recalled by Galen, his bedside manner was far from impeccable: cf. Gal., De sanit. tuenda III 13,1–4: CMG V 4,2, p. 100,27f.; In Hipp. Epid. VI comment. IV 10: CMG V 10,2,2, p. 207,1–10. His influence upon Galen is sympathetically discussed by Mewaldt, pp. 123–127, but the best account of him still remains that of W. A. Greenhill.[1]

The regular suspicion that the doctor was a possible, or even an actual murderer may have arisen partly from a general ignorance of medicine and partly from the legal difficulties involved in proving the negligence of the doctor.[2] Complaints and recriminations about the failure of doctors to effect a cure range from the death-bed cry of Hadrian (Cassius Dio, Hist. LXIX 22) to the humble testimony of inscriptions (CIL III 3355; 14188; VI 30112; ILS 9441; Carmina Latina Epigraphica 94; L'Année Epigraphique 1952, n. 16).

P. 70,26: The tradition that medicine had its origins among the family groups of Asclepiadae at Cos, Cnidos and Rhodes was fully accepted by Galen (e. g. Anat. admin. II 1: II, p. 281,3–5 K.; Meth. med. I 1: X, p. 4,9–11 K.), who lamented the decline from the golden age of the Asclepiadae to the domination of slaves and charlatans (De exam. medico, p. 192,9–15 Dietrich).[3] The Asclepiadae continued to exist on Cos at least until the middle of the first century A. D., when an inscription mentions a relative of C. Stertinius Xenophon as being "the descendant of the Asclepiadae and Heracleidae" (A. Maiuri, Nuova silloge epigrafica di Rodi e Cos, Florence 1925, n. 461), but Galen does not appear to know of their existence in his own day.

P. 72,1: Almost certainly this is a reminiscence of Plato, Republic 608C: τά γε μέγιστα ἐπίχειρα ἀρετῆς καὶ προκείμενα ἆθλα οὐ διεληλύθαμεν. In taking ἐπίχειρα to mean 'reward', Galen is being more Platonic than other later philosophical writers, who replaced the neutral meaning 'recompense' with that of 'punishment': cf. Philodemus, De ira 32: κἄπειτα τῆς προπετείας πικρὰ κομίζονται τἀπίχειρα. The reward consists in the knowledge and acceptance of the truth vouchsafed to the man who observes things rightly and who, through his retirement, is not forced to recant or to compromise his beliefs.

P. 72,3: As well as being an allusion to Demosthenes (De corona 263, ed. Sandys), this metaphor of the hare suits Galen's liking for

[1] In Smith's Dictionary of Greek and Roman biography, London 1854, III, p. 637, s. v. Quintus.

[2] Lucian, Calumniae non temere credendum 13; F. Kudlien, Medicine and popular ethics in Greece and Rome, Clio medica 5, 1970, pp. 97–107; K. H. Below, Der Arzt im römischen Recht, Munich 1953, pp. 108–121.

[3] See H. Schöne, Bruchstücke einer neuen Hippokratesvita, Rheinisches Museum 58, 1903, pp. 62–66.

animal comparisons (cf. Gal., De moribus, p. 25,12, ed. Kraus; and the quotation given by Ibn ʿAḳnin, Halkin, pp. 68f., n. 7; and R. Walzer, GA, pp. 151f.).

P. 72,4: Although the phrase πρὸς – αὐξάνειν may strengthen καί τι πείσεσθαι, it weakens the comparison between the brave man and the coward and takes away some of the force of the metaphor: but, although I should like to remove it from the text, Galen's love of repetition is a strong argument in favour of its retention.

P. 72,11: A traditional theme, as Galen notes, going back at least to Solon, 4,19; to the gnomic poet whose lines lie behind Herodotus, Hist. VIII 3[1]; and to Theognis, 51f.:

ἐκ τῶν γὰρ στάσιές τε καὶ ἔμφυλοι φόνοι ἀνδρῶν
μούναρχοί θ'· ἃ πόλει μήποτε τῇδε ἅδοι.

The sentence structure, as often in this literary treatise, is elaborate and complex: ἤ εἴπερ (l. 9) corresponds to ἤτοι (l. 8), and the verb δύνασθαι (l. 12) to the earlier γενέσθαι (l. 8). For the resumptive μὲν οὖν (l. 10) omitted by A but a common feature of Greek scientific prose, see Denniston, p. 474, and Blass-Debrunner-Funk, § 451,1.

P. 72,15–21: More Platonic reminiscences. συρφετός is found at Hippias 288D, Theaetetus 152C and Gorgias 489C, while ἐν χειμῶνι μεγάλῳ καὶ ζάλῃ πνευμάτων alludes to Plato's famous description of the philosopher who, realising the immense folly and madness of his contemporaries, withdraws from public life to shelter οἷον ἐν χειμῶνι κονιορτοῦ καὶ ζάλης ὑπὸ πνεύματος φερομένου, Republic 496D.[2] This well known passage was admired and copied by many authors of the late second and early third centuries (e. g. Clement Alex., Strom. p. 707; and Porphyry, De abst. I 36) and Marcus Aurelius (Med. IV 3) advocated a philosophical withdrawal, not into a country retreat far from other men, but into self meditation.

The text presents several problems. If καὶ is copulative, rather than emphatic, it should be followed by the infinitive, not the participle, but its omission, in which I follow Schöne, leaves a hiatus which might be considered awkward.[3] A and Nic. offer an easier reading than that of L and M, which corresponds closely to the Platonic model and which I have preferred: on the other hand, it is possible that the reading in L and M was itself changed from that of A by a scribe who remembered his Plato well and who corrected a Galenic variant accordingly.

1 A. W. Verrall, Two unpublished inscriptions from Herodotus, Classical Review 17, 1903, p. 99.

2 Cf. also Theaetetus 174B–175B and Adam's note to his edition of the Republic, Cambridge 1902, II, p. 32.

3 Galen's normal practice in avoiding hiatus was described by J. Marquardt (Scr. min. I, pp. L–LV), but Galen was never as consistent as Marquardt thought (cf. CMG V 2,1, p. 64) and, if the Platonic phrase is a direct quotation, as seems likely, then hiatus may be permitted to stand. Cf. above, pp. 82,5 ἐπάρχου ἐδεῖτο; 92,2 ἀδικίᾳ ἑαυτῶν; 96,21 περαινόμενα οὐκ; 120,15 δύναται οὔτε; 120,22 κοιτωνίτῃ ὅ τι; 120,29 ἐλέγξῃ ἐμέ.

P. 72,22: The argument that the luxury of the rich and powerful was the foundation of social and moral decline was a common theme in satire and diatribe, cf. Seneca, Ep. 76,1–7; Juvenal, Sat. 3; 11, 1–55; Lucian, Nigrinus 61 ff. Maximus of Tyre (Or. 4, pp. 41,16–43,2, ed. Hobein) adapts this commonplace and argues that modern medicine has had to change εἰς δίαιταν ποικιλωτέραν καὶ κρᾶσιν πονηρὰν (τῶν σωμάτων) and from its former simplicity has gained παντοδαπὸν σχῆμα in attending to luxury.

The Basle editors, forgetting that πρεσβυτέρως can occasionally mean 'to a greater extent' (cf. Plato, Republic 548C) followed Nic.'s version (preferentes) and, like the scribe of A, replaced it with περαιτέρω.

P. 72,27: Statues of these notable performers were to be found in many cities, where, if they were located in the public squares, they would be adjacent to the temples and statues of the gods. However, I have found no certain example of such a statue placed within a ritual area, although the evidence collected by E. Rosenbaum suggests that this may be due to chance.[1] Galen's complaints were not unique – Tacitus (Dial. 29) says: "iam vero propria et peculiaria huius urbis vitia paene in utero matris concipi mihi videntur, histrionalis favor et gladiatorum equorumque studia: quibus occupatus et obsessus animus quantulum loci bonis artibus relinquit?" – nor were they heeded, for Ammianus (Hist. XXVIII 4) describes a similar situation some hundred and fifty years later. The popularity of histriones may well have been encouraged by the example of Lucius Verus, who is said to have had a great passion for them (Hist. Augusta, Vita Veri 8,7–11) and who received from Lucian the tract 'On the dance', probably while he was staying at Antioch c. 162.[2] L. Robert (OMS I, pp. 221–226; 654–708) has discussed the widespread evidence for actors and dancers[3]: charioteers and jockeys enjoyed a similar success.[4]

P. 72,28: The neglect of μαθήματα by contemporary doctors and intellectuals is a common theme in Galen (cf. Quod opt. med. sit etiam phil. 1: Scr. min. II, p. 1,7–11 Müller = I, pp. 53,8–54,1 K.), especially in his polemics against the Methodist followers of Thessalus

1 E. Rosenbaum, Cyrenaican portrait sculpture, London 1960, p. 12. A public statue of Antonius Musa, Augustus' doctor, was erected "iuxta signum Aesculapi" (Suetonius, Aug. 59). A. Cameron, Porphyrius the charioteer, Oxford 1973, pp. 185f., plausibly suggests that in sixth century Constantinople statues of charioteers stood on the spina of the Hippodrome alongside those of Hercules and Nike (among other deities): cf. also Martial, V 25.

2 J. A. Hall, p. 19; C. P. Jones, Two enemies of Lucian, Greek, Roman and Byzantine Studies 13, 1972, p. 484, prefers to date it to 164.

3 Cf. also Pap. Oxy. 475; ILS 5186; 5189–91; 5194; J. Bayet, Mélanges de littérature latine, Rome 1967, pp. 439–460; M. Sordi, L'epitafe di un pantomimo, Epigraphica 15, 1953, pp. 104–121; J. E. Spruit, Catalogus van Romeinse acteurs, Meded. v. h. Nederlands Hist. Instituut te Rome 34, 1969, pp. 59–95.

4 Cf. Suetonius, Galba 15; Juvenal, Sat. VII 114, 242; Historia Augusta, Vita Marci 11,4; Vita Veri 6; Cassius Dio, Hist. LXXVII 10; ILS 5287ff.; and A. Cameron, Porphyrius the charioteer, p. 15 and pp. 247f.

(Meth. med. I 1f.: X, pp. 5,1–18,13 K.). It goes almost without saying that it all goes back to Plato, possibly mediated through the Stoics. Seneca (Ep. 88,9–11) makes similar objections to the current practitioners of music, geometry (metiri geometres docet latifundia) and astronomy, and (ib. 21) quotes Posidonius as saying that in the arts commonly held in honour "nulla decoris nulla honesti (τὸ καλόν?) est". Galen's advocacy of the philosophical aspects of music and arithmetic, which comes from Plato (esp. Republic 525–531) and ultimately from the Pythagoreans, was accepted by many other writers of the imperial period like Strabo (Geogr. I 2,3; X 3,9f.) and Athenaeus (Deipnosoph. XIV 616–638). Mathematics, geometry, astronomy and music had been associated together since the days of Pythagoras (Nic. Gerasinus, Intr. Arithm. I 4,1, cf. I 3,4) and were, in Greek theory at least, essential parts of a gentleman's education (cf. K. Deichgräber, Medicus gratiosus, pp. 94, 100–107). Divination was not included in the astronomy recommended by later authors (cf. Strabo, Geogr. I 1,1, 13–15) although its critics, such as Seneca (Ep. 88,14–17) and Sextus Empiricus (Adv. math. 5), professed to regard astronomy as no more than astrology and the casting of horoscopes and Vitruvius (De arch. IX 6,2) knew of a school of astrology founded by Berosus at Cos. It is significant that Plutarch (fr. 147, ed. Sandbach) uses a similar method of argument to Galen's and a similar division of arts into those developed by necessity, those that satisfy luxury, and those that are studied for their accuracy and their purity, in order to justify his support for mantic divination, another method of foretelling the future.

P. 74,3: Both philosophy and demonstrative theory are regarded by Galen as essential for the intellectual well being of the physician and, since ἀποδεικτικὴ θεωρία is a subdivision of philosophy, I take φιλοσοφίαν to be an accusativus pendens. On Galen's claims for demonstrative theory, a method of argument that attains its conclusions by proceeding from true premisses (Inst. log. 11,1: p. 24 Kalbfleisch), see the remains of his treatise 'On demonstration', edited by I. Müller, Abh. d. k. bayer. Akademie d. Wiss. 20, München 1895, pp. 403–478. His aspirations may have been shared by Lucian (Hermotimus 811): ὡς εἴ γέ τινα εὕροις διδάσκαλον, ὃς ἀποδείξεως πέρι καὶ τῆς τῶν ἀμφισβητουμένων διακρίσεως τέχνην τινὰ εἰδὼς διδάξειέ σε, παύσῃ δηλαδὴ πράγματα ἔχων, although, 812, he doubts the competence of the philosophers of his own time to obtain this accurate ἀπόδειξις.

κῦρος is a sound Attic word, used by Thucydides (Hist. V 38,2) and Plato (Gorgias 450E–F): ἡ διὰ λόγου τὸ κῦρος ἔχουσα ῥητορική ἐστιν, and by Galen again at Meth. med. I 5: X, p. 43,11 K.

P. 74,5: The educational dispute between orators and philosophers can be traced back at least to Plato and Isagoras (cf. E. Rohde, pp. 345–347). Galen allies himself vigorously with the philosophers, regarding the Platonic philosopher as his ideal physician, competent to judge medical, ethical and logical problems, and he delivered forceful attacks on sophists and orators (In Hipp. Progn. comment. I 4: CMG V 9,2, p. 205,3–8). For the contemporary background, see B. P. Reardon, pp. 31–42, 64–71, and G. W. Bowersock, pp. 10–12, who makes it clear that the boundaries between the groups were defined more often by personal animosities than by any obvious differences of doctrine.

Unless λογικὴ θεωρία was the description favoured by Galen's opponents, λογικῇ θεωρίᾳ cannot be right, since it is regularly praised by Galen and approved of by Hippocrates (Gal., Quod opt. med. sit etiam phil. 1: Scr. min. II, p. 2,3 Müller = I, p. 54,9f. K.) while the sophists are abused and despised, cf. Gal., De dieb. decret. I 4: IX, p. 789,13–15 K.: τοὺς σοφιστικοὺς λῃροὺς ἑτέροις παρέντες οἷς οὐ τῶν ἔργων τῆς τέχνης φροντὶς ἀλλὰ τοῦ φλυαρεῖν ὥσπερ ἐπὶ μειρακίων διατριβαῖς. On Galen's own definition (De plac. Hipp. et Plat. VIII (1): p. 651,14–16 Ml. = V, p. 651,1–3 K., cf. ibid. II (3): p. 179,6–12 Ml. = V, p. 221,6–8 K.), as arguments depart further and further from true scientific method, so they are called rhetorical and sophistical. The πανουργία of the sophists may well have been a cliché, cf. Plutarch, Lysander 7,5: πανοῦργος καὶ σοφιστής, and above, p. 90,18–20.

P. 74,7: κέγχρος, panicum miliaceum, Linn.[1], is here used colloquially to mean something exceedingly small (cf. Gal., De nat. fac. II 3: Scr. min. III, p. 164,6 Helmr. = II, p. 87,2 K.; De dign. puls. II 2: VIII, pp. 841,8–842,2 K.). Although R. Strömberg cites four proverbial expressions from Galen's writings[2], he omits this despite its similarity to others on his list (pp. 27, 62, 79, and 84). Galen is fond of such saws and proverbs: see E. L. A. Leutsch and F. G. Schneidewin, Corpus Paroemiographorum Graecorum, Göttingen 1839–1841, I, pp. 231 (= Gal., De diff. puls. IV 16: VIII, p. 763,1 K.) and 441 (= ibid. II 4: VIII, p. 577,13f. K.) to which may be added: ὅταν ἐν φρέατι, τοῦτο δὴ τὸ τοῦ λόγου συσχεθῶσι (De diff. puls. II 10: VIII, p. 631,9 K.) and: πόκον εἰς γναφεῖον οὐδεὶς ἀποφέρει (De diff. puls. II 9 and III 3: VIII, pp. 624,6 and 656,6 K.).

P. 74,9–11: Galen ends with a reference to two passages in Plato, although he may have had in mind only the first: Gorgias 464D–E, "If a confectioner, ὀψοποιός, and a doctor were to dispute before an audience of children, or of men as foolish as children, whose judgement of what was good food was to be obeyed, the doctor would die of hunger." and Politicus 289A, where Plato talks of the differences between medicine and cookery. The opposition between these two skills is common in Galen and other writers (cf. Seneca, Ep. 88,18). They use the same material but with different ends in view: ὠφελείας γὰρ ἡμεῖς στοχαζόμεθα τῆς ἐκ τῶν ἐδεσμάτων, οὐχ ἡδονῆς (Gal., De alim. fac. II 51: CMG V 4,2, p. 317,14–18); a doctor differs from a cook as a παιδοτρίβης from a γυμναστής (De sanit. tuenda II 9:

[1] First identified by E. H. F. Meyer, Botanische Erläuterungen zu Strabons Geographie, Königsberg 1852, pp. 44–52.

[2] R. Strömberg, Greek proverbs, Gothenburg 1954, pp. 44 and 72.

CMG V 4,2, p. 63,27ff.); and he complains that the army doctors who had the opportunity of inspecting the bodies of dead Germans (in 169?) gained no greater knowledge than that possessed by cooks (De comp. med. per gen. III 2: XIII, p. 604,13–17 K.).

P. 74,15: The constant appeal to Epigenes to confirm Galen's statements by his own recollections (cf. above, pp. 80,7; 110,13; 124,23; 134,1) may be explained by J. Ilberg's supposition (NJ, p. 285) that this treatise is designed to justify Galen's preeminence and that other witnesses are required to testify to his merits.

P. 74,16: Eudemus was a Peripatetic philosopher from Pergamum and a friend of Galen's father (76,29) who, if διδάσκαλος at 92,26 is to be taken to refer to philosophy rather than to the information just given (cf. 82,12) had taught Galen philosophy: possibly he may be identified with the unnamed pupil of the Peripatetic Aspasius who on his return to his native Pergamum after a long absence taught Galen (Gal., De aff. dign. 8,4: CMG V 4,1,1, p. 28,15f.). He had moved to Rome about ten years before Galen's first visit, i. e. about 152 A. D. Apart from his attendance at Galen's public demonstrations (Gal., Anat. admin. I 1: II, p. 218,6 K.), nothing further is known about him, but this has not hampered speculation. Martini claimed on the evidence of this passage that he was the author of a tract on prognosis[1], and A. Stein identified him with the old doctor from Pergamum who invented the Isis plaster (Gal., Meth. med. VI 6: X, p. 454, 8–18 K.).[2] Wellmann rightly distinguished the two[3], since the philosopher does not appear to have practised medicine and the doctor seems to have lived in Pergamum for most, if not all, of his life. If Lucian disguises real persons under fictitious names in his dialogues, it may well be that Eudemus is depicted as Euthydemus (Hermotimus 750f.), who is involved in a brawl over dinner as a result of his proposition of Peripatetic objections to Stoic belief.

Eudemus' complaint was malaria[4], especially if Galen's treatment of him for bilious attacks occurred now and not later (Gal., De temp. 6: pp. 76,23–77,19 Helmr. = I, pp. 631,6–632,12 K.; and In Hipp. De victu acut. comment. II 29: CMG V 9,1, pp. 187,16–188,19). The many references made by Galen to this case show that it was the most important of his early career, giving him an entrée into the upper reaches of Roman society. Indeed, in view of Eudemus' friends, it is not surprising that after one astonishing success, in which he demonstrated painstakingly and at length his accomplishments in several branches of medicine, he should have become the doctor to senators

[1] RE VI, 1907, col. 905, s. v. Eudemos 12.

[2] PIR² E. 109. His reference to I, p. 613 is an error for I, p. 631 K.

[3] RE VI, 1907, col. 905, s. v. Eudemos 19.

[4] See F. E. Kind, RE XIV, 1930, cols. 833–837, s. v. Malaria. Cf. Gal., De crisib. II 3: pp. 131,12–135,14 Alex. = IX, pp. 649,3–655,6 K., with the comments of R. E. Siegel, Galen's system of physiology and medicine, Basle and New York 1968, pp. 274–277.

and imperial councillors. The power of patronage was universal in the Roman Empire. Rather, the problem is how did Galen, an immigrant from Asia Minor, achieve his friendly relationship with Eudemus so quickly.

Galen's early career is a paradigm of successful social mobility, yet only J. Ilberg (NJ, p. 286) has noted the importance of his friends from Pergamum in assisting his rise. It was not only his medical and philosophical ability, on which he expatiates fully, but also his family connections, made among the leading citizens of Pergamum and Asia, that enabled him to make his mark almost at once in Rome. When he arrived in 162 (cf. below, p. 210), he came not as an impoverished and friendless provincial but as a man of means whose school friends and associates were already there: Teuthras, Apellas, Eudemus, Epigenes and possibly even Glaucon. If he owed his climb up the social ladder to his own abilities, it must be admitted that, because of his family, his education and his wealth, he began his ascent from a higher rung than most other doctors.

P. 74,19: In Attic Greek διάγειν takes the accusative of the time spent, and thus, unless κατὰ is emended to καὶ, a simple palaeographic change, the use of κατά with the accusative is pleonastic, but not necessarily un-Galenic (cf. the repetition of αὐτῶν at 92,33).

P. 74,24: It is clear that the number of the hour, which, according to Galen's precept (De antid. I 5: XIV, pp. 31,10–32,5 K.), should have been written out in full, was first abbreviated and then misinterpreted. If the original was ὀγδόην, as A has it, it is difficult to see why both ἐνάτην and πέμπτην were suggested as alternatives, since the abbreviations ϑ' and ε' can in no way be confused with η', while the fact that the shivering fit occurred at the eighth hour makes ὀγδόην an obvious choice as one of the suspected hours. The similarity in uncial script of ϑ' and ε' suggests that this was the reason for the corruption and that the scribe of A, or of his exemplar, faced with an unintelligible πέμπτην, a good three hours before the suspected hours, made a plausible guess at the right number. But all other indications point to ἐνάτην. As on the previous day, Eudemus is being ultra-cautious, waiting beyond the eighth hour, when the shivering fit might be expected, until the ninth, and only then taking his bath and eating.

P. 76,15: Although Nic.'s "dicens" implies φάσκων, the accusative and infinitive construction agrees better with the reading of the Greek Mss., φάντων; and the position of ὡς οἶσθα is easier to understand if it is within, rather than at the beginning of, the clause, and the genitive πλειόνων is the subject of the genitive absolute, not an adjective agreeing with σιτίων.

P. 76,16: Schöne, who believed that the Mss. reading could be kept, refers to the discussion of W. Havers, Untersuchungen zur Kasussyntax, Strasbourg 1911, p. 118, for evidence that the possessive dative is often used by the medical writers, especially with parts of the body (cf. above, p. 130,28) but the close proximity of ἔφην makes it equally likely that μου was corrupted to μοι, and I have emended accordingly.

P. 76,27: To Eudemus at any rate Galen's early reputation was as a philosopher and his presence at philosophical debates was noted as well as at those of doctors (Gal., De aff. dign. 8,3–7: CMG V 4, 1,1, pp. 28,9–29,12). Under his father's guidance he sat at the feet of the best available teachers of every sect at Pergamum and Smyrna; a pupil of Albinus the Platonist, and one of Gaius; an Epicurean from Athens; a Stoic; and a Peripatetic follower of Aspasius; he was acquainted with some Pythagorean doctrine (ibid. 6,10: CMG V 4,1,1, p. 20,8ff.). In an age full of 'Halbphilosophen' (B. P. Reardon, pp. 31–62), he regarded his own works on philosophy highly (cf. De ord. lib. suor. 2 and 4: Scr. min. II, p. 83,7–23 Müller = XIX, pp. 53,10–54,7 K.; II, pp. 87,24–89,11 Müller = XIX, pp. 58,11–60,8 K.; and De lib. propr. 11–16: Scr. min. II, pp. 115,40–124,5 Müller = XIX, pp. 39,1–48,7 K.), and he discussed many philosophical problems from ethics to logic, the latter affording him the most lasting fame as a philosopher.[1] He summarised many of Plato's dialogues and commented upon them[2], for which he was roundly attacked by Alexander of Aphrodisias, who called him "mule head" (see below, p. 189). Most later references to him are favourable. Athenaeus (Deipnosoph. I 2) says that he published so many philosophical and medical writings as to surpass all his predecessors; Eusebius (Hist. Eccl. V 28,7) ascribes the origins of the Theodotian heresy in part to him[3]; and Damascius (Vita Isid. fr. 244, ed. Zintzen) explains how Marinus, the leader of the Neo-Platonists in the fifth century, dissented from the views of Proclus, his master, to follow the erroneous opinions of Galen and Castricius Firmus on Plato's Parmenides.

P. 78,2: Like his father, Galen also received injunctions from Asclepius in dreams; to write treatises (Gal., De usu part. X 14: II, p. 110,7 Helmr. = III, p. 837,5 K.); to perform certain cures (see below, p. 225); and not to go on campaign against the Germans in 169 (below, p. 211). Other authors such as Lucian (Somnium 5,8), Artemidorus (Oneir. II 70) and Cassius Dio (Hist. LXXII 23,2–4 and LXVIII 10,1–2) received similar divine instruction, and the preface to Lucian's Longaevi (208) suggests that this may have become an acknowledged literary convention. But during this period there is an increasingly more open reliance on dreams and portents in determining

1 See N. Rescher, Galen and the syllogism, Pittsburgh 1966.

2 Much evidence for his services to Plato are collected by R. Walzer, GA, passim; see also A. Müller, Die griechische Philosophie in der arabischen Überlieferung, Halle 1873, pp. 5, 7, 13f., 23–28; P. Kraus and R. Walzer, Corpus Platonicum medii aevi: Plato Arabus I, London 1951; and E. I. J. Rosenthal, Averroes' Commentary upon Plato's Republic, 2nd. ed., Cambridge 1966, p. 12 and index s. v. Galen.

3 Following R. Walzer, JC, pp. 75ff., I believe that the Theodotians worshipped Galen for his logical methods rather than for his textual criticism as B. M. Metzger supposed (The text of the New Testament, Oxford 1964, pp. 150ff.).

conduct (cf. Marcus Aurelius, Med. I 17,9; Cassius Dio, Hist. LXXII 23,1), a sign that this was an age of anxiety, of personal uncertainty even in the midst of prosperity.[1]

P. 78,11: The custom of multiple consultations, which is rare in England today, was one of the ways in which patients could protect themselves against the inadequacies of their own physicians and avail themselves of whatever assistance was at hand. In De examinando medico Galen sets out at length the methods that a patient should use for selecting a doctor and how he should profit from the presence of more than one physician, for, if In Hipp. De off. med. comment. II 7: XVIII B, p. 744,9 K. is believed, the σκέψις ἀκριβὴς ἰατρῶν πλειόνων συνόδου was the usual system of treatment. It had one advantage for the physician. Like Galen here, he could compete on equal terms with the ἄριστοι and gain a reputation by succeeding where others of proven merit had failed (cf. Hipp., De diaet. acut. 44 (11): I, p. 131,10–13 Kw. = II, pp. 316,13–318,2 L.). Galen's refusal to participate in this meeting may not have been as honourable as he suggests, since he evidently relies on his family ties with Eudemus to influence him, and it is just this sort of personal influence that general debates discounted. But unlike the public debates between sophists, where no participant could lose, provided that his exposition was fluent, the consequences of a wrong prescription might bring about the ruin of a reputation as well as the death of the patient.[2]

It seems to have been the custom for doctors to bring their pupils and friends along to these bedside consultations. Philostratus (Vita Apoll. VIII 7) says that over thirty pupils accompanied Seleucus of Cyzicus and Stratocles of Sidon to visit Philiscus and cf. above, p. 68,20. The result was not always happy for the patient. Martial's epigram (V 9) on the man who caught a fatal chill from the cold hands of questing students is a re-working of an old joke found in Menander (Monostich. 659, ed. Jäkel) and Pliny (Nat. Hist. XXIX v, 11): "hinc illa infelix monumentis inscriptio, turba se medicorum periisse."

P. 78,14: Theriac is a general term for a medicine containing many animal substances, especially castoreum and those derived from snakes, which was in fashion in Rome under Marcus Aurelius (Gal., De antid. I 4: XIV, p. 24,14–18 K.). Each doctor would know at least one of the recipes for it, which were composed of a variety of ingredients according to the disease and wealth of the patient, of whom the most famous was Mithridates, king of Pontus, the eponymous user of Mithridation. The distinguished London physician Wil-

[1] E. R. Dodds, Pagan and Christian in an age of anxiety, Oxford 1965, pp. 38–53; G. Strohmaier, pp. 375–379. At De propr. plac. 2, Galen declares that the workings of god are revealed in visions and dreams, acknowledging the god's cure of him in a dream and telling how by signs the god had saved a man from shipwreck.

[2] Cf. J. Kollesch, Arztwahl u. ärztliche Ethik in d. römisch. Kaiserzeit, Das Altertum 18, 1972, pp. 27–30.

liam Heberden, writing in his 'Antitheriaca' (London 1745, p. 4), said that the original mithridatium had all along been used, as well as the deformation of it by Andromachus, and was still prepared by apothecaries according to the recipe of Damocrates, whose Greek iambics were preserved by Galen. The fragments of Andromachus' poem on theriac even became the object of a mediaeval commentary, still unpublished, in a Ms. at Salamanca, Univ. M. 365. Of the two tracts on theriac ascribed to Galen, one dedicated to Piso (XIV, pp. 210–294 K.), the other to Pamphilianus (XIV, pp. 295–310 K.), neither is certainly authentic, although the prosopographical notices in the former are consistent with a date of composition in the late second century.[1] G. Watson, in his unsatisfactory book on theriac[2], expresses surprise that Galen refuses to use theriac here when he had declared it a suitable remedy for quartan fever (De ther. ad Pison. 15: XIV, p. 277,5f. K.). A glance at Jacchinus' commentary would have given him the answer. The cooking effect of theriac, added to the heat generated by the fever as it came to its height, would merely double the effect of the fever, not disperse it (Gal., Meth. med. ad Glaucon. I 12: XI, p. 40,6–10 K.).

P. 78,20: The conjunction of Eudemus' age, quartan fever, the winter season and the fact that the disease had not yet been digested by the humours of the body was very dangerous, especially when a large antidote had been given to stimulate the defences of the body. Galen often stresses the danger of a disease remaining undigested for a long time, for death might follow if the body could not produce a stronger reaction to the disease (In Hipp. Epid. I comment. II 49: CMG V 10,1, p. 74,18–25; In Hipp. Progn. comment. II 31: CMG V 9,2, p. 285,18–23). It was a commonplace of Hippocratic medicine that old men in winter were liable to suffer quartan attacks that were often fatal, the explanation of which was in terms of humoral pathology (Gal., In Hipp. Progn. comment. III 33f.: CMG V 9,2, pp. 357, 10–359,13; In Hipp. Epid. I comment. II 14: CMG V 10,1, p. 56, 23–33).

P. 78,33: Here and at 88,14 and 134,23, the Basle editors added οὖν, following the indication given by Nic.'s "igitur", the preferred version of μὲν οὖν (6: itaque 2: autem 3: quidem 3). But, as H. O. Schröder has shown, CMG Suppl. I, Leipzig and Berlin, 1934, p. 43, with several examples from other treatises, Galen often omits οὖν, especi-

[1] The authenticity of the tract dedicated to Piso is denied by L. Richter-Bernburg, Eine arabische Version der pseudogalenischen Schrift De Theriaca ad Pisonem, Diss. Göttingen 1969, p. 42. I have not seen the edition of the Greek by F. Holtiegel.

[2] G. Watson, Theriac and Mithridatium, London 1966, p. 66. The book, which has very inadequate references, has been strongly criticised for superficiality, especially with regard to the mediaeval herbal tradition, by J. Stannard, Journ. Hist. Med. 21, 1966, p. 430, cf. also M. R. McVaugh, Theriac at Montpellier, 1285–1325, Sudhoffs Archiv f. Gesch. d. Med. u. d. Naturwiss. 56, 1972, pp. 113 to 144.

ally after demonstrative pronouns, and it could well be that the Latin translator regularly turned μέν solitarium by "igitur", cf. also p. 132,24, where μὲν is translated by "igitur". To restore οὖν on the evidence of the Latin alone may be to mistake an idiom of translation for the original text, but the presence of οὕτως here permits an easy palaeographical justification.

P. 80,1–4: A difficult and possibly corrupt passage. Although neither a drug nor a day can be said in strict terms to correspond to a paroxysm, Galen's expression may well be accepted as a shortened form of "corresponding to the drug used in (or "to the day of") the previous paroxysm". Thus, although the words τῷ προτέρῳ παροξυσμῷ are repeated in the next line, there is no compelling reason why they should be removed from the text on grounds of scribal repetition. There are three possible solutions to the problem of the interpretation of this passage, which I give in reverse order of plausibility.

(1) If ἀναλόγου is emended to ἀνάλογον (an easy palaeographic change), it is the drug that corresponds to that used in the earlier paroxysm. But an adjective (or an adjective and noun) must be found to complete ἐπὶ τῆς. The easiest supplement, ἐπιούσης, (cf. Gal., De comp. med. per gen. VII 12: XIII, p. 1022,10 K.) is excluded, unless by this Galen meant that the doctors departed and came again on the next day (the fourth) and gave him the drug, and no suitable numeral for the hour (ἕκτης or ὀγδόης) is immediately compelling. Such an emendation must therefore be rejected, since it creates as many difficulties as it solves.

(2) Nic.'s version "in die proportionali", shows that he assumed that τῆς ἀναλόγου meant "the corresponding day" and that he expanded his Latin to remove any misunderstanding about the meaning of "in proportionali", which, unlike the Greek ἐπὶ τῆς ἀναλόγου, is meaningless by itself. If, then, it is the day that corresponds to that of the previous paroxysm of quartan fever, that day should be the fourth. But, if the day on which the theriac is first given is the first day (p. 78,25), the second attack comes on the second day (p. 80,1), two days earlier than expected, and if the doctors arrive the next morning (ἕωθεν) and give the theriac then, that is the third day, not the fourth. There is nothing to suggest that Galen has omitted a day in his narrative, either by bringing the doctors' arrival forward a day or by failing to indicate clearly that the theriac was given on the fourth, not the third, day. Thus, because the third day does not correspond to the day of an attack of a four day fever, I reject this interpretation, despite the support given to it by Nic.

(3) The last interpretation is that the theriac was given on the third day, at the hour that corresponded to that of the first paroxysm, i. e., at some time in the morning (p. 78,24 f.), shortly after the doctors arrived. This makes good sense, but it may well be doubted whether it is the most obvious meaning of the Greek.

P. 80,11–13: On urinoscopy and its importance for the prediction of the course of a disease, see Gal., De crisib. I 12: pp. 97,12–105,3 Alex. = IX, pp. 594,13–607,2 K.; and In Hipp. Progn. comment. II 26–37: CMG V 9,2, pp. 279,19–290,17. Three small tracts on urinoscopy are ascribed to Galen and are printed by Kühn, XIX, pp. 574–628 K. As can be seen from the series of mediaeval Prognostica Galieni, the concentration upon urine as a sure guide to prognosis flourished for centuries, either under the name of Galen, as in Cambridge University Library Ms. Gg. V 35, fol. 426ʳ (11th cent.), or anonymously, as in Vatican, Regin. Lat. 1324, fol. 66ᵛ (14/15th cent.), whose incipit is: Pronostica urinarum; haec sunt quae in aegrotis vitam aut mortem denunciant futuram.[1]

P. 80,15: For a discussion of the construction and of the use of the aorist participle ἐπισκεψάμενοι, see below, p. 215.

Although the reading of the name in L is possible Greek, cf. the inscription from Pergamum of Iulius Nicodemus ὁ καὶ Νείκων, IGR IV 504, I prefer to believe that καὶ was added by an ignorant scribe who did not know that τε was picked up by καὶ in line 17. L. Sergius Paullus was consul for the first time under Antoninus Pius (CIL VI 253) and cos. II ordinarius in 168 A. D. The date of his urban prefecture, confirmed by CIL VI 1803, is uncertain, possibly c. 170 A. D. Rufinus' Latin version of Eusebius (Hist. Eccl. IV 26) names him as governor of Asia between 164 and 167 A. D., most likely in 164/5 A. D., but since the Greek Mss. and the Armenian version of Eusebius refer to an otherwise unknown Servilius (or Servinius) Paullus, recent scholars have tended to doubt his proconsulate of Asia (especially Birley, Marcus Aurelius, p. 328; Bowersock, p. 83). This passage indicates that he was in Rome during the winter of 162/3 A. D., and the absence of any definite reference to him in Rome after 163 A. D. may well be thought to support the traditional view that depends on Rufinus. I see no reason to identify him with Paullus the orator, mentioned by Galen at In Hipp. De vict. acut. comment. II 29: CMG V 9,1, p. 187,13 and p. 188,13.

P. 80,16f.: ἔπαρχος τῆς πόλεως is the regular Greek version of praefectus urbi. This official, in the Antonine Age usually a senator who had held or was shortly to hold a second consulate, was, among other things, the Emperor's deputy in judicial affairs[2]; Septimius Severus declared that all crimes were within his jurisdiction so long as they were committed in Rome and Italy (Dig. 1, 12, 1, praef.),

[1] A manuscript illustration of Galen examining urine from Dresden Db 92, fol. 293ᵛ, is reproduced by L. C. MacKinney, Medical Illustrations in Mediaeval Manuscripts, London 1965, p. 195, fig. 14, and others are noted in his census, nos. 80,3; 86,85; 94,11; 133,36; and 146,2.

[2] On his powers, see E. Sachers, RE XXII, 1954, cols. 2521–2534, s. v. praefectus urbi; G. Vitucci, Ricerche sulla praefectura urbi in età imperiale, Rome 1956; P. Garnsey, Social status and legal privilege in the Roman Empire, Oxford 1970, pp. 90–100.

although the limit is elsewhere set at one hundred miles from Rome (ibid. 4; Collatio 14, 3, 2).

P. 80,17: Galen calls his male Roman friends either by their cognomen, e. g. Boethus or Paullus, or by their nomen and cognomen, e. g. Claudius Severus (p. 122,12). Only at In Hipp. De artic. comment. II 9: XVIII A, p. 435,13 K., Πλάκινος (= Plancius? Plancinus? or Placidus?) is there a possible parallel, and that very dubious, to Galen's use of the nomen, Flavius, alone, as given by the Mss., and I have accepted Groag's suggestion that the cognomen Βοηθός dropped out.

Flavius Boethus, a Syrian from Ptolemais and later governor of Syria Palaestina, was a great supporter of Galen, who dedicated several treatises to him and who is our sole source of information about him[1]. At their first meeting he is called ὑπατικός, here and at De lib. propr. 1: Scr. min. II, p. 94,20 Müller = XIX, p. 13,4 K., but ὕπατος at Anat. admin. I 1: II, p. 215,6 K. There is no reason to date his consulship precisely to 162/3 A. D., since, as G. W. Bowersock demonstrated, p. 7, n. 1, ὕπατος in a literary text often refers to a consular, ὑπατικός, without implying that he is still in office.

P. 80,18: It was the Aristotelians above all, οἱ τὰς λογικὰς τέχνας μεταχειριζόμενοι, who championed Galen and who welcomed his tract De usu partium (De lib. propr. 2: Scr. min. II, p. 100,21 Müller = XIX, p. 20,16f. K.) for its defence of the logical basis of medical thought against the denials of sceptical philosophers (De usu part. XVII 2: II, pp. 450,26–451,18 Helmr. = IV, pp. 364,15–365,13 K.). On the quarrel between Galen and the Aristotelian Alexander of Aphrodisias, see below, p. 189.

P. 80,19: No reading of the Greek Mss. is acceptable, while the Latin version implies the omission of λείπειν either by the translator in desperation at the corrupt text in front of him or in his Ms. The sense is that Galen's formal prediction made as a result of his prognosis, his prorrhesis, still remained unfulfilled and that Eudemus waited for it to come true. λείπειν, rather than Schöne's ἐκλείπειν, offers an easy explanation of the iotacistic error.

P. 80,24: Among other important friends of Galen should be noted: C. Aufidius Victorinus (In Hipp. De victu acut. comment. III 59: CMG V 9,1, p. 265,22; De diaeta Hipp. in morb. acut. 1: CMG Suppl. Or. II, p. 77,4), whose career has been studied in detail by H. G. Pflaum, Sodales, pp. 41–48; L. Calpurnius Piso, cos. 175[2]; the female philosopher Arria, a close friend of the emperor and wife of the consul and governor of Asia, M. Nonius Macrinus (PIR[2] A. 1115–1116); the anonymous nobleman of Über die medizinischen Namen,

[1] See E. Groag, PIR[2] F. 229; and for the date of his governorship, my article, CQ, p. 169.

[2] Gal., De ther. ad Pison. 1: XIV, pp. 210,1–213,9 K., with the discussion of A. von Premerstein, Das Troiaspiel, Festschrift für Otto Benndorf, Vienna 1898, pp. 261–266, but I am not entirely happy with this identification.

p. 20,4 M.; and possibly C. Pomponius Pollio [1]. That Galen was not the only doctor to have friends in the senate and government is clear from his reference (Meth. med. I 1: X, p. 3,2f. K.) to his opponents' audience, some of which, in the morning after a heavy drinking bout, goes "to the forum and to the courts of no small nation".

P. 80,26f.: The surviving fragments of the treatise that resulted from these demonstrations, 'On the voice and breath', have been capably edited by H. Baumgarten.

P. 82,2f.: On this, admittedly tendentious, evidence, not only human anatomical dissections but even those on animals appear to have been rare in Rome. A knowledge of human anatomy existed at that time at Alexandria, but even here it was probably taught from skeletons rather than from dissections (Gal., Anat. admin. I 2: II, p. 220,15f. K.). This neglect is not surprising, for, as L. Edelstein pointed out (Ancient medicine, pp. 299f.), only the Dogmatic sect and a few eclectics such as Galen insisted upon dissection. The Empirics, for their part, declared that dissection was superfluous since books alone were enough to teach anatomy (Gal., De comp. med. per gen. III 2: XIII, pp. 607,17–608,6 K.).

P. 82,4: M. Vettulenus Sex. f. Civica Barbarus, cos. ord. 157, is an important figure in the history of the Second Sophistic movement. A close friend of Herodes Atticus (Philostratus, Vit. Soph. 537–539; L'Année Epigraphique 1939, 109), he may have known Galen even before 162, if he is the Βάρβαρος ὑπατικός of an inscription from Pergamum (Athenische Mitteilungen 29, 1904, p. 162, line 9; G. W. Bowersock, p. 63, n. 1). A second inscription, from Argos [2], records his services to Lucius Verus in the Parthian War, when he escorted his bride-to-be, Lucilla, to him, but the date of this mission is disputed. G. W. Bowersock, p. 82, thought that Barbarus stayed in Rome until 165 (putting the marriage in 166, as Vita Abercii 44 suggests), but since Galen's last reference to him (p. 98,13) probably comes from summer 163, 'On prognosis' cannot be said to support either this theory or that of T. D. Barnes (Hadrian, p. 72) that the wedding, if indeed it took place, was in 163. [3] The evidence of the Historia Augusta (Vita Marci 9,4), "medio belli tempore", which, taken literally, suggests a date for the wedding in 164, is not opposed by that of Galen and may be accepted until new and better dated testimony supervenes.

[1] See my article, The doctor and the oracle, Rev. Belge de Philologie et de l'Histoire 47, 1969, pp. 37–48.

[2] L'Année Epigraphique 1958, 19. His career has been studied by R. Syme, Antonine relatives, Athenaeum 35, 1957, pp. 306–315, and by H. G. Pflaum, Sodales, pp. 48–50.

[3] His evidence, the omission of Armeniacus from Lucius' titulature on an Ephesian inscription (Jahreshefte d. Österreich. Archäolog. Instituts 44, 1959, Beibl. pp. 257ff., n. 3), is unconvincing because no imperial title at all appears on the inscription and thus there is no dating criterion. For a further argument against 163, see below, p. 190, note 2.

The orthography of proper names is always tricky. I. Müller (Scr. min. II, p. 98, app. crit. on line 22) has set out the problem of the Greek spelling of Lucius. Only in 'On prognosis' is it given with -ευ- rather than with -ου-, although all Mss. of De alim. fac. III 1: CMG V 4,2, p. 336,3 read Λευκανίᾳ. Λούκιος is found at Adv. eos qui de typis scrips. 1: VII, p. 478,15 K.; at De lib. propr. 2: Scr. min. II, p. 98,22 Müller = XIX, p. 18,7 K.; and at In Hipp. Epid. VI comment. IV 10: CMG V 10,2,2, p. 206,17; and the Roman 'u' in Numisianus is represented in Galen by -ου-.[1] Other writers show similar divergencies: Cassius Dio (Hist. LXXI 1,1) and Lucian (Lucius 303) prefer Λούκιος; Plutarch (Cato Maior 24,11, and Otho 5,1) Λεύκιος. Although the form in -ου- is found in more treatises and more Mss. of Galen than that in -ευ-, it may be unwise to standardise the spelling, when other writers differ among themselves and when Galen may not have made up his own mind on the right transliteration. Thus I have retained the Ms. form throughout.

P. 82,4f.: For the campaigns of Lucius Verus against the Parthians, which began in 162 A. D., see Historia Augusta, Vita Veri 6,7–7,10, with the annotations of T. D. Barnes, pp. 70–72. The choice between ἔπ- and ὕπαρχος for Prefect of Mesopotamia (which is not necessarily Verus' official title) is difficult. Both words can mean a provincial governor, see L-S-J, s. vv., and ἔπαρχος is regularly used as the translation of the Latin praefectus, cf. above, p. 80,16. Galen's use of ὕπαρχος at Protr. 5: Scr. min. I, p. 107,25 Marquardt = I, p. 8,5 K. to mean a subordinate official, οἷον ὕπαρχοί τινες καὶ ὑπηρέται τοῦ θεοῦ, thereby emphasising his dependent position, leads me to accept the reading that lies behind Nic.'s version, ἐπάρχου.

P. 82,6: Cn. Claudius Severus, cos. II ordinarius in 173 and a friend of Fronto, is a leading figure in the Second Sophistic movement and may even have delivered public lectures on philosophy before the emperor.[2] He is an easterner in origin, from Pompeiopolis in Paphlagonia, and a member of one of the greatest dynasties of Asia Minor, who married in a second union one of the daughters of Marcus Aurelius. J. Ilberg, NJ, p. 277, followed by PIR[2] C. 1024, accepted this passage as evidence that he was consul for the first time before March 163, and A. Degrassi went further and concluded that he was the same as the suffect consul S]everus who appears on the Fasti Ostienses under the year 160.[3] But a recent attack on this dating has been made by H. G. Pflaum[4], who has argued that, if Severus Arabianus, his father, became consul in 146 suo anno, that is, at the

[1] E. g. Anat. admin. I 1 and VIII 2: II, pp. 217,17 and 660,5 K.; De ord. lib. suor. 3: Scr. min. II, p. 86,24 Müller = XIX, p. 57,8 K.; but cf. the reading Νουμ- adopted by J. Mewaldt at In Hipp. De nat. hom. comment. II 6: CMG V 9,1, p. 70,8 and 10.

[2] O. Murray, Journ. Roman Studies 59, 1969, p. 265.

[3] A. Degrassi, I fasti consolari dell'impero Romano, Rome 1952, p. 132.

[4] H. G. Pflaum, Les gendres de Marc Aurèle, Journ. d. Savants 1961, pp. 29–31.

age of 32 for a patrician senator, he would have been born in 114. On the assumption that he married at 19, his son could not have reached his suus annus before 166, and thus Galen's reference to a consulate before mid-163 is dismissed as an anachronism. But when Galen's other datings are accurate, can we dismiss this one so lightly? H. G. Pflaum's argument is cogent only if all the promotions of Severus and his father are regular. However, if Severus' marriage to Annia Faustina took place in 162/3 (H. G. Pflaum, p. 30) – and it must be admitted that this date is even more uncertain – he may have been advanced to the consulate a few years before his due time as a mark of imperial favour to a son-in-law designate. On either argument A. Degrassi's dating of his consulate is too early, and R. Syme may well be right in suggesting a suffect consulship in 161 for Severus, succeeding Marcus and Verus.[1] J. Ilberg, in an article which has been the foundation of all subsequent studies of the chronology of Galen's life[2], wrongly regards the consular date 163 as fixed and uses it to date Galen's arrival to 162. Twenty five years earlier, NJ, p. 277, he had rightly attacked the problem of the consular date from that of Galen's arrival, and it was unfortunate that he reversed his method of investigation.

P. 82,12: If p. 92,26 is to be taken to mean that Eudemus had been Galen's tutor in philosophy, the words οἷα διδασκάλῳ μὲν can be left to stand: cf. for this use of οἷα De usu part. XII 6: II, p. 197,2 Helmr. = IV, p. 22,1 K.: οἷα παῖς ... ἐμπεσών. The Basle editors omitted καὶ without reason (although Nic. does not translate καὶ . . . καὶ), for the construction καὶ . . . μὲν . . . ἀλλὰ καί is found also at In Hipp. Epid. I comment. III prooem.: CMG V 10,1, p. 126,16. Since I have found no example of Galen's use of καταστυγχάνω with a participle in the sense of τυγχάνω, I have followed the Basle editors in accepting the reading suggested by Nic., κατὰ τύχην.

P. 82,14: Antigenes, one of Galen's Roman opponents, is known only from this anecdote. Unlike other pupils of Quintus, such as Numisianus and Satyrus, he does not appear to have been consulted by Galen in his search for the true teachings of Quintus, whose opinions and discoveries were preserved only among the writings and oral testimony of his students. The literary variation in the references to his two teachers does not involve the conclusion that he spent more time at the feet of Quintus than of Marinus.

P. 82,15: Marinus was the greatest anatomist of the generation before Galen. His writings included twenty books on anatomy, which Galen epitomized to four (Gal., De lib. propr. 3: Scr. min. II, p. 104, 12f. Müller = XIX, p. 25,3f. K.); one on the anatomy of muscles (Gal., De musc. diss. I 1: XVIII B, p. 926,1–3 K.); an introductory tract on anatomy (Gal., Anat. admin. II 1: II, p. 280,2 K.); and he

[1] R. Syme, The Ummidii, Historia 17, 1968, pp. 102f.

[2] J. Ilberg, Wann ist Galenos geboren?, Sudhoffs Archiv f. Gesch. d. Med. 23, 1930, pp. 289–292.

commented upon the Aphorisms of Hippocrates (Gal., In Hipp. Aph. comment. VII 13 and 24: XVIII A, pp. 113,7 and 123,5 K.; cf. In Hipp. Epid. VI comment. V 14: CMG V 10,2,2, p. 287,25ff.). Galen's high opinion of him is clear from Anat. admin. XIV 1: p. 185 Dkw.: Marinus had accumulated no small experience in dissections and it was he himself who had set his hand to and had observed everything that he had explained in his writings. In his great work he had established the record of the bones with the greatest thoroughness and he had laboured to trace all the foramina which perforate the skull and the vertebrae and to exhaust their study, although now and then we may discover him in error; and from De placit. Hipp. et Plat. VIII (1): p. 651,3 Ml. = V, p. 650,7 K.: Marinus revived anatomical observation that had meanwhile fallen into neglect. Not even Hippocrates receives such praise as an anatomist, and, in view of Galen's critical attitude towards other doctors, this is a remarkable tribute to his merits.

P. 82,24f.: For the nominative participle following a dative after an impersonal verb, cf. Lucian, Demosth. Encom. 491: ἀμφὶ γάρ τοι τῶν νυκτῶν ἐξαναστὰς ἔδοξέ μοι . . . ἀπάρξασθαι, and W. Schmid, I, p. 249f.; IV, pp. 114 and 631f. σεμνότης is a favourite virtue among doctors as well as the community at large. K. Deichgräber, Medicus gratiosus, pp. 34 and 74, n. 2, collects some of the references from Galen[1], and his list can be supplemented from many authors (e. g. Marcus Aurelius, Med. I 9,1 and II 5, with Farquharson's notes, Oxford 1944) and from inscriptions (see L. Robert, OMS I, p. 681; Hellenica 13, 1965, p. 222; Revue de Philologie 41, 1967, p. 12, n. 4). A particularly good epigraphic example in honour of a doctor comes from Magnesia ad Maeandrum, Kern 113: T. Claudius Tyrannus is praised because ἀνάλογον πεποίηται τὴν ἐπιδημίαν τῇ περὶ ἑαυτὸν σεμνότητι.

Both genitive and dative are possible with ἐπί (cf. L-S-J s. v. θαυμάζω 5), neither a good Attic usage[2], and although A has the (simpler) pair of datives, I have kept the reading of L and M as displaying variatio, cf. W. Schmid, II, p. 53.

P. 84,1: The phrase δύνειν κατὰ γῆς, repeated in Nic.'s Latin version of De caus. procat. 7,88: CMG Suppl. II, p. 12,28, is a good example of the way in which Galen, unlike the stricter Atticists, was prepared to use colloquial phrases in his writings: cf. 86,16, where ἰάλεμος derives from contemporary speech, see L-S-J s. v.

P. 84,2: All Mss. of this treatise agree in calling Galen's opponent Martianus, but De lib. propr. has the variant Μαρτιάλιος. The corruption of the latter is palaeographically more likely; but Mar-

[1] Add, for the word in a bad sense, De diff. puls. I 1 and II 3: VIII, pp. 494,17; 495,2; and 572,10 K.

[2] The genitive is given by L and M at 90,2, the dative by A: the genitive is found at Gal., De theriaca ad Pison. 2: XIV, p. 217,15 K.; the dative at De loc. aff. V 8: VIII, p. 361,13 K.

tialis is a more common cognomen than Martianus, which is a straight formation from the nomen Martius. But De lib. propr. is based upon only one Greek Ms., and the agreement of several branches of the Ms. tradition in this treatise is enough to counsel against any alteration in the text.[1] He was over seventy when he first heard of Galen, and his claim to be a follower of Erasistratus (De lib. propr. 1: Scr. min. II, pp. 94,23–95,2 Müller = XIX, p. 13,8–12 K.) adds piquancy to the stories of Galen's prognostic cure of Eudemus and of Boethus' wife. Despite Galen's strictures on him, his two books on anatomy were still widely used at least twenty years later (ibid.).

P. 84,7: Galen's cures are often said to have caused amazement among his contemporaries (cf. Gal., De loc. aff. V 8: VIII, pp. 365,10–366,5 K.; De crisib. III 8: pp. 189,18–190,10 Alex. = IX, pp. 737,6–738,6 K.) and they accuse him in turn of relying upon μαντική and premonitions for his cures (Gal., De diff. febr. II 7: VII, p. 354,4–6 K.). Although he ascribes this to their ignorance (De caus. proçat. 3,18: CMG Suppl. II, p. 5,17–23), he does at times make use of such premonitions (De dign. somn.: VI, p. 833,10f. K. and above, p. 134,26f.): καὶ δή τινα μαντικῶς ὑπ' αὐτῆς (sc. τῆς ψυχῆς) προδηλοῦνται. καὶ γὰρ τοῦτο τῇ πείρᾳ μαρτυρεῖται. In this he differs from the Methodists, who believed that to predict the future was the job of a prophet and was thus to be avoided (Gal., In Hipp. Progn. comment. I 1: CMG V 9,2, p. 197,12), a view he attacked in his tract 'On the opinions of Asclepiades' (De nat. fac. I 12: Scr. min. III, pp. 121,24–122,3 Helmr. = II, p. 29,7–11 K.). His opposition to divination was not based upon a denial of its occasional effectiveness but upon its unreliability if exclusively trusted and upon the uses to which it was put. His own prognoses (Gal., Über die medizinischen Namen, p. 21,14ff. M.) were attained by rational calculation, not by acting as a prophet, augur or astrologer, whose predictions did not allow for changing circumstances (Gal., De const. art. med. 17: I, p. 292,2–4 K.). The physician is thus more flexible than the prophet (Gal., In Hipp. Epid. II comment. III: CMG V 10,1, p. 282,10–13), whose predictions only rarely came true. "I have never seen a prophet make a true prediction about an invalid in Rome – and I have never experienced them elsewhere" (Gal., In Hipp. Epid. I comment. III 17: CMG V 10,1, p. 125,25–27). Other doctors were less scrupulous. Iulius Africanus (ed. O. Thevenot and D. Boivin, Veteres mathematici, Paris 1693, p. 296) claims that if a man digs a deep hole, he will be able to discover the future course of a disease and reveal it as a prophet.[2]

[1] See W. A. Greenhill, Smith's Dictionary of Greek and Roman Biography II, London 1854, cols. 942 and 963, s. vv. Martianus and Martilius; W. Kroll, RE XIV (1930), col. 2003, s. v. Martianus. K. Deichgräber's reference, Medicus gratiosus, p. 28, n. 2, to this man as Martilianus is, I suspect, a slip of the pen rather than an attempt to harmonize the two versions.

[2] On the attitudes of doctors in general to prophecy and divination, see G. Stroh-

P. 84,8f.: According to Galen (In Hipp. De vict. acut. I 15: CMG V 9,1, p. 129,1), it was only divination from the flight of birds that conferred the title of μάντις. He does not accept the validity of such divination of the course of a disease (In Hipp. Epid. VI comment. IV 27: CMG V 10,2,2, p. 244,5–23), since to draw inferences from the flight of birds is no part of medicine, except that, as Hippocrates said, fine days are healthier than foul. Indeed, when he records a debate between an Arabian and a Greek bird diviner (In Hipp. De vict. acut. comment. I 15: CMG V 9,1, pp. 129,12–130,17) in which each endeavoured to prove the merits of his case by citing further texts and by producing witnesses of his past achievements, he condemns them only for their folly in applying a rule drawn from a particular case to a general situation (ibid. I 16: CMG V 9,1, p. 131,29–32). He disputes their premisses, not their success. His discussion of divination in the course of his eight volume work on the opinions of Asclepiades (De nat. fac. I 12: Scr. min. III, p. 121,24 Helmr. = II, p. 29,9 K.) has unfortunately not survived.[1]

The speciality of the bird diviner continued to flourish. The Traditio Apostolica, 16, forbade any bird diviner, magus, astrologer, soothsayer, conjurer, maker of phylacteries, etc., from being given instruction or Christian baptism, and several inscriptions record οἰωνόσκοποι (see L. Robert, OMS III, p. 1283; Hellenica 2, 1946, pp. 43–50). The competence of the augur or bird diviner in predicting the future, especially health and sickness, was often noticed by the satirists, e. g. Juvenal, Sat. V 585:

"divitibus responsa dabit Phryx augur,"

and, as A. A. Barb pointed out[2], the tradition of birds, especially eagles and vultures, had a very long history in medico-magical lore. Such magic and divinatory lore, as Galen realised, complemented medicine, it did not replace it, and there must have been many, as in sixteenth and seventeenth century England, who had recourse to it before a doctor and who felt that they derived benefit from it.[3]

P. 84,10: Galen (In Hipp. De vict. acut. comment. I 15: CMG V 9,1, p. 128,15–20) identifies θυτική with ἱεροσκοπία, which he describes as prophecy from the entrails of sacrificial victims. It was practised especially among the Etruscans, where, in the particular form of hepatoscopy carried on by haruspices, it displays some af-

maier, pp. 375f.; L. Edelstein, pp. 239–244; L. Thorndike, A history of magic and experimental science, I, London 1923, pp. 165–181.

[1] For Galen's views on oionoscopy, see further, K. S. Kontos, Athenaion 7, 1878, pp. 246–250, and K. Deichgräber, Ausgewähltes aus der medizinischen Literatur der Antike, I, Philologus 101, 1957, pp. 135–147.

[2] A. A. Barb, Birds and medical magic, Journ. Warburg and Courtauld Institutes 13, 1950, pp. 318–322.

[3] K. B. Thomas, Religion and the decline of magic: studies in popular beliefs in sixteenth and seventeenth century England, London 1971, pp. 209f. The whole section on magic and astrology, pp. 177–388, will be found illuminating (cf. also pp. 623–628).

finity with Babylonian medicine[1], without proving any derivation therefrom.

συμβολική is divination by means of σύμβολα (cf. Gal., In Hipp. De vict. acut. comment. I 15: CMG V 9,1, p. 128,25f.). An early reference to this speciality is made by Xenophon (Mem. I 1,3): ὁ δ' οὐδὲν καινότερον εἰσφέρει τῶν ἄλλων ὅσοι μαντικὴν νομίζοντες οἰωνοῖς τε χρῶνται καὶ φήμαις καὶ συμβόλοις καὶ θυσίαις, where the Rev. C. E. Moberly, in his edition, London 1886, while explaining that the σύμβολον was an omen met by the way, like a wolf or a snake, was moved to warn his Protestant readers against the properties of the evil eye popularly ascribed to Pope Pius IX. This method of divination remained common at least until the time of Iamblichus (Vit. Pyth. 13,62), who wrote περὶ οἰωνῶν καὶ συμβόλων καὶ διοσημιῶν. This explanation of σύμβολον as a chance occurrence must be distinguished from the theurgic practices of late antiquity in which statues of the gods were animated by the draping of σύμβολα, their earthly signs, around them to utter oracles.[2]

Astrological medicine was common[3], especially in Egypt, where the Historia Augusta (Vita Saturnini 8,3) states that "every head of a synagogue, every Samaritan and every Christian presbyter was an astrologer, a soothsayer or a masseur.", which R. Syme connects with the list of magical skills in Juvenal, Sat. III 76f. and VI 553 and 580f.:

"aegra licet iaceat, capiendo nulla videtur
aptior hora cibo nisi quam dederit Petosiris."[4]

One doctor even went so far as to boast of his astrological ability on his tombstone[5]:

ὧδ' Ἐπάφου γέννημα, σοφοῖς ἐπ⟨ι⟩είκελος ἀνήρ
κεῖμαι, Ῥωμαίων σπέρμα πολυκτεάνων
κληζόμενος Δέκμος Σερουίλιος, εἰς ἔτη ἐλθών
ἐννέα που δεκάδων καὶ τρία, ὡς ἔλεγον.

As a result of such benefits gained from astrology Alexander Severus may have given official support to and recognition of astrologers (Historia Augusta, Vit. Alex. 44), but contemporary legal decisions cast doubt on this evidence.[6]

Within the Galenic corpus there is at least one treatise on astrological medicine, the Prognostica de decubitu, for which an Egyptian

1 G. Furlani, Mantica Hittita e mantica Etrusca, Studi Etruschi 10, 1936, pp. 1–12.

2 E. R. Dodds, The Greeks and the irrational, Berkeley 1951, pp. 292f.

3 On astrology in general, see W. and H. G. Gundel, Astrologoumena, Sudhoffs Archiv f. Gesch. d. Med. u. d. Naturwiss., Beiheft 6, Wiesbaden 1966, with the criticisms expressed by M. Plessner, Isis 62, 1971, pp. 397–401.

4 R. Syme, Ammianus and the Historia Augusta, Oxford 1969, p. 61ff.

5 CIL X 1497 (= IG XIV 809). I cannot accept the division of line 1 proposed by W. Peek, Griechische Vers-Inschriften, Berlin 1955, n. 435: ὧδε Πάφου.

6 J. Straub, Severus Alexander und die Mathematici, Bonner Historia-Augusta-Colloquium 1968/9, Bonn 1970, pp. 247–272.

origin was invoked by S. Weinstock[1], and the later version of the mediaeval Prognostica Galieni represented by Montpellier, Faculté de Médecine, Ms. 185 (10/11th cent.), fol. 1r; and Vatican, Reginens. Lat. 1324 (14/15th cent.), fol. 66r, is clearly influenced by astrological ideas.

Although Galen had been informed that Egyptian astrologers had discovered that the phases of the moon affected the course of a disease (Gal., De dieb. decret. III 6: IX, p. 911,14ff. K.) and that planetary conjunctions at a patient's birth determined his future health, he refused to accept their theories entirely. While agreeing that the seasons and the phases of the moon affect the atmosphere, a fact he observed himself, and that astronomical observations in the manner of Hippocrates and Aratus are valuable in predicting the varying course of a disease (Gal., In Hipp. Epid. VI comment. IV 27: CMG V 10,2,2, pp. 244,24–245,4), it is observation of the definite atmospheric changes, not the rough calculation of the number of days unaided by experience, that is to be used in forecasting (Gal., De dieb. decret. III 6: IX, p. 914,3–18 K.). Such ideas on the influence of seasons and climate go back at least to Hippocrates, especially to 'Airs, waters and places', and Galen (ibid., IX, p. 913,10–16 K.) sees himself as representing this tradition when he attacks those who refuse to believe in the effects of atmospheric changes. "If you are unwilling to see this or to believe those who have seen it, you are one of the modern cheapjack sophists who demand that we justify in argument obvious phenomena (i. e. and go no further until this has been done), when in fact they should proceed from clear phenomena to a logical conclusion about what is obscure." This does not mean that he accepted without demur the teachings of the astrologers, far from it. He disclaims all connection with the practitioners of number mysticism (ibid. 11: IX, pp. 934,10–936,16 K.), whose basis, unlike that of astronomy and meteorology, did not rest upon careful rational observation. Whereas some of his contemporaries, like Pamphilus and Xenocrates, were less scrupulous about what they accepted, Galen's reliance upon astronomy[2] and dreams is conditioned by the rational uses to which they are set and by the logical demonstration by which they are tested.

P. 84,18: The dative after θαρρῶν is frowned upon by the Atticists (W. Schmid, IV, p. 180), but is regularly used by Galen: cf. In Hipp. Prorrhet. I comment. III 6: CMG V 9,2, p. 114,22, μὴ θαρρεῖν ὡς καθολικῷ τῷ λόγῳ; In Hipp. Epid. VI comment. I 10: CMG V 10,2,2, p. 32,26: τῇ τῶν οὔρων ἐπισχέσει θαρρεῖν; and III 40: CMG V 10,2,2, p. 181,13f.: μὴ τοίνυν αὐτῷ θαρρήσῃς μόνῳ. It

[1] S. Weinstock, The author of the Ps. Galen Prognostica de decubitu, Class. Quart. 42, 1948, pp. 41ff.

[2] On Galen's knowledge of astronomy, see De plac. Hipp. et Plat. VIII (1): p. 655, 8–15 Ml. = V, p. 654,9–16 K.; De septimestri partu, ed. R. Walzer, Rivista di Studi Orientali 15, 1935, pp. 346ff., and O. Neugebauer, ibid. 24, 1949, pp. 92–94.

was constructions and usages like this that would have led Phrynichus (p. 160, ed. Lobeck) to class Galen with the "unlearned physicians" who loved to commit grammatical solecisms (cf. ibid., p. 152 with ἐπίδοξον, above, p. 136,2).

P. 86,20: The emendation of the Basle editors, τετάχαται, is possibly correct, as the examples collected by I. Müller, Scr. min. II, p. XIX, suggest. But Galen may be using ὁδοὶ τέτμηνται metaphorically, cf. for a literal use of the phrase, Meth. med. X 8: X, p. 633,6f. K.

P. 86,22: Galen followed in the tradition of doctors such as Celsus (Med. VI 18,9: CML I, pp. 295,30–296,22), for whom the habitual bleeding from piles was regarded as a periodic natural cleansing, a purgation, not as a disease, and he advises against the checking of the bleeding since in its turn it will produce an affliction like dropsy (Gal., De nat. fac. II 8: Scr. min. III, p. 180,19–22 Helmr. = II, p. 109, 13–16 K.).

P. 86,24–29: The method of reasoning by elimination is a favourite of Galen, and another good example is found at De praes. ex puls. I 4: IX, pp. 248,19–249,17 K. A hard pulse is brought about by drinking wine or cold water at the wrong time, by eating fruit, and by using a cold bath. The pulse produced by taking wine increases in size, speed and vigour, as well as in hardness: that produced by the other causes only in hardness. The presence of other symptoms indicates that the patient has taken cold fruit and even what the fruit was: e. g. an attack of delirium means vinous fruit. If none of these signs are present and if the pulse increases only in hardness, the condition has been caused by cold water, either drunk or as a cold bath. Cf. also, for the same method of argument, below, p. 194.

P. 88,1: There is no doubt that Galen regularly used διείλεγμαι for the augmented perfect of διαλέγομαι, but can this be also assumed for the aorist and imperfect? L-S-J, p. 400, record only διε- but G. Helmreich showed complete Ms. support for διειλέχθην at In Hipp. De vict. acut. comment. II 53: CMG V 9,1, p. 214,2. The Mss. of 'On prognosis' are divided on this point: L, the oldest and best, has διελέχθη here, at 104,6 and at 114,3, M διει-. A has here a variant, διη-, phonetically equivalent to διει-. Elsewhere, In Hipp. Epid. I comment. III 1: CMG V 10,1, p. 106,28, has διελέγετο, and De aff. dign. 4,13: CMG V 4,1,1, p. 15,3 and De pecc. dign. 5,21: CMG V 4,1,1, p. 59, 30, διελέχθην and διελέχθη. On the whole the evidence is against Helmreich and I have thus kept the spelling of L.

P. 88,2: Galen's case usage after ἀκούειν remains undetermined, cf. CMG V 10,2,3, p. 33: I have retained the genitive here as a variation on the accusative at 86,6.

P. 88,3: It was Aristotle and the Peripatetics who above all defined moral virtue in terms of a mean between two extremes (Aristotle, Eth. Nic. 1106b–1107a), and thus Galen's joke at the philosopher who was immoderately excited has added point.

P. 88,4: If ἡμᾶς is to be retained, it is ironically associative (cf. Giangrande, Revue des Etudes Grecques 94, 1968, p. 62), of which another Galenic example is at De plac. Hipp. et Plat. V (3): p. 424,9 Ml. = V, p. 447,14 K. If this explanation is thought unconvincing, then the simple change to ὑμᾶς should be made (cf. B. Alexanderson, Bemerkungen zu Galens ... De placitis, Eranos 68, 1970, p. 69). A is damaged precisely at the doubtful letter, although the space available favours ὑ more than ἡ, but, even so, its reading can be dismissed, if required, as a scribal conjecture.

The cult of Apollo the healer (iatros) was widespread[1], but Eudemus' exclamation refers to the successful prediction rather than the cure. Note also Galen's opinion in his Commentary on the Hippocratic Oath (Bull. Hist. Med. 30, 1956, pp. 66f.): "Asclepius is said to be the son of Apollo; for the doctor should possess up to a point the gift of divination. No complete doctor can fail to know what is going to happen later." Cf. also above, p. 124,19.

P. 88,16: H. Schöne's emendation is very attractive. There is nothing to suggest that Martianus was among Galen's friends and supporters or that he could have been acknowledged as such, more the opposite if we are to believe Gal., De lib. propr. 1: Scr. min. II, p. 94,26ff. Müller = XIX, p. 13,11ff. K., while, on the other hand, Galen's ideal of the philosopher doctor was not unique. Asclepius was as much a philosopher as a doctor (Gal., Comment. on the Hippocratic Oath, Bull. Hist. Med. 30, 1956, p. 68 and Journ. Asiatique 5, 3, 1854, pp. 247f.; Aelian, frag. 99; O. Weinreich, Antike Heilungswunder, Gießen 1909, p. 113 and p. 129); Julian claimed to follow Zeno, Plato and Aristotle in his teaching (Gal., Adv. Iulianum 4,1: CMG V 10,3, pp. 42,9–43,3); Sextus, the contemporary head of the Empiric sect, wrote philosophical treatises on scepticism[2]; and two doctors mentioned their philosophical abilities on inscriptions. Menecrates of Sosandra is simply ἰ]ατρὸν καὶ φιλ[οσοφ]ον[3], but Heracleitus of Rhodiapolis (IGR III 733) is πρῶτος ἀπ' αἰῶνος ἰατρὸς καὶ συγγραφεὺς καὶ ποιητὴς ἔργων ἰατρικῆς καὶ φιλοσοφίας (cf. also IG XIV 1900, from Rome). Other (non-medical) specialists stressed the philosophical importance of their art: Strabo (Geogr. I 1,18f.) praises the merits of geography; Vitruvius (De archit. I 1ff.) those of architecture; and Lucian, in a deliberate parody (De salt. 35,81), those of dancing. Such a claim could thus have been easily made by Martianus and accepted by his contemporaries.

The word μαρτυρεῖν is also found on several honorific inscrip-

[1] B. Lifshitz, Inscriptions grecques de la côte nord du Pont-Euxin, La Parola del Passato 20, 1965, pp. 478f.; W. M. Calder III, Amer. Journ. Archaeology 75, 1971, p. 328, n. 54.

[2] K. Deichgräber, Emp., pp. 216ff.; F. Kudlien, Die Datierung des Sextus Empiricus und des Diogenes Laertius, Rheinisches Museum 106, 1965, pp. 251–254.

[3] IGR IV 1359; V. Nutton, Menecrates of Sosandra, doctor or vet?, Zeitschr. f. Papyrologie u. Epigraphik 22, 1976, pp. 93–96.

tions to doctors: IGR III 694, from Aperlae in Lycia, describes a doctor as μαρτυρηθεὶς ἐπὶ πάσῃ τῇ τοῦ βίου καλοκαγαθίᾳ, and a female doctor from Tlos is μαρτυρηθεῖσα ὑπὸ τῆς Τλωέων βουλῆς καὶ τοῦ δήμου ἐπὶ τῇ περὶ τὴν ἰατρικὴν τέχνην ἐνπειρίᾳ.[1]

P. 88,20: The street of the Sandalmakers was by Galen's time the centre of the Roman book trade. His story of how he heard a man detect a Galenic forgery up for sale on a stall there (De lib. propr., Praef.: Scr. min. II, p. 91,3–13 Müller = XIX, pp. 8,5–9,4 K.) is parallelled by that of Aulus Gellius (Noct. Attic. XVIII 4,1), who tells how, when he was "in Sandaliario forte apud librarios", his friends unmasked the pretensions of a man who claimed to be the only true interpreter of Sallust still alive.[2] The spelling of the name presents difficulties. The three Latin inscriptions, ILS 3614, ILS 3308 and Bollettino Communale 5, 1877, p. 162, and the Mss. of Aulus Gellius all give the form "Sandaliarius" and thus H. Jordan and C. Huelsen, Topographie der Stadt Rom, I, Berlin 1907, p. 329, n. 17, emended the text at Scr. min. II, p. 91,3 Müller = XIX, p. 8,5 K. and at 94,8 to that of the inscriptions. The Ms. tradition of Galen is not strong, and the presence of an 'm' in Nic.'s "Damarium" can best be taken as indicating a confusion between Λ and Ι in his Greek Ms. or its source, and Jordan and Huelsen's example should be followed here.

P. 88,21: μηδέ, not μήτε, would be the correct Attic form, as H. Schöne saw; but the papyri and later Greek texts show such a confusion between the two that the error could easily have been that of Galen himself rather than of a later scribe.[3]

P. 88,22: It is evident from his commentary on Hippocrates' Prorrheticon I and from his statements at In Hipp. Epid. III comment. I 4: CMG V 10,2,1, p. 13,7–12 that Galen, like Erotian before him (p. 135, ed. Nachmanson), regarded only the first book of the Prorrheticon as genuine. Even on this he had doubts. Its language contained non-Hippocratic words (Gal., In Hipp. Prorrhet. I comment. I 4: CMG V 9,2, p. 13,27ff.) and, although furnishing an accurate record of particular observations, it was wildly wrong (i. e. non-Hippocratic) in its general conclusions from the evidence (ibid. III 7 and 34: CMG V 9,2, p. 115,3–21; p. 148,1–15; In Hipp. Epid. III comment. II prooem.: CMG V 10,2,1, p. 62,6f.). As for those who follow its teaching rather than that of the Prognosticon, the Aphorisms and the Epidemics,

[1] Tituli Asiae Minoris II 2, 595. Cf. Supplementum Epigraphicum Graecum 13, 1956, 526 (from Amisus in Pontus): τέχνης πολλοί μάρτυρές εἰσιν ἐμῆς; Journ. Roman Stud. 57, 1967, p. 41 (Choma in Lycia), a doctor κριθέ[ντα ...] ἀλιτούργητον: and a doctor from Magnesia ad Maeandrum, O. Kern, n. 113, is δεδοκιμασμένος τοῖς θεοῖς κριτηρίοις τῶν Σεβαστῶν ἐπὶ τῇ τέχνῃ τῆς ἰατρικῆς καὶ τῇ κοσμιότητι τῶν ἠθῶν.

[2] The street lay in Regio IV, close by the temple of Tellus and North East of the Forum Pacis, see S. B. Platner and T. Ashby, p. 577.

[3] See Blass-Debrunner-Funk, § 445,1; G. Dalmeyda, ed. of Xenophon of Ephesus, Paris 1926, p. XXXVII.

from which it takes its most valuable portions, they are mere λογιατροί (ibid. I 40: CMG V 10,2,1, p. 59,2–14), doctors in name only. That there is some genuine Hippocratic material in Prorrheticon I is admitted by Galen, but its author has confused it with much of his own invention (In Hipp. Prorrhet. I comment. II 17: CMG V 9,2, p. 67,30ff.). But what of Prorrheticon II? The arguments of Erotian and Galen against authenticity are never stated and thus their force cannot be estimated, but Littré himself, IX, p. 1, believed that the style, irony, common sense and practicality of the tract suggested a connection with Hippocrates. As far as can be known, Galen's criteria for authenticity were never so subjective[1], for he relied upon the treatises generally considered Hippocratic as a basis for checking the others. His main guides are the language, thought and teaching of Hippocrates as expressed in these 'genuine' treatises, and to some extent his belief that what he himself found to be false was written by a physician inferior to Hippocrates. But since in antiquity, as much as now, there was much speculation upon the authenticity of every book in the Corpus Hippocraticum[2] and some doctors based their Hippocratic theories upon books that others considered non-Hippocratic, a simple reliance upon 'accepted writings' was basically dangerous. However, it is fair to praise both Erotian and Galen for using the evidence of language collected in their Hippocratic glossaries in an attempt to determine authenticity objectively: it was their selection of primary data, not their methods, that led them astray.

P. 88,26: All the Mss. of this passage as given in Littré's apparatus, IX, p. 8,2 L., read μαντεύσομαι, but this is not sufficient reason for changing Galen's text. Even after the great editions of Dioscorides and Capito there were many variants in the text of Hippocrates in circulation, some of which were diligently collected and published by Rufus of Samaria.[3] Galen's quotation may derive from one of these variants or, more likely, is a slightly inaccurate reference made from memory without recourse to a text (cf. above, p. 156).

P. 90,1: καὶ ὅς of the Mss. should be retained both here and at 124,9, although asyndeton results there, since it is another example of an archaic or Platonising usage (cf. Phaedo 118A; Protagoras 310D) being retained and employed by Galen.

P. 90,8–92,33: This whole section is a fine example of a well known rhetorical topos: the evils of the city, here contrasted with the friend-

[1] See L. O. Bröcker, Die Methoden Galens in der literarischen Kritik, Rheinisches Museum 40, 1885, pp. 415–438: the references to his lost treatise 'On the genuine and spurious writings of Hippocrates' are given by J. Mewaldt, pp. 111–134; and by M. Ullmann, p. 53, no. 72.

[2] See L. Edelstein, RE Suppl. VI, 1936, cols. 1315–1317, s. v. Hippokrates; G. E. R. Lloyd, The Hippocratic question, Classical Quarterly n. s. 25, 1975, pp. 171–192.

[3] F. Pfaff, Rufus aus Samaria, Hermes 67, 1932, pp. 356–359; Die Überlieferung des Corpus Hippocraticum in der nachalexandrinischen Zeit, Wiener Studien 50, 1932, pp. 67–82.

liness of the small town rather than with the peaceful countryside of pastoral tradition. The antithesis between town and country is a common theme among second century authors. Juvenal (Sat. III), Pliny (Ep. I 9), Martial (Ep. III 38), Tacitus (Dial. 11f.), Dio Chrysostom (Or. 7), Lucian (Nigrinus), all offer variations upon it in different degrees of realism[1], and Galen's interpretation, unique as far as I know and adorned with all the trappings of rhetoric (cf. J. Ilberg, NJ, pp. 287f.), is equally literary and equally stylised. Aristeides (Or. 23 and 24) and Plutarch (Jones, pp. 110–121) may give a truer picture of the turmoil and the hardships of life in the cities of the Eastern provinces – which Galen also notices when he writes with less passion.

P. 90,9: His homeland, Asia Minor and Pergamum, is prominent in Galen's thoughts and affections. Despite his long residence in Rome, he still considers Pergamum his home and often allies himself with its inhabitants in his choice of words. "Among us" is at Pergamum; "our king" is Attalus[2], and, as for the intention of his writings, "I write for Greeks and for those who are barbarian by birth but aspire to Greek pursuits" (De sanit. tuenda I 10,17: CMG V 4,2, p. 24, 22–25). He is indifferent to Rome's achievements. Trajan's new straight roads, with their bridges and cuttings, are mentioned only as a parallel to Galen's own successes (Meth. med. IX 8: X, p. 633, 1–10 K.); and al-Mubaššir, p. 56, associates this with a commendation of the emperors for attending to the welfare of their subjects rather than to bodily desires. He can thus in no way be likened to the eulogistic Aristeides or to Cassius Dio, who combined Roman political traditions with the cultural outlook of a Greek, but he is similar to them in his cultural bias.[3] His literary references are to Greek authors, including such rarities as Cercidas (Meth. med. VI 3: X, p. 406,3 K.), Euphorion (In Hipp. Epid. VI comment. I 29: CMG V 10,2,2, p. 51, 1f. and De septim. partu: Rivista di Studi Orientali 15, 1935, p. 348), and Plutarch (De plac. Hipp. et Plat. III (2): p. 266,3 Ml. = V, p. 300,17 K.).[4] This should not be taken to indicate hostility to Rome, rather as another indication of the expansion of Greek ideas within the oikoumene of the Roman Empire, in which the Greeks shared and for whose culture they could take much credit. After all, Marcus Aurelius wrote his Meditations in Greek, like a Greek.

In legal theory, it is just at this period that the concept of πατρίς/origo begins to play a part in the debate over the demands and obliga-

[1] G. Highet, Juvenal the Satirist, Oxford 1954, pp. 64–68.

[2] H. Schöne, Τὸ τοῦ Τραιάνου γυμνάσιον, Hermes 52, 1917, pp. 107ff.

[3] Cf. the evidence collected by J. Palm, Rom, Römertum und Imperium in der griechischen Literatur der Kaiserzeit, Lund 1959, pp. 130ff.; F. Millar, A study of Cassius Dio, Oxford 1964, pp. 174–192; G. W. Bowersock, pp. 15ff.; and my article in P. Garnsey and C. R. Whittaker, Imperialism in the ancient world, Cambridge 1978, pp. 209–221.

[4] His interest in Jewish and Christian literature is well described by R. Walzer, JC.

tions of citizenship[1] and it was only now that there was a clear ruling that a person domiciled abroad, like Galen, was expected to contribute his share to the services of his native town.

P. 90,15: ὡς ἄν + participle, used in the sense of ἅτε, is a construction rarely discussed in the standard grammars, although common in later Greek prose. It is a favourite usage of Xenophon, see L-S-J, s. v. ὡσάν, and is frequently found in Galen.[2] The ἄν does not indicate potentiality but the unreality of the supposed reason, see Eunapius, ed. Boissonade, p. 587; E. Mayser, II, p. 356.

P. 90,17: As R. Walzer has shown (GA, pp. 160f.), Galen distinguished between those who are naturally good and cannot be corrupted; those who are naturally bad and cannot be improved; and those who are in an intermediate state and who are rendered good by the company and admonitions of the good. To which of the last two categories have we to assign the persons here described by Galen? Are they naturally wicked, as L and M suggest? or are they merely "inclined to wickedness", the reading of A, and thus capable of correction?[3] From line 11, "those who are already wicked", I believe that these are persons already naturally corrupt who find a greater play for their misdeeds in Rome and emulate their fellow criminals. It is the combination of their nature, the many opportunities for crime and their greater knowledge of the ways of wickedness that has increased their corruption, which they had under control at home in the provinces, without mastering it entirely[4]. Although A's reading is plausible, it is much weaker than that of L and M and may well be the invention of a scribe unhappy at the meaning of the second φύσει.

P. 90,20: The anonymity of the city of Rome, where it is impossible for all to know each other, p. 92,30, as in Aristotle's ideal city (Pol. 1326b), is Galen's chief confessed reason for disliking Rome. In De examinando medico (p. 193,8–10 Dietrich) he condemns Rome as a city full to excess with those seeking after gain, where a neighbour may die almost unnoticed and without involving the incompetent doctor in any loss of reputation. In these circumstances the task of choosing a doctor was not easy. In De examinando medico Galen advises his friends to make use first of doctors recommended them by their friends (cf. De puero epilept. cons. I: XI, pp. 357,3–358,16 K.), but such personal knowledge was not always available. Public debate and

[1] D. Norr, Origo, Tijdschrift voor Rechtsgeschiedenis 31, 1963, pp. 530ff.; and my article, JRS, pp. 52–55.

[2] E. g. De dign. puls. II 1: VIII, p. 826,8 K.; De caus. puls. I 9: IX, p. 15,9 K.; De antid. I 1: X, p. 4,5f. K.; Thras. 7: Scr. min. III, p. 39,15 Helmr. = V, p. 815,6 K.

[3] Although the Latin version "malignorum" appears to favour A, little weight can be attached to it, since the translation is here too imprecise to be reliable, whichever reading is adopted in the Greek.

[4] For the construction οὐ μόνον ... οὐδὲ ... ἀλλὰ καί, see R. Kühner and B. Gerth, Ausführliche Grammatik der griechischen Sprache, Satzlehre, 4th ed., vol. 2, Hannover 1955, 2, p. 257.

discussion, although it might reveal some of the incompetents, was never entirely reliable. Pliny (Nat. Hist. XXIX 17) says that a Greekless doctor is not respected by the illiterate and inexperienced, who have greater confidence in a doctor's prescriptions the less they understand them. Nor had a patient any chance of estimating the ability of a doctor who hawked his wares around the city, touting for cases (Epictetus, III 23–27). Unlike the provincial cities, Rome had no system of approved practitioners until Valentinian's law of 368, although some form of registration may have been employed, and thus an invalid had no obvious doctor of merit to engage.[1]

P. 90,22: It is easy to substantiate Galen's claim that great profits could be made in Rome. The fees of imperial doctors were high. Charmis of Massilia (Pliny, Nat. Hist. XXIX 22) charged 200,000 HS for a single cure and one thousand Attic drachmas for less than a pound of one drug[2]. C. Stertinius Xenophon pointed out to Claudius that his city practice brought him in 600,000 HS a year, and had his annual retainer increased from 250,000 to 500,000 HS (ibid. XXIX 7). Alcon, a surgeon fined 1,000,000 HS by Claudius and exiled to Gaul, later returned to Rome to recover that amount within a few years (ibid. 22). Crinas of Massilia (ibid. 9 and 22), despite giving nearly ten million sesterces towards the rebuilding of the walls of his native city, still left more than ten million at his death. Arruntius left thirty million, the same as the combined estate of Xenophon and his brother (ibid. 7). These incomes are far higher than the salaries paid to the top equestrian procurators of the imperial administration, some 200,000 HS per annum, and H. G. Pflaum, CP, p. 43, justly remarks that Xenophon's 500,000 HS a year is not consonant with his position within the administration as "ad responsa graeca", which probably carried an annual salary of no more than 100,000 HS.

But evidence from writers contemporary with Galen or from Galen himself is scanty. The bet of a thousand drachmas (Gal., Anat. admin. VII 16: II, p. 642,8 K.) implies wealth on the part of the contending doctors, but only once does Galen appear to receive a substantial fee, 40,000 HS for his cure of Boethus' wife, above, p. 116,18[3], which, not unnaturally, provoked his opponents to envy. Nor was Rome the only place where wealth could be obtained. L. Staius Rutilius Manilius, archiater at Beneventum, was wealthy enough to become a knight (ILS 6496)[4] and P. Decimus P. lib. Merula, medicus

[1] The law is Cod. Theod. XIII 3,8: see further, V. Nutton, JRS, pp. 61ff. and Archiatri, Papers of the British School at Rome 45, 1977, pp. 191–226.

[2] Gal., De antid. II 4: XIV, pp. 126,6–127,18 K., reading Χάρμις at p. 127,17, cf. p. 128,2 K.

[3] I exclude the estate worth three hundred dinars given him by Qustās, as the tract in which this is mentioned, On the secrets of men and On the secrets of women, trans. M. Levey and S. S. Souryal, Janus 55, 1968, pp. 208–219 [p. 215], is almost certainly falsely attributed to him.

[4] That is, possessing a property census rating of 400,000 HS, which would make him a respectable member of the curial class in his local provincial town.

clinicus chirurgus ocularius at Assisi, after disbursing 119,000 HS in his lifetime, left 800,000 HS at his death (ILS 5369, 7812). At Pergamum the young pupil of Metrodorus would have been rich for life if he had made a particular successful cure (Gal., In Hipp. Epid. II comment. VI: CMG V 10,1, p. 401,6–43), while the expenses of Heracleitus of Rhodiapolis on a temple, statues and games in honour of Asclepius amounted to 60,000 HS (IGR III 732f.). Samiades of Mastaura erected a shrine and sanctuary to Asclepius (L. Robert, Etudes anatoliennes, Paris 1937, p. 256) and doctors holding high office in city and province, a sure sign of wealth, are found throughout Asia Minor; e. g. at Aperlae in Lycia (IGR III 693), at Ephesus (CIG 2987), and at Sebaste in Phrygia (CIG 3872b). Others married their daughters into the highest provincial nobility; e. g. Aquilus of Synnada (Mon. Asiae Min. Antiquae VI 373) and Aurelius Isidorus of Thessalonica (IG X ii 1. 163). At a lower level, a Ptolemaic papyrus suggests that the teaching and practice of the speciality of an ἰατροκλύστης would provide a suitable income until old age. [1]

This section on the desire of immigrant doctors for gain and their general unfitness is a major example of Galen's inconsistency. He attacks foreigners who come to Rome, though he is one himself: he criticises their greed for gold, but rejoices in the money he gets from Boethus. Is this rhetorical nonsense? or a display of thick skinned indifference to the opinions of others? or a sign of Galen's psychological confusion? In trying to solve this problem, we should not forget that moralising had entered into the writing of autobiography at least with Nicolaus of Damascus [2] and such a motif, the revelation of one's own righteousness and virtue, could well have become traditional.

P. 90,23-26: The thought here is that, although provincial doctors know the theory of crime, they are prevented by public opinion from putting it into practice: cf., for this meaning of ἀγύμναστος, Gal., De aff. dign. 10,11: CMG V 4,1,1, p. 37,13; De pecc. dign. 2,8: ibid., p. 44,27; De crisib. II 5: p. 139,23 Alex. = IX, p. 662,7 K.; and In Hipp. Prorrhet. I comment. II 57: CMG V 9,2, p. 98,31. Nic.'s "nudam", which derives either from a mistranslation or from an original γυμνὴν, is doubtfully relevant.

P. 90,25: Since πρός with the genitive only very rarely means 'from all the things', see L-S-J, s. v. πρός A. II, 2, πρὸς ἁπάντων means 'by all and sundry'. If that is so, the participle must depend on the infinitive, not on the indicative, and should be changed to the accusative. The error arose because the participle was thought to depend on the verb in the indicative.

P. 92,1-3: The idea of 'honour among thieves' may go back at least to the argument of Socrates in Plato's Republic, 352C, cf. 361A, where the completely unjust man is characterised by his successful

[1] Pap. London 43, with the comments of R. Rémondon, Problèmes du bilinguisme dans l'Egypte Lagide, Chronique d'Egypte 39, 1964, pp. 126–146.

[2] G. Misch, A history of autobiography, I, London 1950, pp. 309ff.

attempts to avoid detection by doing good to those immediately about him.[1] Galen's notion may also be a version of the well known comparison of victorious generals and sportsmen to λῃσταί writ large: cf. Marcus Aurelius, Med. X 10; XI 18; Aristeides, Or. 24,27.

P. 92,6-10: It may well be doubted whether such sentiments were already in Galen's mind in 163 or were merely later rationalisations to conform with his rhetorical standpoint or even the simple product of a fertile imagination ready to believe as facts ideas that it had suggested to itself at a later date.

Various attempts have been made to identify the stasis, cf. above, p. 116,27. J. Ilberg, NJ, p. 288, supposed that it was the war with Parthia and Armenia that ended in 165, an assumption that provides a good reason for Galen's return in 166, but it is hard to believe that Galen, who wrote on the vocabulary of the Greek historians and comedians, would use a word that carried the technical meaning of 'internal strife' (cf. L-S-J, s. v.) in a more general sense of 'external war'. Nor can Sarton's suggestion of an (otherwise unattested) war between the Pergamenians (sic!) and the Galatians be accepted, for there is no evidence that the Romans allowed such internal disorder to reign unchecked.[2] The true solution was long ago pronounced by W. A. Greenhill, p. 208, as a 'popular commotion'. Even in the apparent felicity of the second century, the speeches of Dio Chrysostom, Or. 38–51, the letters of Pliny, especially Epp. X 58 and 81 ff., epigraphic records of strikes and riots[3], and even Galen's own words (De aff. dign. 8,9: CMG V 4,1,1, p. 30,2 ff.) amply demonstrate the volatility of domestic politics and the ever present threat of an upheaval serious enough to demand Roman intervention. The contemporary orator and historian, Cephalion (Suidas, s. v.), was forced into exile from his homeland because of the hostility of its ruling clique; and the dangers of stasis was one of the major themes of the second-century sophist, Philip of Pergamum, when he addressed the cities of Asia, Europe, Libya and the islands (Epigr. Gr. 8776, from Epidaurus). If 'stasis' was the reason for Galen's departure from Pergamum in 162 (which should not be confused with that from his post with the gladiators in autumn 161), then it could well have been caused by a dispute over his tax immunities, a medico-sophistical quarrel (cf. G. W. Bowersock, pp. 30–42 and 88–100) or, more likely, his political friends at Pergamum were out of favour. But, as D. E. Eichholz saw, p. 60, his sojourn in Rome need not have been caused by the 'stasis', but merely prolonged, especially as in none of his surviving writings does he inveigh against the corruption and villainy of those who forced him to leave Pergamum for

[1] Adam's note to Republic 352 C refers to the development of this idea in Isocrates, Panath. 226.

[2] G. Sarton, Galen of Pergamum, Lawrence, Kansas 1954, p. 20.

[3] B. Baldwin, Lucian as social satirist, Class. Quart., n. s. 11, 1961, pp. 199–208; J. A. Hall, pp. 183 ff.; E. L. Bowie, Greeks and their past in the Second Sophistic, Past and present 46, 1970, p. 24.

Rome. And, after all, any man with ambition, be he doctor or interpreter of dreams like Artemidorus (Oneir. I prooem. and V prooem.: p. 2,18 and p. 301,12 Pack) would make his way to Italy, whether compelled to leave or not.

P. 92,13: There is no need to supply ἐκ after αὐτοὶ to balance line 18, for this is but another example of elegant variation. μαθεῖν gives no sense, for it is the discovery of their crimes rather than their knowledge of that fact that impels them to fly. It may be the result of a scribal conjecture to supply an infinitive after the loss through haplography of διαμένειν.

Excluding imperial doctors, many of whom, like C. Stertinius Xenophon (H. G. Pflaum, CP, no. 16) and the Statilii of Heraclea (J. and L. Robert, Carie, pp. 178f., 201 and 220)[1], came from families of wealth and importance in their native cities, we have little epigraphic or literary evidence for the social origins of Eastern doctors in Rome. As well as the celebrated Asclepiades of Prusa, Themison of Laodicea and Thessalus of Tralles, called the son of a weaver by Galen (De crisib. II 3: p. 137,1 Alex. = IX, p. 657,15 K. and Meth. med. I 2: X, p. 10,4 K.), other doctors came to Rome from Smyrna (IG XIV 967); Tralles (ibid. 1680); Ephesus (ibid. 1755 and 2104); Nicomedia (ibid. 2019); Thyateira (L. Robert, Hellenica 9, 1950, p. 26); Pamphylia (CIL VI 9580); and Nicaea (an unpublished inscription from the Museo delle Terme). Two others arrived as ambassadors of the Lycians: Ameinias of Lydae (IGR III 534), who performed the embassy at his own expense; and Patron, who later settled in Rome.[2]

How many of these doctors ever returned to the peace of their home town is uncertain. I know of 52 doctors with Roman citizenship in the Eastern provinces before 200 A. D., of whom only one who is not an imperial physician, C. Iulius Epianactis f. Mnesicleides of Paros (IG XII 5, 199), possibly gained citizenship in Rome as a result of the supposedly generous grants of Iulius Caesar and Augustus to all doctors residing in the city of Rome.[3] Certainly some of the imperial doctors returned to play a part in the life of their communities. T. Statilius Attalus (J. and L. Robert, Carie, p. 179) and L. Gellius Maximus of Antioch in Pisidia[4] were considerable local benefactors, and presumably it was doctors like them and T. Claudius Tyrannus, who died at his home town of Magnesia ad Maeandrum after imperial

[1] Cf. now, J. Benedum, Statilius Attalos, Medizinhistorisches Journ. 6, 1971, pp. 263–277; I. Russu, Getica lui Statilius Crito, Studii Clasice 14, 1972, pp. 111–128.

[2] IG XIV 1934, cf. G. Kaibel, Epigrammata Graeca, Berlin 1878, no. 546a and p. 220; Tran Tam Tinh, Catalogue des peintures romaines (Latium et Campanie) du musée du Louvre, Paris 1974, figs. 58–63.

[3] Suetonius, Iulius 42; Augustus 59. The list will be found in my unpublished dissertation, The medical profession in the Roman Empire, Cambridge 1970, pp. 266ff.

[4] V. Nutton, L. Gellius Maximus, physician and procurator, Class. Quart., n. s. 21, 1971, pp. 262–272.

service, O. Kern, n. 113, who are dismissed as "those who return after making money".

Corroborative evidence for Galen's sweeping statements is almost entirely lacking, and so his denunciations must be treated with the same mixture of admiration and caution as those of the elder Pliny on the subject of Greek doctors (Nat. Hist. XXIV 4ff., XXIX 11–22).

P. 92,18: Galen's father, Nicon, was an architect by profession who owned several slaves (Gal., De aff. dign. 8,1 and 9,7: CMG V 4,1,1, p. 27,24 and p. 32,6) and a country estate some miles from Pergamum which Galen often visited (Gal., De alim. fac. I 37,2f.: CMG V 4,2, p. 261,6–24; De bon. mal. suc. I 16: CMG V 4,2, p. 393, 1). He was a well known figure among the sophists and rhetoricians who frequented Pergamum then[1] for, although he was skilled in geometry, architecture, logic, arithmetic and grammar, he continued to attend public lectures on philosophy with his son.[2] He has generally been identified with the architect Aelius Nicon[3], who was also a dabbler in verse, but it is equally possible that he is Aelius Nicon's colleague, Iulius Nicodemus ὁ καὶ Νείκων.[4] His father, according to the Arabic biographical tradition, al-Mubaššir, p. 55, had been head of the important guild of carpenters, an office that demanded considerable resources, and his father, Galen's great-grandfather, had been a land surveyor. The family was well off, and, although Galen feebly attempts to deny it (Meth. med. VIII 3: X, pp. 560,4–561,7 K.), Nicon was rich enough to pay for the best possible education for his son straight from birth (cf. Gal., De diff. puls. II 5: VIII, p. 587,3ff. K.). Galen admits that he is one of the εὐγενεῖς, and of the εὔποροι, even of the πλούσιοι, and that he never had to worry about money for books and equipment (cf. De aff. dign. 9,1–19: CMG V 4,1,1, pp. 30–34). He moved in high society: he was a 'therapeutes' at the Asclepieion, a member of an influential cult group, (Gal., De lib. propr. 2: Scr. min. II, p. 99,9 Müller = XIX, p. 19,1 K.), a friend of the provincial high priest, and possibly a member of the city council of Pergamum, if Gal., De aff. dign. 8,9: CMG V 4,1,1, p. 30,3 can be pressed. Even so, we have as yet no record of any large scale benefaction to his city such as was expected of rich citizens (cf. V. Nutton, JRS, pp. 52–56), although he claims to have provided many fellow doctors with drugs, instruments and travelling expenses when they were in need (M. Meyerhof, Autobiographische Bruchstücke Galens aus arabischen Quellen, Sudhoffs Archiv f. Gesch. d. Med. 22, 1929, p. 84). However much he might disguise it and accuse others of entering the medical profession for the tax immunities it could provide (De

[1] See C. Habicht, Die Inschriften des Asklepieion von Pergamon, Berlin 1968, pp. 6–18, and no. 104, where the restoration of Nicon's name is very doubtful.
[2] To the references collected at PIR² A. 226, add A. S. Halkin, pp. 112f.
[3] As by PIR² A. 226: see also H. Schöne, Galeniana, Festschrift H. Usener, Bonn 1891, pp. 90–93; W. Dörpfeld, Athenische Mitteilungen 27, 1902, pp. 29f.
[4] Cf. H. Diller, RE XVII, 1936, cols. 507f., s. v. Nicon.

plac. Hipp. et Plat. IX (5): p. 764,9 Ml. = V, p. 751,5 K.), he belonged himself to a group, the imperial physicians, highly privileged in wealth and status, who were well able to keep on socially equal terms with leading senators.

P. 92,29: To estimate the population of Rome has exercised scholars for centuries without reaching an agreed conclusion, but the most recent study has suggested a total population at this period of just under one million. [1] Pergamum should not be ranked with such provincial cities as rocky Tithorea (Pausanias, X 32,6f.; and L. Robert, Hellenica 2, 1946, p. 105), Augusta Praetoria (pop. c. 10,000), Antioch in Pisidia (pop. c. 6,000–10,000) and Comana in Pisidia (6,300–9,450) [2], and certainly far outnumbered the semi-mystical 5040 citizens advocated by Plato, Laws 737E (cf. Aristotle, Pol. 1265 a). As Galen tells us (De aff. dign. 9,13: CMG V 4,1,1, p. 33,17), its citizen body numbered 40,000 males or, counting women and slaves, 120,000 souls. Far from being the small country town "in which we all know one another", it is one of the metropoleis of Asia Minor at the very height of its prosperity. [3]

P. 92,31: Galen's education was almost the best available at the time. Pergamum and Smyrna were outstanding centres of learning and Galen took full advantage of them. [4] As for Alexandria, its medical reputation was the best in the world: Anonymous, Expositio totius mundi 37, calls it "the foundation of health for all men", and it attracted students from all over the Greek world, e. g. the young man from Adada in Pisidia who died while studying there (IGR III 374). Galen's emphasis on education is continued in De examinando medico (Bull. Hist. Med. 36, 1962, pp. 364f.), where he demands as the first qualification a knowledge of all previous medical theories, which can only be acquired by book learning.

[1] J. E. Packer, Housing and population in imperial Ostia and Rome, Journ. Rom. Studies 57, 1967, pp. 80–95, but the old survey of R. Pöhlmann, Die Übervölkerung der antiken Großstädte, Leipzig 1884, is still the best account available of the social consequences of the growth of Rome.

[2] Figures given by B. M. Levick, Roman colonies in Southern Asia Minor, Oxford 1967, pp. 93f.

[3] For comparative figures, see K. J. Beloch, Die Bevölkerung der griechisch-römischen Welt, Leipzig 1886, pp. 223–260; for Ephesus, D. Knibbe, RE Suppl. XII, 1970, cols. 270–278, s. v. Ephesos; and for Smyrna, C. J. Cadoux, Ancient Smyrna, Oxford 1938, p. 186. Note the qualifications suggested by F. G. Maier, Römische Bevölkerungsgeschichte und Inschriftenstatistik, Historia 2, 1954, pp. 318–351. It is impossible to say how Galen obtained his figures or whether they refer only to inhabitants of the city or included those in the *chōra*.

[4] References to Galen's education are given at PIR² G. 24 (from which delete that to XIV, p. 628 K.). On the background, see G. W. Bowersock, pp. 17–29; R. Herzog, Urkunden zur Hochschulpolitik der römischen Kaiser, Sitzb. d. Preuß. Akademie d. Wiss., phil.-hist. Kl. 1935, pp. 1007f.; C. J. Cadoux, Ancient Smyrna, Oxford 1938, p. 186. I doubt that Galen's words at Anat. admin. I 1: II, pp. 217,17–218,3 K. are enough to prove that he actually attended Numisianus' lectures at Corinth: he may have arrived only to find him already gone. Nor can the other ἔθνη that he visited in his quest for him be identified for certain.

Not everyone agreed that a physician was better able to cure those who knew him. The Sayings of Jesus (Pap. Oxy. 1, cf. Pap. Labib 5,7), which derive from Luke 4,23f., claim that "no doctor effects cures upon those that know him", but this runs counter to most other authors, who preferred to see the doctor in action before entrusting themselves to him.

P. 94,1: Presumably this is the youth last mentioned at p. 78,7 whose case is taken up briefly and then dismissed. This digression on the malice of Galen's Roman enemies ends abruptly and is not linked closely with the general narrative. It is a rhetorical set piece inserted into the middle of the story to give liveliness and variety.

P. 94,5: J. Ilberg, NJ, p. 288, identified Charilampes with the Charilas mentioned as an intermediary by Fronto (Ep. I 4,2), but not enough is known of the imperial familia to confirm this. Another friend of Galen in the imperial household was Euphrates ὁ καθολικός, who obtained for him the post of maker of the emperor's theriac when Marcus was on the Danube[1] (De antid. I 1: XIV, pp. 4,11–5,3 K.) and who may be the same as Euphrates in Marcus Aurelius, Med. X 31.

The importance of this passage in indicating Galen's position in the contemporary debate between the Atticists and other writers is well brought out by W. Herbst, p. 121.[2] Galen, like Sextus Empiricus (Adv. gramm. 234) and Lucian (Pseudol. 24; Lexiphanes, passim), stands for a simplicity of language without resorting to obscure archaisms or to a consistent refusal to admit words not found in Attic writers of the fifth and fourth centuries B. C. Not all doctors avoided such archaisms. Xenocrates (apud Oribas., Coll. med. rel. II 58,54 and 96: CMG VI 1,1, p. 50,28f. and p. 53,19f.) can write: αἱ ἐν Δικαιαρχίᾳ ἐν τῷ Λουκρίνῳ λάκκῳ, which combines an obsolete name, Δικαιαρχίᾳ, condemned as an affectation by Galen (De comp. med. per gen. I 13: XIII, p. 416,2 K., cf. De antid. I 3: XIV, p. 16,1 K.) with a crude Latinism.[3] Galen, who prefers to follow ἡ κρατοῦσα σαφήνεια rather than solecise in Attic (De comp. med. per gen. I 10: XIII, p. 408, 1–6 K.) and to rely on the example of the Ἕλληνες (In Hipp. Progn. comment. III 44: CMG V 9,2, p. 373,15), strives above all for clarity and uniformity, not mixing Greek words with those from other languages such as Syrian, Cilician and Galatian (De diff. febr. II 5: VIII, pp. 584,18–587,1 K.).

The Greek equivalent of Latin technical terms was always a problem for Greek authors accustomed to canons of history writing that excluded innovations.[4] On the one hand, Galen's favoured trans-

[1] Presumably in the early 170s, pace T. W. Africa, Rome and the Caesars, London 1965, p. 215, who puts it in Galen's first visit to Rome.

[2] On the stylistic debate in general, see W. Schmid, B. P. Reardon, pp. 80–96, and U. von Wilamowitz-Moellendorff, Asianismus und Attizismus, Hermes 35, 1900, pp. 1–52 (repr. in: Kleine Schriften, III, Berlin 1969, pp. 223–273).

[3] Galen himself uses λάκκος at De simpl. med. temp. et fac. IX 34: XII, p. 240,14 K.

[4] H. J. Mason, Roman government in Greek sources, Phoenix 24, 1970, pp. 150–159, esp. p. 152.

lation of cubicularius is found on inscriptions and in 'technical' passages (e. g. IG XIV 1664; Acta Alexandr. 3,28=Pap. Gießen 46; Epictetus, I 19,17), although deplored by Phrynichus, p. 252: on the other, σωματοφύλαξ still has a long history before it as an erudite and literary alternative. Cf. John of Epiphaneia (ed. Müller, Fragmenta Hist. Graec. IV, 275): ὃς τῶν βασιλέως ἦρχε σωματοφυλάκων – κόμητα δὲ τοῦτον ἐξκουβιτόρων Ῥωμαῖοι καλοῦσιν. The omission of οἱ ... ἀττικίζοντες is a good example of Nic.'s translation technique, since the words can be turned into Latin only with difficulty and are both irrelevant to practical medicine and of little interest to fourteenth century readers.

P. 94,9: Nothing further is known of this orator. The reading of A suggests that the scribe confused him with the Athenian orator Demades, a suggestion that Rota accepted in his Latin translation. The phrase used to describe the physicians, οἱ κατὰ τὴν αὐλὴν / ἐκ τῆς αὐλῆς (again, elegant variation), is only one of the titles applied to the imperial household physicians. 'archiatros', possibly the technically correct word, appears for the first time in the Roman Empire applied to C. Stertinius Xenophon under Claudius or Nero (H. G. Pflaum, CP, no. 16) and is used by Galen (De antid. I 1: XIV, p. 2,14 K.) of the elder Andromachus and by Erotian (Praef., p. 3,3, ed. Nachmanson) of the younger. Galen is given this title in some mediaeval Mss., Ms. Merton 219, fol. 36^v, and Ms. Wellcome 284, fol. 1^r, and the word becomes standard in the late third century. But even then there are variations: "archiatri inter penetralia regalis" (Cod. Theod. XIII 3,12); "archiatri sacri palatii" (ibid. 14, cf. Revue Biblique, n. s. 6, 1909, p. 104); "archiatri inter palatium militantes" (Cod. Theod. VI 16,1, cf. Sozomen, Hist. Eccl. II 38). The medicus palatinus, attested only by the Historia Augusta, Vita Alex. Severi 42, occurs in a passage of doubtful syntax, meaning and historical reliability and may not be an official title.

P. 94,14: J. Vahlen, in a notable article[1], collected much of the evidence for the importance in classical antiquity of the survival of one's name. Other authors did not share Galen's enthusiasm. Lucian (Navig. 274) said: τὸ μέγα ὄνομα πάντα κατ' ὀλίγον ἀπορρεῖ, and Marcus Aurelius (Med. IV 33, cf. V 33) dismisses the idea curtly: τὸ δὲ ὄνομα ψόφος καὶ ἀπήχημα.

P. 94,22: The identity of Iustus is disputable. F. E. Kind[2] believed that he was the same as the oculist Iustus (Gal., Meth. med. XIV 19: X, p. 1019,9 K.), but the general impression that he was a man of wealth and social standing, something very unusual among oculists, excludes this. I prefer to identify him with the Iustus to whom De partibus artis medicativae was dedicated, a man of affairs rather than a doctor.[3] If an identification is sought with a known

[1] Opuscula academica, I, Leipzig 1907, pp. 351f.
[2] Bursians Jahresberichte 180, 1919, p. 59, followed by L. Petersen, PIR^2 I. 874.
[3] The identification, but of all three persons, was made by E. Wickersheimer, Le

senator of the period between 163 and 166, both C. Curtius C. f. Iustus, legate of Moesia from 157 to 159 [1], and C. Modius Iustus, cos. suffectus in 171 or, more likely, 172 [2], enter into consideration, but it is probable that he is either an unknown senator or merely another of Galen's rich friends from Pergamum.

On the genitive absolute followed by an accusative to which it refers, see Blass-Debrunner-Funk, § 423.

P. 94,25: Galen's narrative of his meeting with the Stoics and Peripatetics is the best example of the links between philosophy and medicine in the Second Sophistic movement. Aulus Gellius (Noct. Att. XVIII 10,8) believed that it was disgraceful for a liberally educated man to be ignorant of health and medicine, and the doctors were pleased to confirm this belief. Athenaeus (apud Oribas., Coll. med. rel., lib. inc. 39,21: CMG VI 2,2, p. 141,5–9), praising the calm old age of a man trained from his youth in logic and philosophy, says, "How the soul rejoices and is uplifted by communion with our predecessors in philosophy and medicine and with the masters of all knowledge, and by constantly entrusting ourselves to them". Even if the links between medicine and philosophy were never as tight as L. Edelstein, pp. 195–203, 349–366, believed, this evidence shows that they continued to exist and to influence both doctors and laymen.

Galen was well acquainted with the theories of both Stoics and Peripatetics, especially in ethics and logic (K. Deichgräber, Medicus gratiosus, p. 73). He had studied under at least one master from each school (above, p. 159; below, p. 189) and treated two of the leading Peripatetics as well as Eudemus: Aristotle of Mytilene [3] and Primigenes of Mytilene (De sanit. tuenda V 11,10–20: CMG V 4,2, pp. 161, 7–162,4). Already by 163 Galen was accustomed to display his ability daily in public (De venae sect. adv. Eras. Rom. deg. 1: XI, p. 194,6 K., cf. 189,1 for the date) either in debating a given theme or in dissecting pigs, goats, apes and even stranger animals, such as the elephant's heart described at Gal., Anat. admin. VII 10: II, pp. 619,16–621,1 K. [4] This practice derives from the Hellenistic custom of doctors giving public lectures and demonstrations in the gymnasium for the benefit of the citizens among whom they resided. [5] By the Roman period, such

médecin Justus, contemporain de Galien, et les écrits portant son nom, Actes du Xème Congrès international d'histoire des sciences, Paris 1964, p. 525.

1 PIR² C. 1613.

2 M. Fluss, RE XV, 1932, col. 2332, s. v. Modius 11.

3 Gal., De consuet. 1: CMG Suppl. III, p. 4,16, with the comments of P. Moraux, Einige Aspekte des Aristotelismus, Archiv f. Gesch. d. Philosophie 49, 1967, pp. 168–171.

4 I do not think that "shortly after Antoninus had begun his reign in Rome" (Gal., Anat. admin. I 1: II, p. 215,6f. K.) can be pressed to mean that he was already in Rome and active by 161. Galen's public demonstrations came to an end in summer 163 (De lib. propr. 2: Scr. min. II, p. 96,7f. Müller = XIX, p. 15,5 K.).

5 Examples are found at Perge and Seleucia, Monumenti antichi 23, 1914, p. 48; at Istros, Bull. Epigraphique 1958, n. 336; at Elatea, Supplementum Epigraphicum Graecum 3, 1929, n. 416; and in the Tauric Chersonnese (ibid., n. 599).

debates could be used deliberately to challenge opponents (Gal., Anat. admin. VII 16: II, pp. 642,3–646,4 K.) and could be declined, either through fear (ibid. II 2: II, p. 283,9–12 K.) or through a snobbish refusal to deal with those who were younger or intellectually inferior (cf. De venae sect. adv. Eras. Rom. deg. 1: XI, p. 194,4–6 K.). They might take place in the open air, at one of the recognised meeting places of doctors, in the theatre (John Chrysostom, Patrolog. Graeca 63, p. 655) or in specially constructed auditoria[1], while at Ephesus there were formal contests between doctors with the list of victors publicly displayed.[2] How much was gained by the populace from these demonstrations is uncertain. Dio Chrysostom's description of a lecture audience (Or. 33,6) does not inspire confidence in its judgement: The doctor sits out in front, surrounded by arrangements and rearrangements of bones; he goes through, describing everything, pores, breaths, excretions. His audience are agape, and are fooled even more than small children.

P. 94,27: 'On prognosis', unlike many other treatises (cf. Anat. admin. I 1: II, p. 217,7–13 K.; De venae sect. adv. Eras. Rom. deg. 1: XI, p. 194,10–15 K.; De lib. propr. praef.: Scr. min. II, p. 92,13–18 Müller = XIX, p. 10,3–7 K.), is intended for public consumption, at least by those whom Galen considers worthy of it, and thus it is more than a collection of personal notes taken down by or directed to a particular group. Galen, who prided himself on writing each treatise to fit its audience or readership (In Hipp. De fract. comment. I 1: XVIII B, pp. 321,1–322,2 K.), here writes in a more literary and allusive manner and employs variation both of style and subject to gain the interest and sympathy of his readers. Even so, he expected his writings to be misunderstood, for they were often written, like books on the mysteries, for initiates alone (De simpl. med. temp. et fac. VII 1: XII, p. 2,3–8 K.), and to be treated as badly as an orphan child among drunkards (De usu part. XII 6: II, p. 197,2 Helmr. = IV, p. 22,1f. K.).

P. 96,3: Galen quotes Homer more than any other non-medical author, both for his general wisdom and for his medical observations.[3] Here in his quotation of a famous line[4] he does not give the reading of

[1] Gal., De venae sect. adv. Eras. Rom. deg. 1: XI, p. 194,14 K.; De lib. propr. 2: Scr. min. II, p. 101,5 Müller = XIX, p. 21,8 K.; Historia Augusta, Vita Alex. Severi 44. No certain archaeological traces of an auditorium survive in Rome, save possibly for the so-called Auditorium of Maecenas (S. B. Platner and T. Ashby, pp. 60f.); for archaeological evidence from Ephesus, see Forschungen in Ephesos, III, 1923, p. 101, and W. Alzinger, RE Suppl. XII, 1971, cols. 1633f., s. v. Ephesos.

[2] See J. Keil, Ärzteinschriften aus Ephesos, Jahreshefte d. Österreich. Archäolog. Instituts 8, 1905, pp. 128–138; P. Wolters, 'Αρχιατρὸς τὸ δ', ibid. 9, 1906, p. 295. On public debate and discussion in general, see E. Rohde, pp. 327ff.

[3] P. De Lacy, Galen and the Greek poets, Greek, Roman and Byzantine Studies 7, 1966, pp. 259–266; cf. also F. Kudlien, Zum Thema „Homer und die Medizin", Rheinisches Museum 108, 1965, pp. 293–299.

[4] It is ascribed to Isocrates in the Gnomologium Vaticanum, 360.

the textus receptus but a variant, προτέρως for πρότερος, confirmed by Nic.'s "prius". Despite A's reading, which is that of the accepted text, I consider that we have another example of a slight misquotation from memory by Galen (cf. above, pp. 156; 176) rather than a phonetic confusion between long and short 'o'.

P. 96,7: Alexander of Damascus, who is treated with such initial deference by Galen, is further described (Anat. admin. I 1: II, p. 218, 6–8 K.) as being, at the time of writing, a public professor of Peripatetic philosophy at Athens. Whether he is to be identified with the Aristotelian scholar Alexander of Aphrodisias, who held a chair at Athens from about 198 A. D. remains an open question. Certainly the Arabic biographers, who had much more of Galen to hand than we have and whose information derived both from the writings ascribed to John Philoponus and from the works of Galen, regarded the identification as certain and referred to Alexander as being "of Aphrodisias and of Damascus".[1] The suggestion is very attractive, for, as P. Merlan has demonstrated[2], Alexander distinguished between two kinds of reality, the sensible and the intelligible (cf. above, p. 98,5) and "with his writings, Platonism staged its comeback within the Peripatos". The objection that if "at the time of writing" refers to the composition of the Anatomicae administrationes, that is, in the late 170s, Alexander of Aphrodisias was not then holding a public chair, is weak, for K. Bardong, p. 615, has shown that Galen was constantly adding notes to his own copy, making cross references and bringing it up to date, and thus the insertion of a reference to an event that may not have occurred before 198 need not affect the date of composition of the work as a whole.

The Arabic biographers have preserved much interesting information on the quarrel between Alexander of Aphrodisias and Galen. They shared the same teacher, Herminos[3], and squabbled for years over philosophical points. Alexander called Galen "mule head" (whatever that means) and said that he had spent eighty years of his life in vain before coming to the conclusion that he knew nothing (Aš-Šahrazūrī, *Kitab rawḍat al-afrāḥ wa-nuzhat al-arwāḥ*, Berlin, Ms. Landberg 430, fol. 33ʳ).

Total certainty about the identification is as yet impossible, but the Arabic evidence is strongly in its favour.

1 See, among others, A. Dietrich, Die arabische Version einer unbekannten Schrift des Alexander von Aphrodisias über die Differentia specifica, Nachr. d. Göttinger Akademie d. Wiss., phil.-hist. Kl. 1964, pp. 92–100; J. C. Bürgel, Averroes 'Contra Galenum', ibid. 1967, p. 283, n. 1; G. Strohmaier, Encyclopaedia of Islam, 2nd ed., Leyden 1974, pp. 129f., s. v. Al-Iskandar al-Afrūdīsi; R. Walzer, GA, p. 98, n. 1.

2 In A. H. Armstrong (ed.), The Cambridge history of later Greek and early mediaeval philosophy, Cambridge 1967, pp. 117–123.

3 Al-Mubaššir, p. 54 and p. 365; Isḥâq ibn Ḥunain, quoted by F. Rosenthal, Isḥâq b. Ḥunayn's Ta'rīḫ al-aṭibbâ', Oriens 7, 1954, p. 79; S. Pines, A refutation of Galen by Alexander of Aphrodisias, Isis 52, 1961, p. 23. On Galen's Aristotelianism, see P. Moraux, Galien et Aristote, Festschr. G. Verbeke, Louvain 1976, pp. 128–146.

P. 96,16: ἀτὰρ οὖν καί is a rare combination of particles, J. D. Denniston, p. 54, and is another display of the flowers of Galen's learning, also at XI, p. 662,4 K. and XIII, p. 314,2 K. It appears occasionally in the works of the Atticists (cf. W. Schmid, III, p. 332) but it is doubtful whether they ever understood the full force of this egregious collocation.

Adrian of Tyre, one of the finest performers of the Second Sophistic movement, is vividly described by Philostratus, Vit. Soph. 585–590. His connection with Boethus' circle is confirmed by the dedication he erected at Ephesus in honour of Cn. Claudius Severus[1] in which he speaks of himself as Μούσαισι μέλων; and by Philostratus (Vit. Soph. 588), who represents Severus as criticising his technique and delivery (cf. Libanius, Or. 64,41). He occupied the imperial chair of rhetoric at Athens in 178 (Vit. Soph. 588), if not earlier, which must have been founded by 176 if Theodotus, its first occupant, held it for two years (ibid. 567; Cassius Dio, Hist. LXXII 31). Adrian was transferred to the imperial chair (from the municipal?) soon after the death of Theodotus by Marcus Aurelius, who relied solely upon reports of his ability (Vit. soph. 587, 591). Finally, as a result of a superb performance before the emperor (ibid. 589), he was promoted to the imperial chair of rhetoric at Rome. On his deathbed, he was appointed ab epistulis graecis by Commodus, who apologised for not having done so earlier. For the problems over the dating of his appointments, see J. A. Hall, pp. 35f., and J. H. Oliver, pp. 80ff.

The phrase οὔπω σοφιστεύων cannot be pressed to indicate that he was already the holder of the imperial (or even the municipal) chair at Athens when 'On prognosis' was written. Rather, as G. W. Bowersock argued, pp. 12ff., it merely denotes a difference between the small town rhetor and the virtuosi professionals with their huge reputations. The sophists are a category within the general class of orators. The importance of Galen's evidence for the attendance of Adrian is that it indicates how an ambitious man would advance his career, even before he performed in public officially, by associating with senators in Rome to gain a reputation and, eventually, preferment.[2] But as Lucian pointed out in De mercede conductis, not all

[1] Jahreshefte d. Österreich. Archäolog. Instituts 40, 1953, p. 14; cf. PIR² C. 1024. See also I. Avotins, The holders of the chairs of rhetoric at Athens, Harvard Studies in Class. Philology 79, 1975, pp. 314f.

[2] C. P. Jones, Two enemies of Lucian, Greek, Roman and Byzantine Studies 13, 1972, pp. 475–487, suggests that Adrian is the object of Lucian's 'Pseudologista', which is very likely, and that the two were at Ephesus on January 3rd., 163, both following Verus from Greece on his way to the Parthian war. But Jones has to place Galen's stay in Rome in 161–164, p. 481, to enable Adrian to be in Ephesus in late 162, although he admits, p. 484, that the meeting could have occurred in January 164, when Verus was at Ephesus for his wedding. Since Adrian appears in Rome in 163, on my chronology, and is not yet a sophist, his argument with Lucian must have been in 164, which agrees with my date (above, p. 65) for Lucius' marriage. Jones also stresses that at the time of his confrontation with Galen, Adrian was no callow youth but aged at least fifty and a man of great experience.

were so fortunate or so capable: poverty and contempt were at least as likely an outcome as prestige and wealth.

P. 96,17: The identification of Demetrius with the Aelius Demetrius mentioned on two inscriptions from Alexandria of this period is almost certain [1], which shows that, like many other sophists, he was a member of the Museum at Alexandria and had other distinguished orators as his pupils. The internationalism of the Second Sophistic movement is well brought out by his association (as a pupil?) with Favorinus, the hermaphrodite from Arles, who, with Polemo, dominated the movement in the time of Hadrian. [2] As we know from Aulus Gellius, Favorinus was deeply interested in medicine. He delivered an oration 'On quartan ague' (Noct. Att. XVII 12) and discoursed in Greek to the doctors of an invalid in Rome, quoting from the first book of Erasistratus' Διαιρέσεις (ibid. XV 3,2, cf. also III 16,8; XII 5,3; and XVIII 10,1f.). Demetrius continued his master's interests and the public displays of rhetoric on themes suggested by his audience, one of the cardinal tests of a good sophist. [3] The works of Favorinus were still influential in the time of Galen, who took the trouble to write three tracts specifically against his opinions: 'Against Socrates' (De lib. propr. 12: Scr. min. II, p. 121,11 Müller = XIX, p. 45,12 K., if the text is sound); 'A defence of Epictetus' (ibid. 11: Scr. min. II, p. 120,6 Müller = XIX, p. 44,8 K.); and 'On the best method of instruction'. [4]

P. 96,21: συλλογίζεσθαι is to draw the correct logical conclusions from the premises and the phenomena that are accepted by all. The difficulty of understanding this passage lies in the genitive phrase οὐκ . . . ἁπάντων: upon what does it depend? Is it a genitive of comparison after μᾶλλον or a subjective genitive after διδάσκαλον, or is the text corrupt as Nic.'s version suggests? I have reluctantly accepted the second explanation, recalling the traditional ability of the Stoics and Peripatetics in logic and dialectic.

P. 96,27–98,4: Galen's experiments on the recurrent laryngeal and intercostal nerves are described at greater length in his De usu part. (XVI 4: II, pp. 386,10–388,11 Helmr. = III, pp. 278,3–281,1 K.) and in De anat. admin. (XI 4 and 11: pp. 81–87, 104–107 Dkw.; XIV 6–8: pp. 203–217 Dkw., and especially in Book VIII: II, pp. 651–706 K.). The recurrent laryngeal branches of the vagus, which supply all the muscles of the larynx save the cricothyrois, enter the larynx from below, passing in close to the lower part of the pharynx, and if they

[1] See, C. P. Jones, A friend of Galen, Class. Quart., n. s. 17, 1967, pp. 311f.

[2] See, PIR² F. 123; E. Mensching, Favorin von Arelate, Berlin 1963; A. Barigazzi, Favorino di Arelate, Opere, Florence 1966; G. W. Bowersock, pp. 35f., 41f., 51f., 90ff.

[3] Cf. above, p. 140,27; Gal., De venae sect. adv. Eras. Rom. deg. 1: XI, p. 194,6 K.; Philostratus, Vit. Soph. 491 and 576; E. Rohde, pp. 332f.

[4] Scr. min. I, pp. 82–92 Marquardt = I, pp. 40–52 K. Now re-edited by A. Barigazzi, Favorino di Arelate, Opere, pp. 179–194.

are ligated (cf. ibid. 4: II, pp. 669,2–670,10 K.), paralysis of the vocal organs ensues. The animal suffers no injury, in contrast to its complete loss of the power of speech when the spinal cord is cut through or to the partial loss when it is half cut (ibid. VIII 7: II, pp. 688,12–689, 2 K.). H. Baumgarten, pp. 114ff., has painstakingly set out the reasons, both philological and anatomical, why the word φάρυγγος here and at 98,24 cannot mean 'pharynx' but corresponds to our 'larynx', a terminological shift that is found throughout Greek medicine, from Hippocrates to John Philoponus.[1]

P. 98,8: Galen always opposes the philosophical ideas of the Academics and the sceptical followers of Pyrrho of Elis (c. 360–270 B. C.), especially in so crude a form as this[2], refusing to trust any sensory phenomenon; since he believed in logical and geometric proof and also that the senses could be trusted at times, especially τὰ ἐναργῶς αἰσθήσει φαινόμενα (De opt. doctr. 4: Scr. min. I, p. 89,3ff. Marquardt = I, p. 48,13ff. K.). But his arguments and examples in De optima doctrina are very traditional (see A. Barigazzi's edition, ad loc.), and his insistence upon the intelligibility of ἀρχαί (De crisib. III 8: p. 190,13–19 Alex. = IX, p. 738,9–16 K.) offers no epistemological proof of what is a simple assertion on his part. His philosophy is as eclectic as his medicine, combining Platonic views on mathematical and logical proof with Stoic and Aristotelian ideas on epistemology, and he is at times prepared to suspend his judgement when he has no criterion of logical proof, as, for example, with the problem of the eternity of the world (De propr. plac. 2).

Since Galen's statement that he would not otherwise have come depends on what he said, φθεγξάμενος, not on what he thought, οἰόμενος, it would be easy to conjecture that Galen originally wrote ὡς . . . ἀφικόμην, which was easily corrupted to ἀφικνεῖσθαι under the influence of the preceding infinitive. But since there are many examples of an indirect statement beginning with ὅτι or ὡς and ending, grammatically wrongly, with an infinitive, even in classical authors,[3] often where a long clause intervenes between the conjunction and the verb, it would be possible to believe that this confusion went back to Galen himself and thus that the text should be allowed to stand.

P. 98,11: The reading of the Mss. suggests that Adrian and Demetrius are opposed to contentiousness in general: but the emphatic position of αὐτῷ in the rest of the sentence, unless it is intended pleo-

[1] The account of J. Walsh, Galen's discovery and promulgation of the function of the recurrent laryngeal nerve, Annals of med. hist. 8, 1926, pp. 176–184, hardly lives up to its grandiloquent title, since it in no way explains the anatomical procedures involved.

[2] Cf. Gal., An in art. nat. sang. contin. 7: IV, p. 727,10f. K.: τὴν Πυρρωνείαν ἀγροικίαν; De diff. puls. IV 2: VIII, p. 711,1–3 K.; De dign. puls. I 2: VIII, pp. 782,1–786,13 K., where he sets out the practical failings of such scepticism.

[3] E. g. Xenophon, Hell. II 2,2; Blass-Debrunner-Funk, § 397,6, p. 205, gives several examples and references to discussions.

nastically to link the two clauses, is very odd, and it is easier to accept the small change suggested by Cornarius and read αὐτοῦ, which is also more consistent with Galen's style. φιλονεικία, certainly for Galen, has both good and bad aspects. At its worst, it is caused by ἀπληστία (Gal., De aff. dign. 7,2 and 9,18: CMG V 4,1,1, p. 24,10 and p. 34,18) and leads to contention for contention's sake (cf. ibid. 3,7: CMG V 4,1,1, p. 22,19; De atra bile 7,3: ibid., p. 85,8; De praes. ex puls. I 1: IX, p. 219,7 K.; and above, p. 128,29). On the other hand, the finest φιλονεικία is to seek to surpass others in the pursuit of σωφροσύνη (De aff. dign. 6,16: CMG V 4,1,1, p. 22,19), but such a use is rare, for the word normally carries pejorative overtones.

P. 98,12: Galen's friends are often called 'philologi', which signifies possession of both logical ability and a wide cultural range, one of the ideals of the Second Sophistic movement. Such a man could distinguish in a moment a genuine from a spurious work of Galen (Gal., De lib. propr. praef.: Scr. min. II, p. 91,9 Müller = XIX, p. 8,12 K.), and regularly attended debates and demonstrations (Gal., De pecc. dign. 5,31: CMG V 4,1,1, p. 62,15ff.), which also indicates their wealth and the amount of their free time they could devote to intellectual pursuits.[1]

P. 98,19: There is no reason to believe that Galen showed both the muscles, the nerves and the means by which the muscles of the thorax were contracted, as the Mss. reading suggests. Nic.'s version, "musculos a quibus constringitur", gives a better reading, but I have followed H. Baumgarten, p. 103, in emending the text in such a way as to explain the presence of τε.

P. 98,24–26: The vocal chords (which actually produce the sound) are attached to the thyroid cartilage in front and to the paired arytenoid cartilage behind, and thus it could easily be assumed that the cartilages produce sound. Even so, it is not τὰ κατὰ τὸν χόνδρον that the passing column of air strikes against but the cartilages themselves within the larynx, and I have emended the text accordingly. If the pharyngeal muscles, which are innervated by the recurrent laryngeal nerve, are damaged, the animal loses even the sound of hoarse rattling: there is still ἐκφύσησις, a sudden rush of air accompanied by the action of the intercostal muscles (Gal., De mot. musc. II 9: IV, p. 459,1–3 K.), but the exhalation is now inaudible.

[1] Cf. also De venae sect. adv. Eras. Rom. deg. 1: XI, p. 194,1 K., where the Ms. reading φιλολόγοις must be substituted for the Basle editors' conjecture, φιλοσόφοις. On its use as a term of approbation, see in general, H. Kuch, Φιλόλογος, Untersuchung eines Wortes von seinem ersten Auftreten in der Tradition bis zur ersten überlieferten lexikalischen Festlegung, Berlin 1965 (Deutsche Akademie d. Wiss. zu Berlin, Schriften d. Sektion f. Altertumswiss. 48); and the examples given by L. Robert, Hellenica 13, 1965, p. 52 and Bull. Epigraphique 1965, no. 180, and by G. E. Bean, Denkschriften d. Akademie d. Wiss. in Wien 104, 1971, p. 25; and, applied particularly to doctors, CIL III 614, IGR III 534, Bull. Communale 56, 1928, p. 300, and an unpublished inscription on a funeral stele from Rome: Naevia C. l. Clara / medica philologa.

P. 98,29: Many others followed Boethus' example of having shorthand writers take down Galen's lectures (Gal., De lib. propr. 1: Scr. min. II, p. 95,24 Müller = XIX, p. 14,15f. K.), and Galen recommended to other doctors the expense of securing and training them (De aff. dign. 9,9: CMG V 4,1,1, p. 32,17). He also often passed on his own lecture notes to be copied for friends who were either absent or intending to go abroad shortly (cf. Gal., De lib. propr. 1: Scr. min. II, p. 96,20ff. Müller = XIX, p. 15,17ff. K.; De venae sect. adv. Eras. Rom. deg. 1: XI, p. 194,17 K.). The consequence of this, as Galen lamented (De lib. propr. praef.: Scr. min. II, pp. 91–93,16 Müller = XIX, pp. 8,3–11,11 K.; De propr. plac. 1: Hermes 77, 1942, pp. 376–379), was the disorganised state of his writings, which reached the general public, for whom they had not been intended, and were then misinterpreted or were forged or suffered serious changes and mutilations.[1]

P. 100,3: On the date of composition indicated by this passage, see above, pp. 49–51.

P. 100,7–104,23: This case and that of the sick slave which is appended to it are important for what they tell us about Galen's clinical methods and about his aims and intentions in prognosis. The steps by which he reached his conclusion that the man and the woman were suffering from a psychological disorder have been summarised by S. W. Jackson in these words[2]: "Starting from the symptoms he first worked towards the identification of a physical disease, but then concluded that such a condition was not present. By this process of elimination, in the second case he came directly to the conclusion that the man's symptoms were the result of mental distress caused by psychological factors. But, in the first case, having concluded that the insomnia was due to a mental disorder, he still considered that there was a problem of differential diagnosis between a depressive state caused by a psychological disturbance and a syndrome of mental distress caused by a psychological disturbance. His final decision was reached upon the basis of further diagnostic interviews in which he systematically tested out a hypothesis."

Galen loved to see himself directly in the tradition of the great doctors of antiquity whose works he had read and admired. The cases that open De venae sect. adv. Eras. Rom. deg. (XI, pp. 187,1–191,7 K.) are deliberately chosen in contradistinction to Erasistratus' observations of Crito and the Chian girl. Here his model was one of the most celebrated romantic tales of the ancient world, the love of

[1] Cf. also A. Henrichs, Didymos der Blinde, Kommentar zu Hiob, Bonn 1968, pp. 12f. On the different shorthand systems in use, see H. J. M. Milne, Greek shorthand manuals, London 1934; R. A. Coles, Reports of proceedings in papyri, Papyri Bruxellenses 4, 1966, pp. 9–27; J. Irigoin, Annuaire de l'école pratique des hautes études 1971/72, pp. 175–182; and H. Boge, Griechische Tachygraphie und Tironische Noten, Berlin 1973.

[2] S. W. Jackson, p. 366.

Antiochus I for Stratonice, whose influence can be traced for over fifteen hundred years in both Western and Oriental literature.[1] But, as J. Mesk argued in his exhaustive study of the literary antecedents and amplifications of this tale[2], the historical kernel, the marriage of Antiochus and Stratonice, and the elevation of Antiochus to co-regent with his father, which could have had an easy explanation in terms of straight politics, was adorned by Hellenistic authors with romantic trimmings to gratify their readership. The basic story is that a young man falls ill through love of his stepmother, the queen; a doctor is called, who diagnoses the trouble, either from the pulse or from the heartbeat of the young man on seeing the woman; after much thought and circumspection he tells the king that his son is in love with his wife; the king, out of love for his son, gives him his wife to marry. But, in the course of telling, variants arose, dramatic touches were added and literary convention speedily replaced and embellished historical fact. As will be shown, Galen does not stick to the traditional version either here or in his later summaries of it.[3]

P. 100,9f.: As Galen expressly notes (In Hipp. Progn. comment. I 4: CMG V 9,2, p. 206,18), his model was Erasistratus' cure of the son of Seleucus I, i. e. Antiochus, but, as all other accounts agree, the object of his affections was not a concubine but his stepmother, Stratonice. Presumably Galen is confusing this with the similar tale of Hippocrates' cure of Perdiccas, king of Macedon, who had fallen in love with the concubine of his father, Alexander (Soranus, Vita Hipp. 1: CMG IV, p. 176,4–11; cf. Marcellinus, De puls. 29–32 Schöne). But the transmission of both stories is doubtful enough and each may involve borrowings from or confusions with the other. Phila, the name of Alexander's concubine, was also that of a daughter of Antiochus and Stratonice, and Lucian, in another variant (De hist. conscrib. 35, wrongly deleted by W. Dindorf as a gloss), says that it was Perdiccas who wasted to a shadow with a passion for his stepmother. It is impossible, and unnecessary, to decide on the historical truth of all the details given in either version of the story.

With two exceptions, all ancient writers ascribe the discovery of Antiochus' passion to the great doctor Erasistratus of Ceos; but as M. Wellmann rightly argued, the date of this incident, 293 B. C., would appear to exclude him as being too young, if the traditional date for his floruit, given by Eusebius (Chron., p. 200 Karst) and

[1] E. Rohde, pp. 55–59; B. E. Perry, The ancient romances, Berkeley 1967, pp. 301f.

[2] J. Mesk, pp. 366–394; D. W. Amundsen, Romanticising the ancient medical profession, Bull. Hist. Med. 48, 1974, pp. 333–337.

[3] At In Hipp. Progn. comment. I 8: CMG V 9,2, p. 218,20, he says that his patient was a man in love with a woman, an error that was soon picked up by the Arabic commentators, e. g. Ibn abī Uṣaibiʿa, *ʿUyūn al-anbāʾ*, II, p. 128,15, ed. Müller: see also E. G. Browne, Arabian medicine, Cambridge 1921, pp. 85–88; and R. Walzer, GA, pp. 48–59.

Jerome (p. 131 Helm) as 258/7, is correct.[1] Valerius Maximus, V 7, whose source cannot be later than the reign of Augustus (31 B. C.–14 A. D.), offers a choice between Erasistratus and Leptines, an otherwise unknown mathematicus, while Pliny (Nat. Hist. VII 123) ascribes the diagnosis to Erasistratus' father, Cleombrotus of Ceos, the private doctor to Seleucus, although elsewhere (ibid. XXIX 5) he has Erasistratus himself. M. Wellmann, for whom the whole incident was historical, believed that the action of a less well known father was transferred to his more famous son, and J. Mesk agreed, but P. M. Fraser, in an erudite paper[2], has recently revived the view that in fact Erasistratus was the doctor and that the traditional date given by the chronographers should be dispensed with. His reliance on the even later testimony of Plutarch, Appian, Julian, Syncellus and, especially, Suidas to prove that it was Erasistratus and no other who performed the diagnosis amounts to little more than a counting of heads, not an evaluation of the source, for one tradition is likely to have been common to all these authors. The alternatives given by Valerius Maximus and Pliny, the two earliest authors to tell the story, suggest that the name of the wise man was originally unknown and could be changed according to the taste or the information of the narrator. Indeed, if Erasistratus was court physician at the time, as Fraser argues, it is very difficult to see why his father and, still more, the mysterious Leptines should have been introduced. Erasistratus may have practised at Antioch, but this tale is hardly strong enough to contradict the impression given by Celsus and Galen that his major work was carried out at Alexandria, and certainly does not prove the theory of Fraser that he lived and worked only under the Seleucids.

P. 100,10f.: The Greek Mss. and Nic., who depends on a similar Greek text, give little sense, unless τοὺς σφυγμοὺς is to be taken as an internal accusative with σφυζουσῶν. An easy solution, which I have adopted, is offered by a comparison with Gal., In Hipp. Progn. comment. I 8: CMG V 9,2, p. 218,18f.: οὐ μὴν οὐδ' ὥς τινες ἔγραψαν, ἐρωτικὸν σφυζουσῶν ᾔσθετο τῶν ἀρτηριῶν τοῦ νεανίσκου: I delete τοὺς σφυγμοὺς as a gloss incorporated into the text, with the subsequent alteration of the accusative τὰς ἀρτηρίας . . . σφυζούσας into the genitive.

P. 100,13: The reason why Galen could not say was that Erasistratus believed in a different working system of veins, arteries and pulses from Galen.[3]

[1] M. Wellmann, Zur Geschichte der Medicin im Alterthum, Hermes 35, 1900, pp. 380f.; and RE VI, 1907, cols. 333f., s. v. Erasistratos.

[2] P. M. Fraser, The career of Erasistratus of Ceos, Rendiconti dell'Istituto Lombardo, Sez. di Lettere, 103, 1969, pp. 518–537. G. E. R. Lloyd, A note on Erasistratus of Ceos, Journ. Hellenic Studies 95, 1975, pp. 172–175, while rejecting Fraser's contention that Erasistratus did not dissect at Alexandria, accepts the story as good evidence of his activity at Antioch.

[3] See Gal., De diff. puls. IV 2: VIII, p. 703,4–9 K.; De usu resp. 1: IV, p. 471,7f.

P. 100,15: Chartier's emendation (τινος for τῆς) would have been acceptable had not the woman already been mentioned at p. 94,22.

P. 100,18f.: The reluctance of the man or woman to tell of their symptoms is an integral part of the romantic tradition. J. Mesk (pp. 380ff.) connects it with the silence of Phaedra in Euripides, Hippolytus 279 and 393f., but there is otherwise little to suggest that the wife of Iustus was entering the terminal stages of love-sickness and wished to die before reveal her secret.

P. 102,1–104,23: By his actions here and by his statements at In Hipp. Progn. comment. I 4: CMG V 9,2, pp. 206,1–209,6, Galen attacks those who, like the poets (cf. Sophocles, fr. 619 Nauck), ascribed the onset of the disease to something θεῖον, a θεήλατος νόσος, and he insists that the disorder is psychosomatic (cf. above, lines 10–12; Gal., In Hipp. Epid. III comment. II: CMG V 10,1, p. 208,17–37). "He conceived of emotions as diseases of the soul, and also thought of them as causative factors that might have various deleterious effects. They might harm the pneuma and thus weaken the soul, and he included them among the causes of fever. And he mentioned strong emotional states as interfering with attention and so causing the memory to fail to register actions and events that occurred during such a state."[1] Mental states, anger, pleasure, grief and fear, are revealed by the pulses first of all (Gal., De crisib. II 13: p. 162,4–8 Alex. = IX, p. 697,1–5 K.; De caus. puls. IV 1–5: IX, pp. 156,1–161,9 K.; De praes. ex puls. I 4: IX, p. 250,6–17 K., Introd. in puls. 12: VIII, p. 473,4 K.), even before they produce fever through their influence on the action of the heart (Gal., De diff. febr. I 4: VII, p. 283,7–16 K.), but, as he remarks, above, p. 104,20–23, there is no pulse peculiar to love, only the same pulse as signifies any mental disturbance.

P. 102,14: It is difficult to know which of the many pantomimes called Pylades is mentioned here, since the name was passed on from generation to generation. He is generally identified with L. Aurelius Augg. lib. Pylades, hieronica, the pupil of P. Aelius Aug. lib. Pylades, pantomimus hieronica, recorded on an inscription from Genoa (ILS 5185), whose superiority to his master was championed by such an expert as Fronto (Ep. I 2). Presumably he was manumitted by Lucius Verus, a connoisseur of such performers (cf. Historia Augusta, Vita Veri 8,10f.; and ILS 5187–5191). He may also be the same as L. Aurelius Aug. lib. Pylades, the leading pantomime of his age, honoured with ornamenta decurionalia by Puteoli for his affection and benefactions towards his native town, probably in the 180s (ILS 5186), and as Theocritus Augg. lib. Pylades, pantomimus, honoured by the

K.; ibid. 2: IV, pp. 473,6–484,9 K.; J. F. Dobson, Erasistratus, Proc. Royal Society of Med. 20, 1927, pp. 825–832; I. M. Lonie, Erasistratus, the Erasistrateans and Aristotle, Bull. Hist. Med. 38, 1964, pp. 426–463; C. R. S. Harris, pp. 195–233.

[1] S. W. Jackson, p. 371; cf. O. Temkin, On Galen's pneumatology, Gesnerus 8, 1951, pp. 180–189.

most splendid cities of Italy with the ornamenta decurionalia, to whom an inscription was set up in Milan after his death.[1] If this great solo dancer was still alive in 193, he may well have been the Pylades commanded to appear before Julianus after the death of the emperor Pertinax (Cassius Dio, Hist. LXXIII 13,1), although this may be a younger dancer.[2] There is no doubt that these dancers were figures of great social and cultural importance in Rome and Italy (cf. above, p. 154) who could gain great wealth from their career.

P. 102,16: As in some versions of the Erasistratus' story, the confirmation of the love-sickness comes from taking the pulse; in others it comes merely from placing a hand over the man's heart.

P. 102,20: Nothing more is known about Morphus; and, if the third of the dancers refers to the tritagonistes rather than to one of the three stars who took the leading roles or the solo parts, it is not surprising that Galen leaves him nameless, for the third part player was the least important of the solo dancers.

P. 102,32: Galen normally uses the active form συμβουλεύειν to mean 'advise' (cf. above, p. 104,2; CMG V 10,2,3, p. 215) and it would be easy to emend to συνεβούλευσα μὲν, picked up by ἐπεὶ δὲ (p. 104,2), but it is possible that Galen used the middle form here to avoid hiatus and for the sake of variation.

P. 104,11: ἐπιλογισμός, inductive reasoning, was particularly stressed by the Empiric sect, almost to the exclusion of the deductive reasoning favoured by Galen (cf. Gal., De sectis 5: Scr. min. III, pp. 11,8–12,8 Helmr. = I, pp. 77,17–79,6 K.; De experientia medicinali, passim).

P. 104,20: For the construction, cf. Gal., De nat. fac. I 12: Scr. min. III, p. 121,21f. Helmr. = II, p. 29,4–6 K.: καὶ ἀνδρεία καὶ φρόνησις καὶ σωφροσύνη καὶ ἐγκράτεια λῆρός ἐστι μακρὸς; and II 3: ibid., p. 159,5f. Helmr. = II, p. 80,6f. K.: λῆρος οὖν μακρὸς ἅπασα πόρων ὑπόθεσις εἰς φυσικὴν ἐνέργειαν; De loc. aff. II 9: VIII, p. 116,17f. K.: λῆρος ἂν εἴη μακρὸς ὁ περὶ τῶν ἀλγημάτων λόγος; and De dign. puls. II 2: VIII, p. 860,1 K.: λῆρον εἶναι μακρὸν δόξαι τοὺς τοιούτους λόγους.

P. 104,24: From this point on, the illustrative episodes become more and more disconnected and are strung together without any attempt at integration into a well structured treatise. The cure of the son of Boethus, which comes precisely in the middle of 'On prognosis' is its humorous highlight, being placed with the medically interesting cures of the wife of Iustus and of the wife of Boethus on either side. L. Jacchinus in his commentary, p. 71, suggested two reasons for the wit and humour of this section. First, Galen wished to amuse his friends and readers; and, secondly, he wanted to avoid the im-

[1] ILS 5195: see also, Th. Mommsen, Tre inscrizioni Puteolane, Römische Mittheilungen 3, 1888, pp. 79–83.

[2] As R. Hanslik thinks, RE XXIII, 1959, cols. 2083f. s. v. Pylades.

pression of making a great discovery, for he shows not so much his superiority in medicine as his careful observation and commonsense. This case also exhibits his obedience to the Hippocratic precept: μηδὲν εἰκῇ, μηδὲν ὑπερορᾶν (Epid. VI 2,12: V, p. 284,1 L., cf. Hipp., De off. med. 1: II, p. 30,2–7 Kw. = III, p. 272,1–5 L.; and Gal., In Hipp. Epid. VI comment. II 27: CMG V 10,2,2, pp. 91,1–92,14), that the doctor should use all his senses in diagnosing the course of a disease, and that he should consider everything, including the patient's environment, when taking the pulse, especially of a new patient (Gal., Synops. de puls. 16: IX, pp. 474,12–475,2 K.). Two other cases of Galen's may fittingly be compared with this: that of a Sicilian doctor and friend of Glaucon in late 162 / early 163, when he used his observations of all the objects and signs of activity in the sick-room to make an accurate prognosis (Gal., De loc. aff. 5: VIII, pp. 361,12–366,5 K.); and his confrontation with the wealthy drug-addict whose secret drug-taking was clear to Galen as soon as he observed his tongue and took his pulse (Gal., De praes. ex puls. I 1: IX, pp. 218,8–220,3 K.). These and the remaining cases in 'On prognosis' display Galen the clinician, able to cope with almost any disease and quick to react to the slightest hint that would lead to a solution of whatever medical problem he was considering. Many of his cures, as L. Jacchinus saw, demanded only commonsense and shrewdness of observation – which many of his dogmatic opponents may have lacked – and they offer a contrast to the literary, polemical and theorising Galen of the first half of this tract. Thus Galen's narrative here, as well as relaxing the tension, successfully masks a transition between the two parts and prepares the reader for the sequence of cures that is to follow.

P. 106,1f.: A difficult and probably corrupt passage, of which Nic.'s version may represent a different Ms. reading, or, more likely, an attempt by the translator to make some sense out of some very dubious Greek. Unless we have another example of Galenic pleonasm, the first τὸν οἶκον should be excluded as either a gloss or a repetitive error in transcription. Both M and the abbreviation in L suggest that the room in question was the boy's, and thus I have emended the first participle from the masculine to the feminine κοιμωμένην, for it would make little point to say that the boy slept in his own room. If the asyndeton is considered harsh, καὶ may be added before κατὰ. There is still the problem of ἀποκεκλεισμένον ἔνδοθεν to be faced. If the mother remained within the room, she could hardly prevent people from coming to see the boy, and p. 108,3–5 may imply that the door was locked on the outside. But it could be that the door was only locked when she went away (p. 108,3–5) or at night when she was sleeping and that it was locked "from the inside" (the most natural meaning of the Greek). But in classical Greek it is normally a person, not a building, that is ἀποκεκλεισμένος (Lysias, Or. 1,17: Demosthenes, Or. 59,41), but the word can be applied to gates (Herodotus, Hist. I 150), temples (ibid. II 133) and cities (Aristophanes, Lys. 487), and so it is possible that here it is the room, not the boy, that is locked up.

P. 106,5: A similar chance assembly of spectators encountered on the way is mentioned at p. 138,18f., and may be compared with the crowd who followed Attalus when he came to treat the (already dead) Theagenes of Patras (Gal., Meth. med. XIII 15: X, pp. 909,10–916,2 K.).

P. 106,12: This is the earliest undisputed occurrence of the feminine noun βάθρα, meaning 'seat'. Almost certainly it is the neuter plural, βάθρα, not the feminine singular, that is given by Pollux (Onomasticon X 48) to correspond with the βαθρίδια of Aristophanes, frag. 513; and editors of Plutarch since Bernardakis have preferred his emendation, ἀποβάθραν, which derives from the parallel passage in Thucydides, to the simple βάθραν of the Mss. of Moralia 347b. L-S-J cite as the first certain example an inscription from Egypt (Sammelbuch griech. Urkunden 402), dated to 274 A. D., in honour of Sarapis ἐπὶ τῇ βάθρᾳ, and, in literature, John Lydus (De Mag. I 3): βασιλεύς ἐστιν ὁ τῶν ἑαυτοῦ ὑπηκόων πρῶτος ψήφῳ ἐπιλελεγμένος ἐπὶ βάθραν τινὰ ὥσπερ καὶ κρηπῖδα (βάθρα M: βάθραν O corr. [18th cent.] and edd.). Nic.'s 'sedilia' translates both the neuter and the feminine forms and should not be used as an argument for emending βάθραι to the more common βάθρα, especially when this section contains several choice technical terms, rarely, if ever, found elsewhere.

P. 106,13f.: From the manner of Boethus' introduction of Galen to his wife, we may deduce that this case fell in the first part of Galen's first stay in Rome, probably in mid – or late 163, especially as, for the most part, the cases are described in the chronological order in which they occurred, cf. below, p. 217.

P. 106,19: Chartier, followed by Kühn, added ἵνα μὲν before ὅπως, unnecessarily, for the optatives δηλώσειεν and διδάξειεν in this complicated sentence depend on ὅπως in line 14.

P. 106,27: Once more Galen demonstrates his familiarity with the writings of earlier doctors, which was, he claimed, more extensive than any his teachers could recall (De exam. med., Bull. Hist. Med. 36, 1962, p. 364; al-Mubaššir, p. 55).

P. 106,28: Kühn's omission of μοι after ἐκελεύετέ merely sidestepped the difficulty. Did Galen always use the construction with accusative and infinitive after κελεύειν, or did he slip occasionally into the Koine usage of dative and infinitive (cf. W. Schmid, I, pp. 33f.; II, p. 205; III, p. 309; IV, p. 180)? The former construction is found without exception in the Epidemics (cf. CMG V 10,2,3, p. 134, ten examples) and also in general in 'On prognosis', but the dative is found here, at 128,23 and 130,17; at De praes. ex puls. I 1: IX, p. 220,17 K.; and at De sanit. tuenda II 11,29: CMG V 4,2, p. 67,37 (where two Mss. have the accusative), and thus I am reluctant to follow Cornarius and emend to με, preferring to consider that both constructions were used by Galen himself, although in general he favoured the Attic form.[1]

Note also how Galen half-humorously accepts the suggestion that he is about to perform a mantic cure and chooses his words to fit the expectation of his audience, μάντευμα, τὸ τοῦ μάντεως θέσπισμα (cf. L. Jacchinus, p. 71).

P. 108,2: Nothing further is known of the life and career of Flavius Cyrillus apart from this incident.

P. 108,4: On the different spellings of γλωττόκομον in Galen and on its relevance to the stylistic debate with the Atticists, see W. Herbst, p. 76. The meaning required here, the box of a lock into which the key is inserted, is not given by L-S-J; see also A. Gaheis, Das römische Tür- u. Kantenschloß, Jahreshefte d. Österreich. Archäolog. Instituts 26, 1930, Beibl., pp. 231–262, who gives several photographs of ancient locks.

P. 108,18: The text as given by all the edd. (ταραντινίδος) indicated that the only place that had escaped investigation was a small object lying on his mother's ταραντινίς. It is surely strange that amid so much precise detail of the bedroom fitments the actual hiding place of the food should alone remain vague and that another word in the sentence should be a hapax legomenon. The abbreviations of L and M place an acute accent on the iota but say nothing of the form of the ending and Nic.'s version implies that the noun was in the nominative, not the genitive: "erat hoc parvum quoddam ("aliquod" Nic.[ce]) capitis amictum ("cohopertorium" Nic.[c]: "coopertorium" Nic.[e]: "-ersorium" Nic.[v]: "i. e. fasceolum" add. Nic.[a]) matris eius (om. Nic.[cev]) superiacens in cathedra." The suggestion of N and Cornarius that the rare word ταραντινίδιον recurs here (also at 100,21) can swiftly be accepted, although the precise meaning of the word is uncertain: probably it is a light wrap or a scarf made from Tarentine byssus. The addition of τὸ after τοῦτο would make the identification more precise, but it is not essential. The result of my investigation of the Mss. at this point is thus that the word ταραντινίς can now be confidently expelled from the standard lexica.

P. 108,22f.: Nic.'s version omits εἰ and places a stop after δηλοῦν, a simple but unnecessary emendation, since ἀλλὰ is used idiomatically following a conditional clause to mean "at any rate" (see J. D. Denniston, pp. 11f.). But it is the person of the verb that must be changed, from the first person to the third, after ὁ σφυγμός, which gives the required contrast with κἀγὼ (line 24). Although Nic.'s "sic coniecturavi" implies that οὕτως stood in his text before ἐμήνυσα, the fact that he does not translate the next sentence leads me to believe that his text was not sound enough to be relied upon here.

P. 110,1–4: The sense of Galen's explanation is that a person in a situation of stress cannot refrain from showing signs of mental agitation

[1] Cf. the similar confusion in Longus, discussed by G. Dalmeyda in his edition, Paris 1934, p. LV.

(for ἴσχειν meaning κατέχειν, simple verb for compound, see above, p. 62). ἐπιδείκνυσθαι is a technical term for making a public display of one's abilities, especially in rhetoric, and πλεονέκτημα has its later Greek meaning (cf. L-S-J, s. v.) 'superiority', either of body, as in a wrestling match, or of intellect, as in court. None of these examples apply to Cyrillus, whose agitation is caused by a guilty conscience. Thus ἐγκαλούμενός, 'being accused', does not go with the infinitives that depend on μέλλων but is independent of them. The sentence then falls into two parts; the mental agitation shown by a boy before a contest, when older competitors have long since conquered their nerves, and that shown by any defendant, be he young or old, faced with a charge: cf. Gal., De praes. ex puls. I 1 (IX, p. 219,17f. K.): ὁ δ' οὐθ' ἑτοίμως ἀπεκρίνατο πρὸς τοῦτο καὶ τὴν τῶν ἀρτηριῶν κίνησιν ἀνώμαλον (ἀνωμάλου Kühn) ἴσχεν ὡς ἐπ' ἀγωνίᾳ. I suspect that, once again, Nic.'s version represents the best that he could do to make a corrupt text intelligible.

P. 110,9: The very rare word προσεπιλογίζεσθαι emphasises Galen's mastery of reasoning from all attendant factors, taking everything (προσ-) into consideration as well as the physical signs of the patient's illness. For this, intelligence rather than erudition was required. Cf. Gal., De praes. ex puls. III 4: IX, pp. 357,2–361,9 K., where Galen says that, during the great plague of 165 and after, the advice of the intelligent layman was often more valuable in diagnosing fevers because of his common sense and experience than that of any doctor.

P. 110,16–18: The Greek Mss. and the Latin version here differ considerably. If αὐτὸ refers forwards to ἓν οὖν ὄντως θαυμάσιον "You heard this particular case ...", it may be allowed to stand, but it would be simpler to emend to αὐτὸς, "I have you as a witness in that case, and other witnesses for many others, and you heard about them from my patients". It is also hard to decide whether there is an ellipse of ἐστι in the Greek Mss., which Nic. filled out with "monet non tacere"; or whether the words οὐ σιωπήσω stood in the Greek and were omitted by a careless scribe who skipped the last words of a long sentence, having already wrongly written ἐποίησα. I have doubtfully preferred the former explanation, against the example of the Basle editors.

P. 110,18: F. Sezgin thought that Boethus' wife was the same as the Queen Filātus (or Filānus) at whose request the treatise 'On the secrets of women' was written[1], but even if this identification is accepted, it tells us very little, for the tract, in the form in which it survives, is assuredly spurious.

P. 110,19f.: The date is indicated vaguely by ἤδη (line 20) and more precisely by θέρους ὥρᾳ (p. 114,14), if this is not a gloss. Galen is now

[1] F. Sezgin, Geschichte des arabischen Schrifttums, III, Leyden 1970, p. 127; cf. M. Ullmann, p. 61, and M. Levey and S. S. Souryal, Galen's "On the secrets of women" and "On the secrets of men". A contribution to the history of Arabic pharmacology, Janus 55, 1968, pp. 208–219.

established among the doctors (ἤδη would appear to rule out 165 and 166 if Galen expected his readers to be impressed by his speedy success) and well regarded by Boethus' household, for his commands (p. 112,20–22) are instantly obeyed. Summer 164 seems a more likely date than 163, although that cannot be ruled out: certainly, the cure of Boethus' wife postdates that of his son, but neither can be securely dated to within a year.

The case of Boethus' wife is the most puzzling of all those described in 'On prognosis'. From the symptoms described by Galen, a vaginal discharge, a hard swelling in the area of the womb which became spongy to the touch after a fainting fit and an evacuation of watery fluid, it would indeed be possible to suspect an incomplete abortion[1], but Galen, who was a sound clinician, expressly denies this, and his word should be believed. The fact that the patient recovers in a fortnight rules out a carcinoma of the uterus, ovary or Fallopian tubes, and the fact that fluid escapes (through the vagina?) without causing any lasting damage to the bladder, the vaginal wall or the rectum excludes also the very rare condition of a hydatid cyst in the uterus. The best diagnosis may be that the woman was suffering from a pelvic abscess, from which the pus can be thick or thin, greenish yellow or watery. The disease begins with a vaginal discharge, which is typical of salpingitis leading to a pelvic abscess: the patient gets worse and the belly swells, as would be expected with the distension of the bowel as the abscess collects: collapse follows, which could well be explained by a prolonged fever and dehydration and then the emission of the fluid as the abscess bursts and discharges. The discharge lasts for nine days, and recovery is complete within three weeks, a time scale suitable for a pelvic abscess even today. The change from a drying treatment to heating the cold temperament of the body (p. 114,10–13) can be explained by the change in the patient's condition from sweating attacks to shivering from rigors, which resulted from the gross infection.[2]

That a modern diagnosis of the patient's condition can be made is a tribute to Galen's accuracy of observation and to his readiness to change his method of treatment if it proved unsuitable at first. But neither his information nor his treatment is as extensive as a modern physician would like, and the identification of the disease with a pelvic abscess remains only a possibility. ῥοῦς γυναικεῖος, the feminine flux, is defined ([Gal.], Def. med. 301: XIX, p. 429,1 K.) as the attraction of excess humours into the uterus, which are then discharged over a period of time. Soranus (Gynaec. III 43: CMG IV, p. 122,7ff.) presents the views of earlier authorities on the subject before passing

1 Cf. the case of the woman with an incomplete abortion, summarised from De exam. medico by Maimonides, Aphorisms XIII 21, ed. Basle, 1579, pp. 480f. – unless this is a Renaissance forgery, cf. above, p. 57.

2 I am grateful to Mr. P. A. F. Chalk, F. R. C. S. for his patience with my importunings: the identification proposed in the text is his.

on to his recommended treatment, carefully distinguishing between the various types of humour and differentiating the female flux from the menstrual discharge, as do Galen (De sympt. caus. III 11: VII, p. 265,11 K.; and De alim. fac. I 18,4: CMG V 4,2, p. 244,13) and Archigenes (apud Aetius, Tetrabibl. XVI 65). Galen assigns its cause to the retention of superfluous moisture under the skin, especially when the abdomen is chilled, which displays itself in the excretion of blood (De loc. aff. V 7: VII, p. 354,3 K.), and to the disturbance of the ἀποκριτική δύναμις (De sympt. diff. 6: VII, p. 80,2 K.). Like unhealthy sweats, it reveals itself by a wormlike pulse (Gal., De caus. puls. III 17: IX, p. 154,4f. K.; De praes. ex puls. II 9: IX, p. 313,5 K.; Introd. de puls. 11: VIII, p. 473,5 K.), and if unchecked, may easily end in dropsy (Gal., De nat. fac. II 8: Scr. min. III, pp. 180,19–181,6 Helmr. = II, pp. 109,13–110,7 K.). It was not unknown for a fainting fit to follow such a discharge, especially if, as in this case, the evacuation was considerable, less so for a convulsion, but both were very bad signs (Gal., In Hipp. Aph. comment. V 56: XVII B, p. 852,6–15 K.), and, if the woman was pregnant, the uterine discharge indicated that the foetus could not be healthy (ibid. 60: XVII B, p. 859,3–10 K.).

Hippocrates (De nat. mul. 90: VII, pp. 408,18–410,3 L.) advocated the use of drying and astringent substances: wine, river crabs, a drying pessary and, if the flux persisted, a drying fumigation and a styptic pessary. Soranus (Gynaec. III 44: CMG IV, pp. 123,19–124,6) followed his example, indicating, among others, warm poultices and hot, light foods (including lentils, cf. Gal., De alim. fac. I 18,4: CMG V 4,2, p. 244,13) and, if the disease was chronic, dressings and ointments that could tone up and strengthen the body, including massage with bare hands. Galen agreed with this, adding a potion devised by Apollonius (De comp. med. sec. loc. IX 6: XIII, p. 295,10–14 K.) and the treatment given here. All the generally accepted treatments were included by Oribasius, and through him they were continued in later Greek medicine (cf. above, pp. 52f.).

P. 110,20: With the phrase ταῖς συνήθεσι μαίαις cf. τοῖς συνήθεσιν ἰατροῖς (p. 76,22; Gal., In Hipp. De off. med. comment. II 7: XVIII B, p. 744,16f. K.). Well over sixty μαῖαι or obstetrices are recorded upon inscriptions of the Roman imperial period, some serving within a wealthy household (e. g. CIL VI 4458, 6325, 6647), others independently in a city (e. g. CIL VI 9477; Monumenta Asiae Minoris antiquae VII 566). In general their social status was low. Only rarely are they found taking any part in public life (cf. a member of a mystery cult at Cyme in Aeolis, Jahreshefte d. Österreich. Archäolog. Instituts 14, 1911, Beibl., pp. 133–140) or even commemorated with a portrait relief.[1] There were even male gynaecologists: see Soranus, Gynaec.

[1] A sign of moderate wealth: I know of only three certain examples; from Ostia (G. Calza, La necropoli del Porto di Roma, Rome 1940, pp. 248–251); from Trier (E. Espérandieu, Recueil général des bas-reliefs, statues et bustes de la Gaule

III 3: CMG IV, p. 95,6ff.; and IG XII 5, 199, from Paros, but their numbers must never have been high.

The requirements laid down by Soranus for his ideal midwife (Gynaec. I 3f.: CMG IV, pp. 4,12–6,11) do not appear to us to be particularly exacting – she must be literate, intelligent, possessed of a good memory, hard working, respectable, without any defect of her senses, nimble, hardy, and with soft hands and long fingers – but they were rarely achieved (cf. the amusing tale of the Egyptian astrologer and the barmaid-cum-midwife told by Eunapius, Vit. Phil. 21, ed. Giangrande).

P. 112,1: As Guinther, Cornarius and Rota made clear in their translations, ἐποίουν is first person singular, not third person plural, which impairs the validity of the Basle editors' πραττ⟨όντ⟩ων. The resulting hiatus rules out πράττον⟨τι⟩, and thus πράττον⟨τος⟩ or, if Nic.'s version ("his gestis") is trusted, τούτων πραττ⟨ομέν⟩ων must both be considered. But the example of another constructio ad sensum at 82,24 above advises caution.

P. 112,16: The confusion between οὔτε . . . οὔτε and οὐδὲ . . . οὐδέ is common in writers of the Roman imperial period and it is unwise to alter this to a more Attic form, cf. Eunapius, ed. Boissonade, pp. 169f. and Xenophon of Ephesus, ed. Dalmeyda, p. xxxviii.

P. 112,17: The reason for this parenthesis, as Galen himself states (De comp. med. sec. loc. VIII 1: XIII, p. 121,17 K.) is that the upper part of the belly was called variously καρδία and στόμαχος and thus Galen is here defining his terms precisely. Similar parentheses are found at Meth. med. VIII 5: X, p. 573,8f. K.; De venae sect. adv. Eras. Rom. deg. 9: XI, p. 242,14 K.; In Hipp. Progn. comment. III 35: CMG V 9,2, p. 360,16f.: none should be removed from the text on the suspicion of being a gloss.

P. 112,20: Nard, or spikenard, nardostachys jatamansi D C, Valerianaceae, was valued especially in the treatment of diseases of the stomach, belly and womb. Dioscorides (De mat. med. I 7,3f., ed. Wellmann) says that the various types of nard: δύναμιν δὲ ἔχουσι θερμαντικήν, ξηραντικήν, οὐρητικήν, ὅθεν κοιλίαν τε ἱστᾶσι πινόμεναι καὶ τὰς ἐκ μήτρας ῥύσεις προστιθέμεναι . . . εἰς ἐγκάθισμα φλεγμονὰς μήτρας ἰῶνται. It was often made into ointment for use: Dioscorides (ibid. 62) mentions at least two methods of manufacture and Galen (Meth. med. XI 16: X, p. 791,5–10 K.) praises the variety produced originally only at Laodicaea ad Lycum, and notes the special kind made from the leaves and the spike alone to gratify the whims of rich Roman women (De sanit. tuenda VI 10,8f.: CMG V 4,2, p. 18,20–22; Meth. med. VIII 5: X, p. 574,2 K.). Ointment of nard was a traditional way of strengthening a weak stomach (Gal., Meth. med. VII 4: X,

Romaine, Paris 1907–1955, n. 4363); and from Istanbul (N. Firatli and L. Robert, Les stèles funéraires de Byzance gréco-romaine, Paris 1964, n. 139, pl. 35 and pp. 175ff.); to which may be added the female statues from Velia (La Parola del Passato 25, 1970, pp. 280, 283 and fig. 7).

p. 466,7 K.), even if, as here, it was not always successful. Because of its property of drying, warming and toning up the affected part, Galen advocates rubbing it in with warm cloths to stop a discharge from the belly (Meth. med. VIII 5: X, pp. 572,17–573,2 K.). The compiler of the Syriac Book of Medicine (p. 326/376, ed. Budge, cf. J. Schleifer, Riv. di studi Orientali 20, 1942, p. 393), who gives two recipes for oil of nard, recommends that for diseases of the womb it should be used as an unguent and injected or applied to the vulva with a pad of soft rag or wool. Although unguent of nard was normally used by itself, as here, it could form the base of other ointments, as for that composed by Asclepiades the pharmacist for Aquilia Secundilla (Gal., De comp. med. sec. loc. VII 12: XIII, p. 1031,13 K.).

The plant and its leaves were imported (cf. J. I. Miller, pp. 88–92, 116), but there is no evidence that the oil or unguent manufactured from them was produced outside the Roman Empire. At first a luxury at 300 denarii a box (Mark 14,5), spikenard was reduced in price to 100 denarii a pound in Pliny's day (Nat. Hist. XII 26,44) with the increase in trade with India, but it never lost its cachet of luxury (cf. Historia Augusta, Vita Heliogabali 24,1).[1]

P. 114,21: Pitch was a good heating substance (Dioscorides, De mat. med. I 72,5, ed. Wellmann), moderately warming (Gal., De comp. med. per gen. IV 6: XIII, p. 709,16 K.) and drying the body rather than heating it (Gal., De simpl. med. temp. et fac. IX 19: XII, p. 101,9–12 K.). It is recommended for stomach chills (Gal., Meth. med. VII 7: X, p. 501,15ff. K.), since, when placed upon the stomach, it disperses internal hardnesses without introducing blood into the affected area.

Resin was also used as a drying agent. Dioscorides (De mat. med. I 70,1f., ed. Wellmann) praised the resin of the mastich highly for its property of stopping discharges from the womb, staying wandering fluxes and stimulating urination. A pitchy resin (Dioscorides, ibid. 70,3f.) or a mixture of pitch and resin (Gal., De comp. med. per gen. IV 6: XIII, p. 709,10ff. K.; ibid. VII 9: XIII, p. 995,10ff. K.) shared in the qualities of both its constituents: when the mixture was applied to the affected parts and rubbed in well, its heat drew the excessive moisture to itself, thus ending the flux (Gal., De diff. febr. II 15: VII, p. 385,1ff. K.); cf. also M. Levey, pp. 269 and 276; A. Weisenberg, pp. 466ff.

P. 114,21f.: Although the properties of honey, that it dried and warmed the body, and cleansed and dispersed impurities, were well known in antiquity (Dioscorides, De mat. med. II 82, ed. Wellmann; Gal., De sanit. tuenda III 38: CMG V 4,2, p. 381,9–11; Meth. med. III 6: X, p. 203,5 K.; De simpl. med. temp. et fac. VII 9: XII, p. 70,

[1] Both nard and oil of nard are mentioned on Diocletian's edict of prices, ed. S. Laufer, Diokletians Preisedikt, Berlin 1971, 36, 50 and 98, but unfortunately the figure for their costs has been lost.

13–18 K.; De comp. med. sec. loc. VIII 2: XIII, p. 21,2 K.), I can find no other example of honey being used on its own as an unguent except in the passages in Oribasius and his successors that derive from this. Even J. Pereira, who declares that it is occasionally employed as an emollient and demulcent in inflammatory affections (II 2, p. 764), would scarcely have considered coating his Victorian patient all over with honey. The medical value of this treatment is questionable, for a pelvic abscess once discharged is cured without further treatment, but it must have boosted the morale of the patient considerably to be given this novel cure and would only have increased Galen's own reputation for daring and wisdom. It was a grand gesture which, if it succeeded, enhanced his glory; if it failed, the patient was not harmed and another cure might be suggested.

P. 114,25: The remedies tried by Galen in no way assist a modern diagnosis of the disease, for neither here nor in his reference to the hydragogic drug (p. 116,3f.) does he specify the treatment used.

P. 116,5: Asarabacca, bacchar or wild nard, Asarum europaeum L. Aristolocheae, was found in Crete, Pontus, Phrygia, Illyricum and the region of Italy inhabited by the Vestini, that is, the present day provinces of Ascoli Piceno and Teramo (Dioscorides, De mat. med. I 10, ed. Wellmann). It has the property of stimulating urination and of warming the body (ibid.) and of thereby converting the offending humours into urine (Gal., De comp. med. sec. loc. IX 279: XIII, p. 155,8 K.; ibid. X 611: XIII, p. 277,15 K.), and was considered particularly good for the purgation of menses (Gal., De simpl. med. temp. et fac. V 22: XI, p. 775,2–10 K.) and for an inflamed womb (ibid. VI 63: XI, p. 840,6–10 K.); cf. A. Weisenberg, p. 87; M. Levey, p. 227; M. Grieve, I, pp. 63f.

Celery, Apium graveolens L. Labiatae, also stimulates urination when taken neat or in a decoction (Dioscorides, De mat. med. III 64, ed. Wellmann; Gal., De sanit. tuenda V 9,1: CMG V 4,2, p. 152,26; De alim. fac. II 51: CMG V 4,2, p. 316,10–23; De simpl. med. temp. et fac. IX 6: XII, pp. 118,17–119,3 K.). When taken with asarabacca it is especially potent in stimulating urination, in thinning the humours and in drawing to the kidneys all that is watery, thin and serous in the blood (Gal., De simpl. med. temp. et fac. V 13: XI, p. 747, 6–17 K.); cf. M. Levey, pp. 324f.; and M. Grieve, I, p. 182. L. Jacchinus (p. 76) praised Galen because, of the types of drug known to him for purging menses, one drawing blood into the veins of the uterus, the other attenuating the flow of blood, he correctly chose the second.

P. 116,7–9: The difficulties of rendering Galen's meaning into modern terms are great, especially since he is often confused over the internal organs of women and their relationship with one another, which he at times derives by analogy with those of men or even of animals (cf. D. Nickel, CMG V 2,1, pp. 101–106; C. R. S. Harris, p. 290).

P. 116,11f.: The soft flesh of rock fish enabled them to be digested easily and to disappear in sweat without harming the kidneys (Diphilus, apud Athenaeus, Deipnosoph. VIII 355a–357; Gal., Meth. med. VIII 2: X, p. 537,9 K.; De alim. fac. III 29,9: CMG V 4,2, p. 370,5–9 and I 1,8: CMG V 4,2, p. 204,18–20, repeated at De consuet. 2: CMG Suppl. III, p. 16,5; De sanit. tuenda VI 11,4f.: CMG V 4,2, p. 190,30; In Hipp. Aph. comment. II 18: XVII B, p. 489,12f. K.). Taken together with the flesh of mountain birds, it was an important part of a diet designed to thin out and remove accumulations within the body and to speed digestion (Gal., De sanit. tuenda IV 4,82: CMG V 4,2, p. 115,16f.; De victu atten. 8,55: CMG V 4,2, p. 441,20–24).

P. 116,18: On Boethus' gift of 400 aurei (= 40,000 HS) in relation to other known fees, see above, pp. 179f.

P. 116,20: ἕτοιμος followed by τό and the infinitive is a poetic flosculus. Although a similar construction is found after a few other adjectives (cf. Schwyzer-Debrunner, II, p. 371), the only other example with ἕτοιμος is Sophocles, El. 1079. That such a usage formerly in poetry and highly rhetorical prose should now occur in bald narrative is typical of Greek prose of this period.[1]

P. 116,22f.: This chronological reference sets this case before the ending of the Parthian War in 166, but is too imprecise to help in settling its date.[2] L and M give the name of the Parthian king as ending in -έσου, Nic. in "-esi", but coins of the Parthian monarchs have -άσου and Cassius Dio and other historians offer -αίσου (cf. H. Furneaux, ed. of Tacitus, Annals, Oxford 1891, on Ann. XII 14,8). I have altered the spelling of Galen's Mss. to conform to the latter variant.

P. 116,25: The Ionic ἐς for εἰς here, at p. 70,4 and at p. 118,5 may be a delicate reference to the Hippocratic writings and is entirely consonant with the stylistic reminiscences of Galen (cf. De uteri dissect. 10,13: CMG V 2,1, p. 56,7) and of many other doctors of the second century.[3]

P. 116,28: A visit to Campania along the Via Appia would not be considered unusual, for many Romans of importance had villas there[4] and Galen knew the region well.[5] An earlier imperial physician, C. Stertinius Xenophon, and his brother had obtained land there and had given money to rebuild the walls of Naples (Pliny, Nat. Hist. XXIX 7),

[1] See P. Aalto, Studien zur Gesch. d. Infinitivs im Griechischen, Annales Academiae Scient. Fennicae 80,2, Helsinki 1953, pp. 28–74.

[2] On Lucius' activities abroad, see T. D. Barnes, pp. 70ff. and A. R. Birley, Marcus Aurelius, pp. 160ff.

[3] Cf. Lucian, De hist. conscrib. 24f.; J. and L. Robert, Bull. Epigraphique 1962, n. 374; ibid. 1970, n. 667; and K. Deichgräber's discussion of the first century doctor Aretaeus, Aretaeus von Kappadokien als medizinischer Schriftsteller, Abh. d. Sächs. Akademie d. Wiss., phil.-hist. Kl. 63,3, 1971, pp. 18–29.

[4] See J. H. D'Arms, Romans on the Bay of Naples, Cambridge, Mass., 1970, pp. 73–164.

[5] E. g. Gal., De sanit. tuenda VI 11,3: CMG V 4,2, p. 190,25; In Hipp. Epid. VI comment. VIII: CMG V 10,2,2, p. 461,40 (Cumae); Meth. med. V 12: X, pp. 363,1–373,2 K., reading ⟨Σ⟩ταβίαι for Ταβίαι (etc.).

and, before them, Antonius Musa, doctor to Augustus, enjoyed a considerable reputation throughout Campania.[1]

P. 116,31: The Subura, the low lying area behind the Forum, between the Esquiline, the Viminal and the Quirinal, now partly traversed by the Via Cavour, was one of the most unhealthy parts of the city and was inhabited only by the poor or by the criminal. It was a great trading centre ('fervens Subura', Juvenal, Sat. XI 51) with many shops (Martial, VII 31,9) offering wares of every kind and origin (ibid. VI 66; X 94; XI 61 and 78) and owned by shifty dealers, hence Galen's choice of κέρκωψ, a derogatory word from Old Comedy. The transcription of the word Subura in Greek is uncertain[2]: the Mss. of Dionysius of Halicarnassus, Ant. IV 14,1, have Σουβ-; but Σιβ- is given by those of Appian, Bell. Civ. I 58,261; of Plutarch, Mor. 287 A; and by four inscriptions (Corpus Inscriptionum Iudaicarum 18, 22, 67 and 380), and I have emended the corrupt Βηβούρας of the Mss. to conform with them.

P. 116,31f.: This shows that Galen was living independently, not as a member of the household of a wealthy patron like Lucian's 'hired scholars'; cf. also above, p. 126,27.

P. 118,2: Does this mean that his servant returned to Asia, Galen's πατρίς, via Sicily, or that he reached his own home by that route? I hesitantly prefer the first interpretation. Galen goes along the Via Appia direct to Brindisi while his servant sails along the West coast of Italy, touching Sicily, before making for Pergamum. This passage may well be the source of the tradition, given by Barhebraeus (Chron., p. 54, ed. Budge) that Galen died in Sicily on his way to Jerusalem.

P. 118,4: Once at Brindisi Galen had a choice of two routes to Pergamum, either direct to Durazzo/Dürres and thence along the Via Egnatia to Thessalonica; or South to the Corinthian Gulf, Athens and then across the Aegean to Asia. From line 9, where Galen sails past Cassiope, the North-East point of Corcyra, he must have taken the second route, on which he was accompanied for part of the way by an irascible merchant from Gortyn (Gal., De aff. dign. 4,9–23: CMG V 4,1,1, pp. 13,9–15,5). From Athens he would have gone directly to Miletus, Ephesus or Smyrna and then overland to Pergamum, rather than by land through Thessaly to Macedonia, Lemnos and Alexandria Troas, as some have thought[3]. The statement at De simpl. med. temp. et fac. IX 2: XII, p. 171,11–15 K., that he had traversed the whole of Macedonia before reaching Philippi on his second visit to Lemnos fits a journey along the Via Egnatia more than one through Thessaly, and W. A. Greenhill (p. 208) was right to conclude from this that Galen paid a second visit to Pergamum, possibly in the 190s.

[1] J. H. D'Arms, Romans on the Bay of Naples, p. 149, n. 153.

[2] R. Valentini and G. Zucchetti, Codice topografico della città di Roma, Rome 1940, p. 103.

[3] A. Stein, PIR² G. 24; followed by G. W. Bowersock, p. 62. I have discussed the problem of the routes at CQ, pp. 166ff.

P. 118,16–22: In three sentences Galen passes over the events of three years, which makes a reconstruction of his activities in that period from this passage and from the account in De lib. propr. 1. 2: Scr. min. II, pp. 96,17–19; 98,11–15 Müller = XIX, pp. 15,13–16; 17,15–18,1 K., extremely hazardous.

If 118,16 is correct, Galen left Rome by August 166, the date of Lucius Verus' return (Historia Augusta, Vita Marci 12,8; Vita Commodi 11,13; ILS 366), and I have tentatively suggested that his flight is to be dated to early or mid-summer 166.[1] Given this fixed date, his cure of Eudemus, which occurred at the middle of winter some three years before, when Lucius Verus was on campaign (Gal., De lib. propr. 1: Scr. min. II, p. 96,17–19 Müller = XIX, p. 15,13–16 K.; above, p. 82,4f.), can be placed in 162/3 and thus, as this cure was made during his first winter in Rome, we can date Galen's arrival in Rome to 162. From this, we may deduce from Gal., De lib. propr. 1: Scr. min. II, p. 96,5–7 Müller = XIX, p. 15,3–5 K., which refers to his arrival in Rome in his thirty fourth year, that he was born in August/September 128 or 129 (for the month, see Gal., De comp. med. per gen. III 2: XIII, pp. 599,10–13; 600,10–15 K.).[2] But the year 128 is ruled out by Gal., De lib. propr. 2: Scr. min. II, p. 97,6f. Müller = XIX, p. 16,6f. K., which puts his return home to Pergamum at the age of thirty seven, i. e. not later than September 166, which does not allow him much time to get from Rome to Pergamum, and so Galen's date of birth can be fixed at August/September 129.[3] His activities between reaching Pergamum and receiving the imperial summons are all subsumed in the words: εἰχόμην τῶν συνήθων (De lib. propr. 2: Scr. min. II, p. 98,11f. Müller = XIX, p. 17,16 K.). Although J. Ilberg assumed that Galen spent his time in attending to patients and writing his treatises[4], it is likely that he also carried out scientific visits to Cyprus (Gal., De simpl. med. temp. et fac. IX 11: XII, p. 220,1–7 K.; ibid. 21: XII, p. 227,4–6 K.) and to Lycia (ibid. IX 10: XII, p. 203,3–8 K.).

P. 118,17: If the Historia Augusta is right (Vita Marci 12,13), trouble with the Germans began even before Lucius' return, but, although a fifth imperial salutation is recorded on a diploma dated May 5, 167 (CIL XVI 123) and on coins of 168 (Coinage of the British Museum, M. Aurelius, CXXII, pp. 148ff.), Marcus and Lucius were still in Rome in January 168 (Fragmentum Vaticanum 195) and set out later in the year. After a brief campaign North of the Julian

[1] V. Nutton, CQ, p. 159; I reject there the suggestion that he left Rome to avoid a plague brought back from the East by the army.

[2] V. Nutton, CQ, p. 160; where the problem of the evidence of Gal., In Hipp. De artic. comm. I 22: XVIII A, p. 347,14–16 K., which puts his arrival in 161, is discussed.

[3] V. Nutton, CQ, p. 160.

[4] J. Ilberg, Wann ist Galen geboren?, Sudhoffs Archiv f. Gesch. d. Medizin u. d. Naturwiss. 23, 1930, p. 291; cf. V. Nutton, CQ, pp. 169f.

Alps (ILS 1098, 1100) they returned to Aquileia for the winter of 168/9.[1]

P. 118,22: Galen made his way from Pergamum to Alexandria Troas, Myrina, Thessalonica and then along the Via Egnatia to the Adriatic (Gal., De simpl. med. temp. et fac. IX 2: XII, p. 171,11–15 K.; cf. V. Nutton, CQ, pp. 167f.). Both G. W. Bowersock (p. 63) and A. R. Birley (Marcus Aurelius, pp. 213f.) assume that he was recalled to deal with the plague that was raging in the army at Aquileia, but Galen's words at De lib. propr. 2: Scr. min. II, p. 98,23f. Müller = XIX, p. 18,8f. K.: ἐπιβάντος οὖν μου τῆς Ἀκυληίας κατέσκηψεν ὁ λοιμὸς ὡς οὔπω πρότερον, imply that the plague either coincided with or followed his arrival. Even if Birley is right to connect with the plague and with Galen's recall the death of Sergius Hestiaeus, the personal doctor of the consular and general Servilius Fabianus[2], this does not help in dating Galen's arrival. Nor, since there were other doctors in attendance on the emperor (above, p. 126,17; Gal., De antid. I 1: XIV, p. 4,3 K.), is it likely, pace Birley, that the emperors' return to Rome was made on the advice of Galen alone (who was then left behind in camp to face the rigours of the winter by himself).

P. 118,23: The month of Lucius' death is uncertain (cf. Historia Augusta, Vita Marci 14,7f.; Vita Veri 9,10f.). Galen's reference to midwinter is too imprecise to help decide between late 168 (cf. T. D. Barnes, p. 73) or early 169. Lucius suffered a stroke similar to one he had had shortly after his return to Rome in 166 (Fronto, Ep. II 6) while he was on the road between Concordia and Altinum, the latter being specifically mentioned by two late authors (Aur. Victor, Caes. 16,9; Chronographer of 354, Monum. Germ. Hist., Auct. Antiq. IX 147). He was buried in the Mausoleum of Hadrian in Rome (ILS 369) and was given divine honours, the title of "divus" (ILS 370) and a special order of priests, the sodales Antoniniani Veriani, to perpetuate his memory.

P. 118,25: We do not know how or when Galen returned to Rome, except that it was not before the end of winter but before October (?) 169, when Marcus left Rome to continue his campaign in the North against the Germans (Gal., De lib. propr. 2: Scr. min. II, pp. 98,26–99,7 Müller = XIX, p. 18,11–17 K.). Galen, who does not seem to have been a man of great physical courage or to have enjoyed his winter at Aquileia, ascribes the emperor's acceptance of his refusal to accom-

[1] The chronology of these campaigns is much disputed: cf., for the view adopted here, A. R. Birley, Marcus Aurelius, pp. 201–234; and, The invasions of Italy in the reign of Marcus Aurelius, Provincialia; Festschrift für R. Laur-Belart, Basle and Stuttgart 1968, pp. 214–225; I. G. Nagy, Bemerkungen zur Deutung der Stelle H. A. Vita Marci 14, Acta Antiqua 16, 1968, pp. 343–350; J. H. Oliver, p. 82, n. 38. I am less happy about the reconstruction proposed by J. Fitz, Der Markomannisch-quadische Angriff gegen Aquileia und Opitergium, Historia 15, 1966, pp. 336–367, who dates the events of the war a year earlier.

[2] IG XIV 2343, together with the photograph and discussion by P. Caracci, Medici e medicina in Aquileia romana, Aquileia Nostra 35, 1964, p. 95 and pl. 6.

pany him to his high moral character (ibid., p. 98,18 Müller = XIX, p. 18,3f. K.), which was χρηστός, φιλάνθρωπος, εὐγνώμων, μέτριος, ἥμερος and πρᾶος (cf. M. Aurelius, Med. XI 13; XII 5; V 32; I 16; VII 63, for these adjectives).[1] But in De lib. propr. he reveals the strategem by which he obtained his 'leave of absence', an appeal to the veto of his ancestral god Asclepius (cf. above, p. 183), whose commands Marcus himself was prepared to accept without question (Med. V 8,3; cf. I 17,9). Is Galen's silence here an indication that he was a little ashamed of his action and wished to disguise his cowardice by giving all credit to the emperor?

P. 118,27: Galen's insistence that Marcus in 169 believed that his campaign would be short (cf. De lib. propr. 2: Scr. min. II, p. 99,13 Müller = XIX, p. 19,4f. K.) supports A. R. Birley's view that the siege of Aquileia by the Marcomanni took place in 170 (Marcus Aurelius, pp. 222ff.), not in 169, as J. Fitz thinks (Historia 15, 1966, p. 343).[2]

P. 118,30: As doctor to the young Commodus (born August 31, 161) Galen accompanied him around the imperial residences, probably including Lavinium, Lanuvium, Tibur and Antium, but there is no evidence that he went with him on his visit to the front some time between 170 and 172[3] or when he left to join his father on May 19, 175 (A. R. Birley, Marcus Aurelius, p. 258). His post was similar to that of P. Aelius Aug. lib. Epaphroditus, magister iatroliptes puerorum eminentium Caesaris nostri (CIL VI 8981), who attended to the gymnastic exercises of the young Marcus Aurelius, Lucius Verus and their friends, in that he treated not only young members of the imperial family but also their close friends.[4]

P. 118,31: 'On prognosis' is our only source of information about Peitholaus, who is described as a κοιτωνίτης (cubicularius) at 120,21 (either of Commodus or the emperor or, less likely, of Sextus) and τροφεύς (nutritor) of Commodus here: cf. also F. Grosso, pp. 118ff., for a discussion of the education of the young Commodus.

P. 120,1: K. Bardong, pp. 633–637, assigns to this prolific period of Galen's life at least twenty three treatises, including the first commentaries on the Hippocratic Corpus, but many of his philosophical writings, which J. Ilberg (Schriftstellerei IV, p. 611) believed were

[1] K. Deichgräber, Medicus gratiosus, p. 44, wrongly assigns to Antoninus Pius the reference made to M. Aurelius' short hair at Gal., In Hipp. Epid. VI comment. IV 10: CMG V 10,2,2, p. 206,16ff. D. E. Eichholz's dating of Galen's refusal to spring 169 (p. 61) is at least three months too early on my chronology.

[2] On the summoning of troops from the East in 169, see C. P. Jones, The levy at Thespiae under M. Aurelius, Greek, Roman and Byzantine Studies 12, 1971, pp. 45–48.

[3] G. Barbieri, Nuove iscrizioni di Marsala, Kokalos 7, 1961, pp. 16–22.

[4] There is nothing to support the hypothesis of R. E. Siegel, Galen's system of physiology and medicine, Basle and New York 1968, pp. 12 and 16, that Galen treated without success Annius Verus, who died of an ear tumour in late summer 169 (Historia Augusta, Vita Marci 21,3–5).

written now, have been shown by R. Walzer (GA, pp. 67ff.) to date from the last years of Commodus or even the first years of Severus, at least in the form in which we now have them.[1]

P. 120,2: Marcus Aurelius did not return to Rome until late autumn 176 (Cassius Dio, Hist. LXXI 32,1) and celebrated his triumph over the Germans on December 23, 176 (A. R. Birley, Marcus Aurelius, pp. 269f.). Galen's tactful reference to the German war hides the revolt of Avidius Cassius in 175 and a visit to Egypt and the Eastern provinces that lasted from August 175 to mid-176.

P. 120,9: The identity of this person and of Sextus, line 16, was for long in doubt. It was J. Ilberg (NJ, p. 296) who first argued that "the son of Quintilianus" and Sextus were one and the same, and C. Cichorius, no mean student of prosopography, swiftly concluded that the patient was none other than the younger of the Quintilii, Sextus Quintilius Condianus.[2] There the matter rested until A. Stein struck at the weakness of this theory[3]: that it did not correspond to the text of Kühn, which called Sextus "son of Antoninus". His alternative was to confess ignorance of the identity of the first man and to claim that Sextus, whose case is described at 120,16–126,2, was Commodus. The first objection to this hypothesis is that no member of the imperial family is known to have been called Sextus, although A. R. Birley, the latest follower of A. Stein, supposed that it was a nickname given Commodus by his sisters and recorded by Galen, since the treatment took place under the supervision of Peitholaus, his sister and her husband (Chiron, p. 468). The second objection is that the cure of Commodus, the παῖς of 126,14, is clearly differentiated from that of Sextus – and it obscures Galen's point to call the same man consistently first Sextus and then Commodus. Thirdly, if the case of the other son of Quintilianus is so important that Epigenes can remember the theory that lay behind it, it is strange that it is not mentioned in any surviving work or at any other place in this treatise.[4] Lastly, two stylistic points: ἐξ αὐτοῦ, as it stood in Kühn's text, had little meaning; and the connecting οὖν at line 16 had nothing to connect with.

The way to the correct solution was begun by J. Kollesch, pp. 57–61, (unfortunately not used by A. R. Birley), who pointed out that the words 'son of Antoninus' were not to be found in L. Indeed, they are to be found in no Greek Ms. but were taken over by the Basle

[1] For further criticisms of Bardong, see D. W. Peterson, Observations on the chronology of the Galenic Corpus, Bull. Hist. Med. 51, 1977, pp. 484–495.

[2] C. Cichorius, Sextus bei Galen, Neue Jahrbücher f. d. klass. Altertum 15, 1905, p. 604.

[3] PIR[2] G. 24. Cichorius' view had been accepted by A. Stein's colleague, E. Groag, at PIR[2] C. 1024.

[4] A. R. Birley, Chiron, p. 464, n. 3, supposes that "the son of Quintilianus" is possibly the same as the young man whose case is described at Gal., De crisib. II 9: pp. 151,17–153,7 Alex. = IX, pp. 680,16–683,10 K., but that case tells nothing about prognosis. In fact Epigenes is asked to recall the prognostic theory given in Book III of De crisib., passim, and apply it to the case of Sextus.

editors from the Latin, as was the name Κυιντιλιάνου, which replaced Κοϊντιαλίων, for the compendium at the end of the word in the Mss. represents a genitive plural, not a singular. We must first dispose of 'son of Antoninus' (or Antonius, as the Latin Mss. read), which would, if accepted, compel us to believe in A. R. Birley's nickname theory. This is not difficult, for there is nothing elsewhere in this section to suggest that the emperor was his father rather than a friend of the family and, more importantly, the Latin Mss. at 126,14 call Commodus "son of Pitholaus". If one identification of the Latin Mss. is accepted, a similar argument can be produced that Commodus was indeed the son of Peitholaus – or that that was the boy's nickname – and that the second should also be accepted.

The case for Sextus Quintilius grows stronger. If the simple palaeographic change is made from ἐξ αὐτοῦ to Ἕξστου, meaning is restored and an antecedent is found for the lonely οὖν of line 16. Nor is there any difficulty about the emendation of Κοϊντιαλίων to Κοϊντιλίων, or about the plural form. As J. H. Oliver pointed out, pp. 66–72, the elder pair of Quintilii, coss. 151, are called the Quintilii without any mark of differentiation, and their sons, who bore the same names as their respective uncles[1], are thus distinguished by the appropriate addition of υἱῶν.[2] It is interesting to note that the epitomators of Cassius Dio (Hist. LXXII 6,4 and 7,1) also refer to the younger Sextus Quintilius Condianus simply by his praenomen Sextus.[3]

Sextus Quintilius Condianus, son of Sextus Quintilius Maximus, cos. 151, and himself consul in 180, is a more suitable candidate for Sextus than his cousin Maximus, cos. 172, as in 169 (cf. below, p. 216) he would probably be aged around twenty one, some eight years younger than his cousin. He was forced to commit suicide to escape the wrath of Commodus (Cassius Dio, ibid.), but popular legend, remembering his ability and learning, asserted that he was still alive and a false Sextus appeared before the emperor Pertinax in 193.[4]

P. 120,12: Geometry, as well as offering a training in logic, was often recommended by Galen and in the pseudo-Hippocratic literature

[1] Cassius Dio (Hist. LXXII 5,4 and 6,1) is decisive proof that Maximus II was the son of Condianus I and that Condianus II was son of Maximus I. The account of them and their fathers given by R. Hanslik, RE XXIV, 1963, cols. 985f., s. v. Quintilius, nn. 23, 24, 26, and 27, is hopelessly confused, and, ibid. 1268, s. v. Quintilianus, we are told that this phantom is a "Zeitgenosse des Galen". I have discussed the case and the identity of Sextus at greater length in: Sextus or Commodus?, Chiron 3, 1973, pp. 429–437.

[2] J. H. Oliver, Arrian and the Gellii of Corinth, Greek, Roman and Byzantine Studies 11, 1970, pp. 335ff.

[3] Some Mss. at LXXII 5,3 read Κυιντιλιάνους for Κυιντιλίους.

[4] The commemoration of a procurator officii Quintiliani, i. e. an imperial agent in charge of the confiscated property of the family, at the Asclepieion of Pergamum, Altertümer v. Pergamon, VIII 3, no. 44, need not indicate that the Quintilii had property there, since the post may have been held in Rome. On their agricultural interests, see K. D. White, Roman farming, London 1970, p. 29.

for its value in assisting the understanding of the mechanics of bones (cf. [Hipp.], Ep. 22; K. Deichgräber, Emp., p. 89, n. 5; Medicus gratiosus, pp. 100 and 103). Such a training in geometry and dialectic could only have been obtained by a man whose family was already wealthy.

P. 120,18: Although Galen normally refers to his tract 'On crises' as Περὶ κρίσεων (cf. line 11 and the indexes to CMG), the examples cited by I. Müller (Scr. min. II, pp. XXXVf.) and by J. Ilberg[1] are enough to show that in the Mss. at least, and probably in Galen's own usage, the book titles were not fixed, and so I have not changed the readings here and at 126,4 and 132,29 to conform with standard practice (cf. Gal., In Hipp. Aph. comm. IV 29 and 36: XVII B, pp. 694,13 and 713,8 K.).

P. 120,26: Elsewhere (In Hipp. Epid. I comment. III 2: CMG V 10,1, p. 112,21) Galen declares that he has never seen a seven day fever although he has made observations from his youth. Hippocrates claimed to have observed five, six, and seven day fevers, but Diocles and other empirics denied this. Gàlen, who has seen only dubious examples of five day fevers, there refuses to accept Hippocrates' evidence for seven and even nine day fevers without wishing to exclude altogether the possibility that they exist. For the varied construction of present and future infinitives, see below, comm. to p. 124,1.

P. 122,2: Galen devoted one whole treatise to the virtues of barley gruel (De ptisana: CMG V 4,2, pp. 455–463) and spent most of another discussing how it should be prescribed (De diaeta Hipp. in morb. acut.: CMG Suppl. Or. II, pp. 76–111). He preferred giving barley gruel throughout an acute illness to making the patient fast on certain days in accordance with the Methodists' mistaken view of the Hippocratic doctrine.[2]

P. 124,1: The use of the present instead of the future participle becomes more and more common in Late Greek prose, especially when the context indicates clearly enough that it is being employed in a future sense. Thus both here and at line 25 a present participle is coupled with one in the future, both after πέμπειν to give elegant variation. This use of the present participle, which can be traced back to Thucydides (Hist. VII 25,9: ἔπεμψαν ἀγγέλλοντας) is often found with verbs whose futures are awkwardly contracted (cf. E. Mayser, II 1, pp. 170–174; Blass-Debrunner-Funk, § 339,2C). Similarly, since the aorist participle does not always carry the connotations of an event in past time but also represents a single rather than a continuous action, the aorist participle κομίσαντα may be retained at 136,24, again after πέμπειν, instead of emending it to the future. Where a future sense can easily be implied, a present or aorist infinitive instead of a future may be employed (cf. above, pp. 78,31, 82,26, and 124,10) or to give elegant

[1] A review in Berliner Philologische Wochenschrift 13, 1892, pp. 7–11.
[2] Cf. also E. Darmstädter, Ptisana, Archeion 15, 1933, pp. 181–201.

variation (above, p. 120,26).[1] The construction with the aorist participle after a verb meaning 'to come' is found three times in 'On prognosis', at 80,15, 102,19, and 138,22, and at Gal., De loc. aff. V 18: VIII, p. 361,16 K. (ὃν ἥκω τε θεασάμενος ἄρτι) and, although rare in Attic authors, becomes increasingly more common as the use of the future declines, cf. Blass-Debrunner-Funk, § 339,1.

P. 124,13f.: Why should Peitholaus tell the details of the illness of Sextus to the emperor? and why should Severus have some sort of charge over the young man? For A. R. Birley, Chiron, pp. 465f., it was because he was the emperor's son, but, as J. Kollesch pointed out, p. 60, there is no reason why an imperial servant should not take an interest in the cure of the son of a friend of the emperor by a doctor whom he knew well, or why a close friend of the family, such as Severus, should not see to the young man's health in the absence of his father. The fact that here Peitholaus merely questions Galen and passes on information to the emperor, as contrasted with his action in the case of Commodus (above, p. 130,20–29), is a further argument against identifying Sextus with Commodus. This passage may help to resolve the problem of the date of Sextus' illness. Unless δεδηλωκέναι applies to a letter – which seems unlikely – we must believe that, since Peitholaus informed the emperor within a fortnight, at most, of Sextus' illness, Marcus Aurelius was still in Rome, i. e. that this case falls in 169, for a later date, post 176, is excluded by the age of Condianus, born c. 148. E. Groag had long ago concluded that the Quintilii brothers were abroad together in Greece as governors from 169[2], but a new inscription from near Dascyleion, Zeitschr. f. Papyrologie u. Epigraphik 21, 1976, pp. 77f., reveals that Sextus Quintilius Maximus was in fact governor of Asia in 168/169, probably in 169, after the death of Lucius Verus.

P. 124,20–22: There is no doubt that some of Galen's philosophical opponents were as violently opposed to him as his medical ones (Gal., De pecc. dign. 3,9: CMG V 4,1,1, p. 48,5–13), since, in particular, his attacks were directed, like those of Lucian and other satirists, at the Cynics, who taught ignorant lads untruths with a solemn countenance (ibid. 12–24: CMG V 4,1,1, pp. 48,23–52,11). This objection of Galen was not new (cf. Appian, Mithrid. V 28) and formed the basis for a well known joke against philosophers that was enshrined in Roman Law as a judgement of Antoninus Pius (Modestinus, Dig. 27, 1,6,8): "I have not specified a restricted number of (immune) philosophers (since philosophers are few), for I think that they should make a voluntary contribution for the good of their cities from their super-

[1] This construction, which is a late development, should not be invoked in correct Attic prose, see J. Madvig, Adversaria critica I, Copenhagen 1870, I iv, pp. 155–184.

[2] E. Groag, Die römischen Reichsbeamten von Achaia, I, Vienna 1939, pp. 128ff.; but cf. J. H. Oliver, p. 69, who places their administration in Greece only after the invasion of the Costoboci in 170 or 171.

abundance of wealth: if they complain about their property, then it is clear that they are not true philosophers" (and thus not entitled to tax immunity).

P. 124,26–31: The sentence οὐ γὰρ – κρίσεως following γενησόμενον (line 26) as in L and M is not an explanation of their visits; for even if they had known Galen's prediction, they would have come to see its fulfilment. Placed after ἀπέβη, as the Latin version has it, it explains their misguided railery, since they had not heard of his qualification of his original prediction. As for ἔφασαν ἑπομένην ἐναλλάξ, its meaning is doubtful and the asyndeton harsh: Nic.'s omission suggests either that he failed to understand it or, probably, that this is a marginal gloss incorporated into the common source of L and M, which from now on is more and more corrupt and interpolated.

P. 126,14: Since in the story of the illness of the young Commodus Marcus Aurelius is not mentioned, the slight change suggested by Nic.'s "in peregrinatione", from ἐπι- to ἀποδημίαν could be accepted, but the sentence is still troublesome. Either αὐτοῦ or ἐκείνου or both must refer to Marcus Aurelius, Commodus' father, but the choice is difficult. ἐκείνου refers to the first mentioned of a pair, so here it should look back to αὐτοῦ, but since Marcus has not been mentioned since 120,2 and Commodus since 118,30 the use of the pronoun is very abrupt. It could, possibly, refer to Commodus and intensify 'boy' or 'Commodus', but this strains the Greek and also leaves untouched the problem of ἐκείνου an odd pronoun to introduce the emperor. In that case αὐτοῦ is a scribal error, a misreading of a compendium for τοῦ αὐτοκράτορος. If the reading of the Greek Mss. is retained, then ἐκείνου will refer to Commodus, αὐτοῦ to the emperor, but the problem of the abruptness of the pronoun still remains.

P. 126,17: The use of the word συναπεδήμησαν (cf. above, p. 128, 5) shows that this case took place either after the emperor's return to Rome in autumn 176 or in the short period in 169 when he and Galen were there together. If the latter, then the cases are more or less in chronological order throughout, which may be a point in its favour: if the former, then it will explain why the doctors who accompanied Marcus on campaign had a much better knowledge of his natural condition than Galen. But it should not be forgotten that Galen could only have had a few weeks at most with the emperors at Aquileia, certainly not long enough for Galen to claim a complete knowledge of his patient's constitution. His praise of Galen and his joy at finding a true physician and philosopher (above, p. 126,28) could apply equally to 169 or to 176/7. A table of cases with the evidence for their dates is as follows:

1	Eudemus	Winter 162/3 (p. 78,22, cf. p. 210)
2	The youth with fever	Autumn 162 (p. 78,4)
3	The servant of Charilampes	Spring 163 (p. 94,5)
4	Diomedes the orator	Spring 163 (p. 94,8) [p. 187)
5	The anatomical debates	Spring/Summer 163 (p. 94,19, cf.

6	The wife of Iustus	Summer 163 (p. 94,22)
7	The slave steward	?
8	The son of Boethus	Summer/Autumn 163 (p. 106,13)
9	The wife of Boethus	Summer 164/5 (p. 110,20)
10	Sextus Quintilius Condianus	Summer 169 (p. 216)
11	Marcus Aurelius	Summer 169 or 176/7 (p. 126,17)
12	Commodus	173–175 (p. 126,15, cf. p. 224)
13	The youth with an excess of blood	?
14	The youth with the intermittent pulse	170–178 (p. 138,13)

P. 126,20: Aloe, aloe vera L., Liliaceae, was often used for its astringent properties (Dioscorides, De mat. med. III 22, ed. Wellmann; Gal., De alim. fac. I 40: CMG V 4,2, p. 214,11), especially in stomach disorders (Gal., De sanit. tuenda V 9,5: CMG V 4,2, p. 153, 5–10; ibid. VI 7,21: CMG V 4,2, p. 182,16ff.; ibid. VI 10,16: CMG V 4,2, p. 188,12f.; Pliny, Nat. Hist. XXVII 16). It is still recommended as a purgative or a stomach stimulant (cf. M. Levey, p. 297; M. Grieve, I, pp. 26–29). We hear more of Marcus Aurelius' daily draught of theriac from Gal., De antidot. I 1: XIV, p. 4,1ff. K., but I remain unconvinced by modern arguments that he was a confirmed drug addict.[1]

P. 126,28–128,8: The text of these two sentences presents several problems. Unless Dr. Giangrande's suggestion that περὶ τὴν ἕω is a pleonastic expansion of ἕωθεν is accepted, the phrase must be condemned as corrupt. Certainly, the harsh hiatus ἕω ἑωρακότων is against it as well as providing a reason for the introduction of ἕω into the text. From 126,19 I have emended to περὶ τὴν ὀγδόην ὥραν, which would then be the second of the two occasions mentioned at line 5. The Latin tradition, adopted by the Basle editors, offers a different sequence of events from the Greek: three doctors see the emperor, only two of whom take his pulse, the other being Galen, who remains silent. In the Greek, three doctors see the emperor and take his pulse twice, Galen neither takes his pulse nor offers an opinion. But Galen's introduction to this case, 126,16–19, suggests that he was not one of the doctors who had accompanied the emperor and had seen his fevered condition, and thus that he cannot be the same as the third doctor in the Latin version, who saw the emperor earlier but who did not take his pulse. Galen was only called in when the illness grew worse, at dusk, at the lighting of the lamps[2], much later than 2 p. m., the eighth hour of their second visit. The reading of the Greek Mss. gives consistent and better sense (with the slight change of τότε to ὅτι, line 5) and should be retained.

[1] T. W. Africa, The opium addiction of Marcus Aurelius, Journ. Hist. Ideas 22, 1961, pp. 97–102; E. C. Witke, Marcus Aurelius and mandragora, Classical Philology 60, 1965, pp. 23f.

[2] For this phrase, cf. also Gal., Meth. med. XI 16: X, p. 792,16 K.

P. 128,11–13: Galen believed that in a stomach disorder brought on by food that was excessive as well as chilling, the pulse was infrequent, slow, small and weak (Introd. in puls. 12: VIII, p. 490,1–7 K.; De caus. puls. IV 23: IX, pp. 197,18–200,13 K.). When the stomach is burdened by excessive food, the pulse is not smaller and weaker, swifter rather than more frequent, as Archigenes thought (Gal., De caus. puls. III 16: IX, pp. 150,12–152,13 K.), but unequal and irregular, containing both vigorous and weak beats.

P. 128,18–20: Cf. the means used to warm Marcus Aurelius with those employed in the cure of the wife of Iustus (above, p. 114,19–26). Not only would this treatment be suitable for an emperor but its cost would be appropriately high (cf. Gal., Meth. med. VIII 5: X, p. 574, 2–6 K.; De sanit. tuenda VI 10,8–9: CMG V 4,2, p. 18,20ff.), for he made no bones about preparing his drugs according to the wealth of his patients (Gal., De simpl. med. temp. et fac. X 22: XII, p. 299, 9–18 K.; and De comp. med. sec. loc. I 5: XII, p. 458,2–9 K.; ibid. VI 2: XII, p. 909,9–11 K.), although he drew the line at satisfying a patient's desires in order to obtain a bigger fee (Gal., In Hipp. Epid. VI comment. IV 8: CMG V 10,2,2, p. 198,21, cf. ibid. V 13: CMG V 10,2,2, p. 283,15f.).

P. 128,25: Sabine wine, a thin dry wine, was especially good for stomach disorders (Gal., Meth. med. VII 6: X, p. 483,5 K.; De sanit. tuenda IV 6,19: CMG V 4,2, p. 121,31) and pepper, piper longum L., piperaceae, was an effective calefacient (Dioscorides, De mat. med. II 159, ed. Wellmann), especially in stomach chills (Gal., Meth. med. ad Glauc. I 14: XI, pp. 55,3–56,12 K.). See also J. I. Miller, pp. 80–83; M. Levey, pp. 371f.; M. Grieve, II, p. 627, who recommends its use as a febrifuge.

P. 128,28: This is high praise indeed from a man who was himself a philosopher and acquainted with medical theory.[1] ἐλεύθερος is a favourite word both of Galen (cf. CMG V 4,2, p. 474; De venae sect. adv. Eras. Rom. deg. 1: XI, p. 193,8 K.[2]), and of the Stoic Marcus Aurelius, for whom it represents a philosophical ideal only rarely attained, the wisdom of the sage that brings spiritual and moral liberty (Med. I 18,4; II 22; III 6; IV 3; V 7; VII 67; VIII 1). Galen achieves his ambition of being recognised as both doctor and philosopher[3], and it is even more gratifying to him, and outwardly less self-assertive, that the praise comes from a man of irreproachable qualifications, the philosopher-king.

1 Med. II 22; cf. I. H. Leopold, De vocabulis medicis apud M. Aurelium obviis, Sertum Nabericum, Leyden 1908, pp. 233ff.

2 R. F. Kotrc, in his edition of this treatise, Ph. D. Diss., Washington 1968, p. 237, identifies Teuthras "who chose a life of freedom" with Telephus of Pergamum; wrongly, for Teuthras, who went to school with Galen, cannot be the same as the aged grammarian of Gal., De sanit. tuenda V 4,15: CMG V 4,2, p. 144,3; and ibid. 12,28: CMG V 4,2, p. 167,24.

3 Cf. above, p. 192 and note 2.

P. 128,29f.: That love of a reputation and of money leads doctors to stray from the true paths of virtue is almost a Galenic commonplace (De plac. Hipp. et Plat. IX (5): p. 764,11–15 Ml. = V, p. 751,6–13 K.; In Hipp. De vict. acut. comment. I 16: CMG V 9,1, p. 132,20–23; De crisib. II 2: p. 129,10–15 Alex. = IX, p. 645,10–15 K.; De caus. procat. 1,2: CMG Suppl. II, p. 1,12ff.; Quod opt. med. sit etiam phil. 2: Scr. min. II, p. 4,13–21 Müller = I, p. 57,9–16 K.; ibid. 7,11ff. Müller = I, p. 61,3ff. K., to say nothing of his advice in his ethical writings, cf. CMG V 4,1,1, pp. 142f.). But while it may be unfair to accuse Galen of φιλοχρηματία, his concern for his reputation, to which this tract bears witness, offers at least the suspicion of φιλοδοξία.

P. 128,33: Archigenes, a famous doctor of the time of Trajan (fl. 110 A. D.) and a native of Apamaea in Syria, was the most celebrated of the Eclectics. He was well versed in earlier medical theory and was competent to correct and to develop the writings of his predecessors (Gal., De comp. med. sec. loc. II 1: XII, pp. 534,5–535,4 K.). He published a treatise on the pulse, on which Galen wrote a commentary (Gal., De lib. propr. 5: Scr. min. II, p. 111,6f.[1] Müller = XIX, p. 33,9f. K.): it appears to have contained a number of minute and subtle distinctions, many of which have no real existence, and were for the most part the result rather of a preconceived hypothesis than of actual observation; the same may be said of the arrangement he proposed for the classification and diagnosis of fevers.[2]

P. 130,1: ἐπισημασία is more specific than attack: as Galen defines it, it is the first clear display of the symptoms of a disease (De morb. temp. 6: VII, p. 426,5f. K., cf. W. Herbst, p. 130). Thus by being able to diagnose a disease when its symptoms are only just beginning to appear, he can impose caution on those who are about to prescribe a method of treatment that might prove dangerously wrong. The word does not apply only to the symptoms of an attack of fever but to any disease, especially one that can be discerned as a result of a change in the pulse rate (cf. Gal., De praes. ex puls. II 1: IX, p. 273, 7ff. K.).

P. 130,2f.: The problem of whether the systole, the contracting movement, of the arteries is perceptible or not is treated at length in Gal., De dign. puls. I 3–7: VIII, pp. 786,13–806,11 K. and summarised in Synops. de puls. 5: IX, pp. 443,11–444,8 K. Agathinus, the tutor of Archigenes, denied that the contraction was perceptible, thus contradicting the opinion of Herophilus, and Galen found it difficult to decide between authorities whose contributions to the development of medicine were equally valuable. To solve this dilemma, he first practis-

[1] Reading κρίσιν for χρῆσιν at line 7 (10), as suggested by J. Ilberg, Schriftstellerei I, 1889, p. 221.

[2] See M. Wellmann, RE II, 1896, cols. 484ff., s. v. Archigenes; F. Kudlien, Untersuchungen zu Aretaios von Kappadokien, Akademie d. Wiss. u. d. Lit., Abh. d. geistes- und sozialwiss. Kl. 1963, 11, pp. 1174–1182; and C. R. S. Harris, pp. 251–257.

ed to gain a finer and more sensitive touch and then read the works of the earlier physicians in order to compare their findings with his. He read that Herophilus and his followers asserted that it was perceptible, but that the Erasistrateans and Athenaeus and his followers (including Agathinus) held divided opinions among themselves. His own masters (Satyrus, Pelops and Julianus) had no clear diagnosis of what a systole was, and their experience and authority almost convinced him that Agathinus was right. But then he suddenly discovered the truth by his own experience of taking pulses – it shone out like a fire suddenly lit by rubbing wood together – and from then on he had no need of other witnesses or authorities. He was, however, prepared to admit that not all pulses could be perceived (De dign. puls. I 5: VIII, pp. 797,13–798,6 K.), and that, even when a pulse was normally perceptible, it did not always continue to be so, and that pulses differed in this among themselves. In the later sections of De dign. puls. I (4–10: VIII, pp. 790,11–818,14 K.) he tried to show how pulses were to be perceived, the best method of taking the pulse, the best place to do so, and the best patient upon whom to practise, so that the systole could become one of the ἐναργῶς φαινόμενα and command unqualified acceptance, thereby becoming available for use in the diagnosis of a disease. In this he was correct, for a modern writer also concludes that the rapidity of the systole has often caused it to be overlooked and that it can be missed unless the whole attention is given to its perception.[1] Many of Galen's observations on the pulses clearly derive from his practical experience, and his large volumes on the subject, which are the most uncongenial of all to read, were intended for a practical, clinical purpose, the diagnosis and prognosis of ill-health. Even if their logic-chopping becomes tedious, especially in De diff. puls., they reveal another aspect of Galen, his care and persistence in seeking out and writing down data from his clinical cases and in training himself until his touch and perception were adequate for that purpose.

P. 130,11: We know little about the childhood illnesses of Commodus.[2] S. Reinach wished to connect a jewel from the Abbey of Silos, inscribed ΣΑΛΒΩ ΚΟΜΜΟΔΩ ΦΗΛΙΞ ΦΑΥΣΤΕΙΝΑ, with the great plague [3], but the words could apply to any illness or, possibly, they may represent a version of a standard vow for the safety of a member of the imperial family (cf. CIL VI 632: Felici imperatori omnia felicia. salvo Commodo felix familia). L. Jacchinus, p. 81, notes that Galen treats this illness as an ephemeral fever, taking Commodus to the bath, the standard remedy (Meth. med. ad Glauc. I 3: XI, pp. 14,11–15, 11 K.), and permitting him to take wine (ibid.).

[1] W. Ewart, Heart studies, London 1894, p. 80, cited by C. R. S. Harris, p. 409; see also Harris, pp. 405–409, and K. Deichgräber, Galen als Erforscher des menschlichen Pulses, Sitzb. d. Deutsch. Akademie d. Wiss. 1956, 3, Berlin 1957, pp. 17 to 25.

[2] Pace R. Walzer (JC, p. 9), who assigns this incident to a date after the accession of Commodus, sc. 181.

[3] S. Reinach, Revue archéologique 39, 1901, p. 121.

P. 130,12: Like Commodus, Galen was a regular visitor to the palaestra (cf. Gal., De diff. puls. II 9: VIII, p. 624,11–13 K.; In Hipp. De artic. comment. I: XVIII A, pp. 348,11f.; and 401,15ff. K.) and treated many injuries brought on by irregular training and by over-exercise (e. g. Gal., Anat. admin. II 4: II, p. 298,17ff. K.; ibid. VII 13: II, p. 632,7 K.; Meth. med. IX 4: X, p. 608,7ff. K.; ibid. X 3: X, p. 671,15 K.; De venae sect. adv. Eras. Rom. deg. 6: XI, p. 227,4 K.; In Hipp. De artic. comment. I: XVIII A, pp. 346,1–351,10 K.).

P. 130,13: On πρίν + genitive, a Koine construction, see W. Bauer, Wörterbuch zu d. Schriften d. Neuen Testaments, ed. 5, Berlin 1958, p. 1391.

P. 130,21: Since I have found no other example of a medicament composed of apples and wax [1], the reading of Nic., I retain the reading of L and M, especially as the mixture of sumach and honey is recommended by many authors for diseases of the mouth and tongue (Celsus, Med. VI 11,5: CML I, p. 286,25; Dioscorides, De mat. med. I 108, ed. Wellmann; Pliny, Nat. Hist. XXI 123 and XXIV 92; Gal., De simpl. med. temp. et fac. III 14: XI, p. 574,16 K.). Elm-leaved sumach, rhus coriaria L., Anacard., is still used as an astringent and as a styptic (M. Grieve, II, p. 781, cf. M. Levey, p. 285), and honey is recommended by J. Pereira, II 2, p. 764, as "a vehicle for the application of other more powerful agents to the mouth and throat, especially in children", and by A. Weisenberg, p. 401.

P. 130,22: For the composition of hydromel (two parts water, preferably rain water, to one part honey) and its properties, see Dioscorides, De mat. med. V 9, ed. Wellmann, and for the medicinal properties of roses, ibid. I 99,1f., ed. Wellmann; and Pliny, Nat. Hist. XXI 121–125. The same remedy is noted by Galen used by a gardener with tonsillitis (De comp. med. sec. loc. VI 2: XII, p. 905, 10f. K.). A. Weisenberg (p. 500) declares, "Der Rosenhonig wird bei Kindern zur Reinigung des Mundes mit oder ohne Zusatz von Säuren oder Borax benutzt", while M. Grieve (II, p. 688) says, "Honey of roses, official in the U. S. Pharmacopoea, is prepared from clarified honey and fluid extract of roses. It is considered more agreeable than ordinary honey and somewhat astringent. In olden days honey of roses was popular for sore throats and ulcerated mouths and was made by pounding fresh petals in a small quantity of boiling water, filtering the mass and boiling the liquid with honey."

P. 130,29: The identity of Annia Faustina has troubled many scholars. A. Stein was not alone in believing that this was Commodus' mother, Faustina II [2], although he was rightly surprised at the circumlocution, συγγενὴς οὖσα τῷ αὐτοκράτορι ἔγγιστα. His surprise was certainly justified, for it is a very coy expression for Marcus' wife, unless it is intended as a tactful reference to her after her death in

[1] On the uses of wax in medicine, see now R. Büll and E. Moser, RE Suppl. 13, 1973, cols. 1385f., s. v. Wachs.

[2] PIR² G. 24; F. Grosso, p. 120.

176. A. R. Birley (Chiron, pp. 465f.), on the other hand, argued strongly for the emperor's eldest daughter, Annia Galeria Aurelia Faustina, the wife of Cn. Claudius Severus, the friend and supporter of Galen, but several objections can be raised against this. (1) Galen's expression is equally odd whether it applies to Marcus' daughter or to his wife: (2) she is accompanied by a Methodist doctor, an opponent of Galen: (3) her compliments to Galen are ironical and tendentious: (4) Galen regards her intervention as harmful to his cause. If Annia Faustina is the wife of Severus, her attitude towards Galen differs greatly from that of her husband – although this is perhaps not a conclusive argument against identification. The correct solution was propounded by J. Ilberg (NJ, p. 296), who preferred to identify her with the emperor's cousin, Annia Fundania Faustina, wife of T. Pomponius Vitrasius Pollio, cos. II, 176, for whom the roundabout description would be more suitable than for a wife or daughter.[1]

P. 132,4: The significance of Peitholaus' remark becomes clear at line 9, for Annia Faustina has brought with her a Methodist doctor, a follower of the therapeutic doctrines of Thessalus of Tralles.

The tradition on Thessalus is uniformly hostile, and it is almost impossible to separate truth from fiction in Pliny's and Galen's accounts of his origins and his beliefs.[2] It is probable that he came from a family connected with the woollen industry of Tralles, but this tells us little of his wealth or background, since, as the prosperity of that city depended upon wool, it is impossible to say whether his family were weavers or factors. We may also accept Pliny's grudging admission that he was the leading physician of the age of Nero (Nat. Hist. XXIX 9), without having to believe that his letter to the emperor indicated that he was an imperial doctor.[3] The idea of a three day period, i. e. the recurrence of a disease on alternate days, went back at least to Themison of Laodicaea[4] and was developed further by Thessalus, who was especially careful about the second day after the onset of the disease (Caelius Aurelianus, De morb. chron. II 1,60; 13,157 and 184). Galen frequently makes great play with this dogmatism (e. g. De crisib. II 3: pp. 135,24–136,11 Alex. = IX, p. 656,1–15 K.; De caus. procat. 3,21: CMG Suppl. II, pp. 5,32–6,9; Meth. med. IV 4: X, p. 264,4ff. K.; ibid. VIII 3: X, p. 561,7 K.; ibid. X 3: X, p.

1 The same identification is made by H. G. Pflaum, La valeur de l'information historique de la Vita Commodi, Bonner Historia-Augusta-Colloquium, 1970, Bonn 1972, p. 223.

2 His doctrines have been tentatively assembled by Th. Meyer-Steineg, Thessalos von Tralles, Sudhoffs Archiv f. Gesch. d. Med. u. d. Naturwiss. 4, 1910, pp. 89–108; and by H. Diller, RE 2 VI, 1936, cols. 168–182, s. v. Thessalos. The standard account of Methodism is now that of L. Edelstein, Ancient medicine, pp. 173–191.

3 Cf. M. Wellmann, Beiträge zur Geschichte der Medizin im Altertum, Hermes 65, 1930, pp. 322–331.

4 Caelius Aurelianus, De morb. acut. I 16,155; cf. R. Fuchs, Aus Themisons Werk über die acuten und chronischen Krankheiten, Rheinisches Museum 58, 1903, pp. 67–114.

671,6ff. K.; Meth. med. ad Glaucon. I 2: XI, p. 6,15 K.) but, as L. Edelstein insisted (Ancient medicine, pp. 572f.), he is being grossly unfair. Under Soranus and his successors Methodism adapted itself more flexibly to new ideas and influences (cf. Gal., De sectis 9: Scr. min. III, p. 26,19–24 Helmr. = I, p. 98,5–10 K.), yet Galen still confined his most violent attacks, as in Meth. med. I, passim, to the Methodists of the previous century. His opposition may not always have been based upon purely medical grounds, for his personal dislike of Methodists attached to the imperial household and in positions of influence, like Statilius Attalus, who may be the unnamed doctor here, could easily have led him to assail the tradition that they represented.

P. 132,11–14: As Galen stressed (De diaeta Hipp. in morb. acut. 6,6–9: CMG Suppl. Or. II, pp. 96,5–98,1), he was following the Hippocratic precept, "The patient must not be starved of nourishment on the first days of his illness" (Hipp., De diaeta acut. 39 (11): I, p. 128,20ff. Kw. = II, p. 306,13ff. L., cf. ibid. 26 (8): I, p. 122,2–6 Kw. = II, p. 278,8–11 L.).

P. 132,21: Faustina's sarcasm is less than clear when she associates Peitholaus' timidity or hesitation with his shrewdness. On one interpretation, his shrewdness is mere cowardice, a slavish subjection to the theories of Galen, but this does not suit adequately her apparent respect for Peitholaus. The second interpretation, which I have followed in my translation, is that the tutor's shrewdness is manifested in a reluctance to accept the views of others and thus that his ready acceptance of Galen's advice – for Peitholaus is portrayed by Galen as his eager defender – is further proof of Galen's abilities. On either version the insult is oblique and it is possible that the text itself is corrupt and that either δειλίαν should be emended – δήλην is a possible, although not entirely satisfactory, emendation – or the whole clause ὡς . . . αὐτοῦ should be deleted as a gloss on ἀκριβέστατος.

P. 132,28: The position of ἔναγχος, within Galen's discourse, indicates that the three tracts were written shortly before Galen reported to Peitholaus rather than, as K. Bardong, pp. 609f., had argued, just before 'On prognosis' was composed. At the latest, the three would have been written in May 175 (cf. A. R. Birley, Marcus Aurelius, p. 258, for the date of Commodus' departure from Rome), and the many tracts that precede them in Bardong's list, pp. 635–637, of works written between 169 and 176, even if the Hippocratic commentaries are to be dated later, make it unlikely that the cure of Commodus occurred much before 174.

P. 134,3: Although Hippocrates used the term σφυγμός and knew something about the art of the pulse, he does not appear to have developed any consistent theory about it or made any clinical use of it or even to have transferred the meaning of σφυγμός from that of the throbbing of inflamed parts of the body to that of all the movements of the arteries (Gal., De diff. puls. I 2: VIII, p. 497,13–17 K., cf. C. R. S. Harris, p. 50). Thus Galen can justly claim in his books on pulses to be extending and expanding the teachings left only in outline, at best, by Hippocrates.

P. 134,10: The debate on the propriety of venesection was vigorously conducted for several years. J. Ilberg (Schriftstellerei III, p. 181) placed it in the early 170s, but, as can be seen from De venae sect. adv. Eras. Rom. deg.: XI, pp. 187–249 K., it was already alive in the middle years of the 160s.

P. 134,27: The only other example adduced by the Thesaurus Linguae Graecae, II, col. 937, for the use of δεῖσθαι in the sense of 'fear', Plutarch, Mor. 217A, is based upon a doubtful Ms. reading, and most modern scholars have read ⟨αἰ⟩δεῖσθαι. I have therefore no hesitation in accepting Ludwig Dindorf's emendation here; cf. the reading of M at 118,27: πεῖσθαι for πεῖσαι.

P. 134,30–136,3: Dreams and hallucinations were regularly used by Galen and other doctors, from the pseudo-Hippocratic De victu IV (VI, pp. 640–663 L.) onwards, in their diagnosis of a patient's condition. Rufus of Ephesus (Quaest. med. 5,28–31: CMG Suppl. IV, p. 34,13–29, cf. pp. 78f.) mentions three examples of dreams that had a bearing on the course of a disease; and Galen, although his opinion of other practitioners who rely on them is characteristically low, also made use of dreams himself. But, unlike the author of De victu IV, who demanded an almost universal validity for dreams (IV 86: VI, p. 640,8–11 L.), Galen restricted the importance of diagnostic dreams to indicating deficiencies, excesses and qualitative changes of the humours (De dign. ex insomn.: VI, p. 835,11–14 K.), although he also accepted as valid the prescriptions sent to him in a dream by Asclepius (De simpl. med. temp. et fac. XI 1: XII, p. 315,12 K. = Subfig. emp. 10: K. Deichgräber, Emp., p. 78,28; De lib. propr. 2: Scr. min. II, p. 99,20f. Müller = XIX, p. 9,11f. K.; cf. above, p. 159) without going to the extravagant lengths of some of his contemporaries such as Aristeides.[1] At In Hipp. Epid. I comment. III 1: CMG V 10,1, pp. 108–109,5 he gives a few examples of the right interpretation of dreams, very much in the schematic manner of Rufus and Artemidorus: a man who dreams of rain has a surfeit of watery humour, of cold phlegm if he dreams of snow, ice or hail. His contemporary, Artemidorus of Daldis, writing on the meaning of snakes in dreams (Oneir. II 13: p. 127,11 Pack), declares that a snake portends illness and misfortune, and it would not be difficult on Galen's humoral theory to deduce that a red snake meant an affliction caused by an excess of blood. But it is important to note how Galen combines this schematic explanation with his own observation of the colour of

[1] On dream healing in the ancient world, see O. Weinreich, Antike Heilungswunder, Gießen 1909, esp. pp. 76–136; C. A. Behr, Aelius Aristeides and the sacred tales, Amsterdam 1968, pp. 171–204; and for its use in modern medicine, J. A. Hadfield, Dreams and nightmares, Harmondsworth 1967, p. 9.

the man's nostril, thereby giving the bystanders the choice of deciding how he came to his prognosis.

P. 136,18–22: The ease with which an issue of blood from the right or left nostril can be predicted is further stressed by Galen at Meth. med. ad Glaucon. I 16: XI, p. 68,15–18 K.; and De crisib. III 11: p. 210,17–20 Alex. = IX, p. 766,4–7 K. A Hippocratic basis for this doctrine can be discovered at Prorrhet. I 125: V, p. 554,3 L.; Prognost. 7: I, p. 84,10–16 Kw. = II, pp. 126,12–128,4 L.; and in the case study of the illness of Lycinus the grammarian from Cranon, Epid. IV 37: V, p. 180,4 L., together with Galen's commentary upon the first two passages, CMG V 9,2, pp. 144,2–146,6; and pp. 249,7–250,8.

P. 136,22: The Basle editors' insertion of ὀλίγον before χρόνον, following Nic.'s 'modico tempore', is unnecessary, since the noun by itself can mean "for a short while", cf. L-S-J, s. v. χρόνος 3a and Gal., De simpl. med. temp. et fac. IX 34: XII, p. 240,10 K. If an adjective is still thought essential – although on balance I think not – then βραχὺν is better than ὀλίγον as it avoids hiatus after παραμεῖναι.

P. 136,27: Oxycraton, a mixture of sour wine and water, was recommended by Galen as an agglutinative and cooling substance that reduced the flow of blood (De simpl. med. temp. et fac. I 31: XI, p. 435,13–16 K.; ibid. 33: XI, p. 439,16 K.). Hydromel, whose composition is described above, p. 222, is also a cleansing, drying and styptic agent especially useful in stemming a flow of blood (Gal., Meth. med. ad Glaucon. II 10: XI, p. 129,7–16 K.), and Galen also recommends (ibid.) that after the imposition of the styptic a fresh sponge dipped in a mixture of vinegar and honey should be applied gently. The differences between oxycraton and hydromel are slight, and although it might be expected that Galen would apply hydromel both to the nostril and to the forehead of the patient, as Nic.'s version suggests, this need not have been so and Galen could easily have varied the treatment a little, as the reading of L and M shows, depending on the part of the head to which it was applied. Thus, although some doubt must remain about the correct reading, cf. L. Jacchinus, p. 82, I have retained that of the Greek Mss.

P. 138,3: Galen prescribes cupping to stop a nasal haemorrhage also at Meth. med. II 3: X, p. 316,1–7 K., and De hirudin. 2: XI, p. 319,13–16 K. and ibid. 3: XI, p. 321,5f. K. The reason is that the warm excessive blood which produces swellings, if retained in the body either escapes through the nose or lodges in the lower abdomen, from which it can be extracted by cupping. A reduction in the volume of blood at one place helps to stabilise it at the other.[1] Cupping was a recognised part of a doctor's activities and several portrait reliefs of

[1] Gal., De crisib. III 3: p. 170,13–19 Alex. = IX, p. 708,1–9 K.; ibid. 15: pp. 210,17–211,5 Alex. = IX, p. 766,4–17 K.

doctors display a cupping glass upon them to indicate the doctor's professional skill.[1]

P. 138,8: The word ἀπόσκημμα describes the movement of humours from one part of the body to another as opposed to an ἔκκρισις, the rejection of peccant humours by the body (cf. Gal., De crisib. III 11: p. 207,14–17 Alex. = IX, p. 761,10–13 K.), and it fits uneasily into the description of symptoms of crisis. The simple change to ἀποστήματα, abscesses, corresponds both to the required sense, to Nic.'s version ("apostases") and to the parallel list at p. 70,2–5 (cf. the similar palaeographic confusion in some of the Mss. of De crisib., loc. cit.). Nor is there any medical difference between παραφορά and παραφροσύνη, and I have again followed Nic.'s version ("cataforas") and the earlier list and emended to καταφορὰς, which distinguishes between a fit of lethargy and one of delirium.

P. 138,14: The case of the young man with the intermittent pulse not only is of great medical interest but also shows how Galen can change and develop his earlier theories as a result of his clinical experience. He discusses the causes of an intermittent pulse at length in his treatises on pulses, chiefly at De diff. puls. I 11: VIII, pp. 525,15–526,3 K., where he defines it as due either to the prolongation of the period of rest after the beat or, less often, to the reduction of the diastole almost to nothing. At De praesag. ex puls. II 4: IX, pp. 280,10–287,7 K. and ibid. 6: IX, pp. 294,14–297,14 he ascribes it to a blockage of the arteries by either coagulated or excess humours or to pressure exerted upon the arteries by a swelling or a tumour (ibid., pp. 280,10–281,18 K.). He doubts whether recovery is possible if two or more beats are missed, since this brings about a loss of movement or paralysis and then death (ibid., p. 282,11–17 K.; p. 284,12–16 K.; cf. L. Jacchinus, p. 83), but he is sure that a gap of a single beat is not necessarily fatal, especially in a child or an old man (a true observation), whose natural pulse faculty is weak and thus easily interrupted by a slight, non-fatal ailment (ibid., pp. 282,17–284,9 K.). An intermission in a group of pulses, which does not deprive the arteries of movement completely, is thus less dangerous than one in a single pulse which produces momentary paralysis (ibid., pp. 296,12–297,14 K.). Both are almost always fatal to the man in the prime of life (among whom this man should be counted) because the thing responsible for the intermission must be very great to counteract the healthy force of his pulse beats. Besides making a careful distinction between an infrequent pulse beat, from which recovery is easy, and the near-fatal intermission, Galen gives a series of examples of the pulse beats in particular diseases, but he gives none of a patient who has survived this intermission in the prime of life, and he always assigns its cause to something that is never present in a natural state of health (ibid., p. 286,8–12 K.).

[1] Examples, with photographs, will be found in E. Berger, Das Basler Arztrelief, Basle 1970, pp. 63–85.

The treatises on the pulses were written in the early 170s, when the effects of the great plague were still visible in Rome (Gal., De praes. ex puls. III 3f.: IX, p. 341,7–9 K.; ibid., p. 359,4ff. K.), and they form a summary of his clinical findings up to that point. In this case, which was noted down, if not actually observed, seven or eight years later[1], there is no suggestion that the man is an invalid, for his sweating is caused by his intermittent pulse (cf. Gal., De caus. puls. II 4: IX, p. 288,4–15 K.), or that his condition is unnatural, far from it. Galen accepts it as something totally natural and therefore harmless, and his diagnosis thereby marks an improvement on what he had said earlier when he had rejected the occurrence of this possibility. As the reaction of the other doctors shows, not all of them were prepared to accept Galen's explanation immediately, and so, when he later came to write his Commentary upon the Prognosticon, he briefly reported his conclusion that an intermittent pulse was not fatal, provided that it was natural, and referred his readers to this treatise for a proof from his own experience (In Hipp. Progn. comment. III 42: CMG V 9,2, p. 369,19–25). Clearly, therefore, as a result of the discoveries he made during his own clinical practice Galen was prepared to alter or add to his own theories and to be flexible where flexibility was needed.

P. 138,18: It is obvious from line 22 that the youth was not with his master but lying sick at home, and so the genitive of L and M must be emended following the Latin ("egressi") to the nominative, as Rota correctly saw.

P. 138,22: Does Galen commit the solecism of ἅπτεσθαι followed by the accusative instead of the genitive? Ms. A, which may have been corrected by an emending scribe, always has the genitive, but L and M, and presumably their exemplar, have the accusative singular here and at 76,4 and 10, and at 90,3, where A has the genitive plural. The Latin translation is unreliable because, although the genitive plural is usually translated by the plural "pulsus", at both 80,13 and 86,3, where the Greek Mss. have the plural, it has the singular, "pulsum". It may be significant that it also has the singular where L and M have, but this may only indicate that the confusion goes back a long way. Since I have found no other examples of the accusative after ἅπτεσθαι in the writings of Galen, I have emended the text here to τῶν σφυγμῶν and I ascribe the error to the common confusion in the Mss. between ο and ω (cf. above, pp. 100,16; 120,21; 130,26; 134,5. 11; 138,8).

P. 138,30: Galen's pulse doctrines, of which he was extremely proud, differentiated pulses by size, speed, vigour, frequency, pressure, equality and regularity (Introd. in puls. 2–6: VIII, pp. 455,1–458,18

[1] If these cases are described in the chronological order in which they occurred, cf. above, p. 217, this must date either from 170 or, accepting a late date for Galen's cure of Marcus Aurelius, we must put it in 176/7. The fact that it is not mentioned in the treatises on pulses suggests a date in the mid- or late 170s.

K.), much as a Western physician is expected to do today (cf. C. R. S. Harris, pp. 397–431). He avoided many of the over-refinements introduced by authors such as Archigenes and in general followed the views and theories of Herophilus (cf. De dign. puls. III 3: VIII, p. 911,16 K.; ibid. IV 3: VIII, p. 956,2–13 K.; De caus. puls. I 8: IX, p. 22,9–14 K.; De praes. ex puls. II 3: IX, p. 278, 8ff. K.). Although his ideas on the cause and effect of pulses are hampered by his acceptance of erroneous beliefs about the circulation of the blood, the relationship between the arterial systole and the expansion of the ventricles, and the part played by the heart as a pump, many of his observations on the connection between the indications given by pulse beats and certain physical and mental states are accurate and valuable. It is important to remember that, in the absence of modern mechanical aids to diagnosis[1], the pulse was for Galen the principle guide to prognosis since it was the clearest sign of the activity of the vital force within the body (Gal., De praes. ex puls. I 1: IX, p. 208,10ff. K.; ibid. 11f.: IX, pp. 420,16–421,6 K.). Thus in his writings on pulses he set out his doctrines and his methods at greater length and in greater detail than a modern physician would do, in order that his readers might derive the greatest benefit and instruction from his knowledge and appreciation of changes in the pulse and of their significance.

P. 140,5–8: The words αἰσθανομένους – τρισὶ were copied by the scribe of y's exemplar (or of L's, if M is a copy of L) from the succeeding tract, De temp. morb. 2: VII, p. 411,3–6 K. The other words represent a marginal instruction and correction.

P. 140,22: The Latin version indicates that the Greek text it represents had ῥυθμόν, not ἀριθμόν. In favour of the Latin is the diagnosis of pulses by rhythm proposed by certain doctors, notably Archigenes (Gal., De diff. puls. II 4: VIII, p. 577,2f. K.) and Herophilus (Gal., De praes. ex puls. II 3: IX, p. 279,6 K.), and the fact that in his discussion of the anomalies among pulses (De diff. puls. I 30: VIII, pp. 558,3–565,12 K.) Galen talks a great deal about rhythm but never about number. But he believed that a diagnosis of pulses according to their rhythms was useless and indeed superfluous, for it was essential only to know the swiftness or slowness of the pulse beat and the length of the rest (Synops. de puls. 7: IX, pp. 431,17–432,4 K.), and his definition of rhythm confined it to the relationship between the beat and the rest (De diff. puls. I 30: VIII, p. 559,13f. K.; ibid., p. 561,10–13 K.; cf. C. R. S. Harris, p. 403). Thus the omission of a single beat cannot be said on Galen's terms to occur at different rhythms, and so Nic.'s reading must be rejected.

But what, then, is the meaning of ἀριθμός? Galen often speaks of anomalies coming either in a single diastole or in a group of beats

[1] Marcellinus, 260ff., ed. Schöne, describes a clepsydra used by Herophilus for timing pulses: cf. H. Diels, Antike Technik, 2nd ed., Leipzig 1920, p. 27, n. 4.

(above, p. 138,29; cf. De caus. puls. I 3: IX, pp. 65,8–68,6 K.; De praesag. ex puls. II 4: IX, p. 280,2–6 K.; Introd. in puls. I 10: VIII, p. 523,1f. K.) and he defines similar pulses not only by the similarity one with another but by their similarity when considered as a group of pulses (Introd. in puls. 6: VIII, p. 458,6–16 K.; De diff. puls. I 9: VIII, p. 522,1–3 K.). The particular group varies in each case according to the number of pulse beats it contains, and an unusual beat can occur anywhere within the group, provided that if the pulse is to be regular, the anomalous beat falls always at the same place in the group. Since both Marcellinus (De puls. 383–398, ed. Schöne) and Galen (De praes. ex puls. II 4: IX, p. 287,2–7 K.) mention a pulse that intermits after three, four, five or even more beats, both regularly and irregularly, I take ἀριθμός to mean the number of beats that form a group (σύστημα) of pulses. The pulse of the young man was irregular, since the missing beat fell at different places within the group and after different numbers of beats.

P. 140,25: The attribution to Isocrates of this story does not guarantee its authenticity, for such gnomic utterances might well be attributed to any famous teacher or philosopher.[1] It fits what we know of Isocrates, who was distinguished from the contemporary rhetoricians by "the relatively small emphasis he placed upon rules and by his insistence on the importance of practice".[2] If this is a genuine fragment of Isocrates – and I know of no other reference to it –, it may well come from the collection, Ἰσοκράτους ἀποφάσ⟨ε⟩ις, made by Philiscus of Miletus[3], but it agrees with Galen's own views on the importance of practice and hard effort in the creation of the ideal physician: the medical student should be very hard working so that he can devote himself night and day to the study and practice of the sciences (De const. art. med. 7: I, p. 244,12ff. K.).

An almost exact parallel to this story is provided by Galen's description of another case in which he astonished many other doctors by predicting a stomach upset when they were confused and divided over the right interpretation of the patient's symptoms.[4] At first Galen refused to answer their requests for an explanation of his prognosis, saying only that no one takes a single flock of wool to the fuller, and thus insinuating that their learning was insufficient to permit them to understand his prognostic theory. After a few days, during which he predicted a haemorrhage from the left nostril, an

[1] Cf. Gnomologium Vaticanum, nos. 355–365, ed. Sternbach; G. Strohmaier, Ethical sentences and anecdotes of Greek philosophers in Arabic tradition, Correspondances d'Orient 11, 1970, pp. 463–471.

[2] M. L. Clarke, Higher education in the ancient world, London 1970, p. 30. See also, R. Johnson, Isocrates' method of teaching, American Journ. Philology 80, 1959, pp. 25–36; F. A. G. Beck, Greek education, London 1964, pp. 252–300.

[3] Suda, φ 360, s. v. Φιλίσκος, and Pap. Oxyrrhyncus 2944, with the comments of E. G. Turner, The papyrologist at work, Greek, Roman and Byzantine Monographs 6, 1973, pp. 12f.

[4] Gal., De diff. puls. III 3: VIII, pp. 656,1–657,14 K.

ear abscess and other similar ailments – and proceeded to cure them –, he was again pressed to explain the theory behind his actions. Once more he refused, quoting to his friends the words of a comic poet:

οὔτε στρεβλὸν ὀρθοῦται ξύλον
οὔτε γεράνδρον μετατεθὲν μοσχεύεται.[1]

P. 142,2: The emendation of Schöne given in the text is to be found in his marginalia, but, in a later article, Verschiedenes, Rheinisches Museum 73, 1924, he offered the palaeographically superior change of εἰς for πρὸς. But, although the phrase then corresponds to λέγων εἰς τὰ προβαλλόμενα (above, p. 96,18), Schöne's second version involves an uncouth hiatus and I have therefore preferred his first one.

P. 142,14: I have deliberately left to the last any discussion of the meaning and purpose of prognosis in ancient and Galenic medicine so that the reader of this text and commentary may draw his own conclusions from the evidence of Galen without any modern gloss or interpretation. In this way he can estimate how far this treatise succeeds as a work of medical instruction, how far it is in itself a sufficient guide to prognosis, and how far it offers a rational theory for it.

Hippocrates defined prognosis as the knowledge of past, present and future events, for a knowledge of the future, if it was to prove valid and therefore useful, depended on an exact knowledge of the past and present conditions of the patient (Hipp., Progn. 1: I, p. 78,3–5 Kw. = II, p. 110,2f. L.), although Galen asserts that the discovery of the past from the present is only necessary for the man who wishes to display in public his proficiency in the art of prognosis (Gal., In Hipp. Progn. comment. I 11: CMG V 9,2, p. 203,3–10). For Galen, prognosis is important as an aid to diagnosis (cf. Gal., De crisib. III 2: p. 168,23–25 Alex. = IX, p. 705,7–10 K.), that is, to the identification of the patient's illness and its possible cause, to the establishment of its duration and its outcome, death or recovery, and hence an aid to its cure (Gal., De const. art. med. 17: I, p. 289,2f. K.; Adv. eos qui de typis scr. 3: VII, p. 488,8–12 K.; De praes. ex puls. IV 11: IX, pp. 417,16–418, 16 K.). In all cases, the prognosis is made from the morbid conditions which will indicate the kind of illness and the extent of the patient's strength or weakness. The nature of the illness is diagnosed from the location of the symptoms and from the condition of the part of the body where they are found, the strength of the patient from the elemental mixture of the solid and liquid constituents of the body. If the patient can resist the disease at its maximum severity, he will recover; if not, he will certainly die. Prognosis assists therapy, not only because it enables the doctor to identify the illness, but also because the knowledge of the likely outcome will help the doctor to treat his patients better. If he knows the course the disease

[1] T. Kock, Comicorum Atticorum fragmenta, III, Leipzig 1888, Comic. adespot. 182: γερανδριὸν Kühn.

will take if things continue as they are, he can attempt to defeat it by altering the patient's regimen or bodily condition; and, similarly, if recovery is predicted if all continues to go well, the doctor can refrain from any additional treatment (cf. Gal., De const. art. med. 17: I, pp. 291,11–292,5 K.). But it is essential that the information and the observations should be accurate, and for this practice and experience are needed (Gal., De crisib. I 13: p. 105,8–11 Alex. = IX, p. 607, 8–12 K.; ibid. III 5: p. 183,4–7 Alex. = IX, p. 727,3–7 K.).

Hippocrates also saw prognosis as an exercise in public relations: a doctor who was good at it was more trusted by his patients and by announcing his forecasts before they were realized he would avoid the responsibility for the death of any of his patients (Progn. 1: I, pp. 78,3–79,8 Kw. = II, pp. 110,2–112,11 L.). Undoubtedly, as L. Edelstein insisted[1], prognosis came to be used to impress diffident clients with the doctor's ability, but this was never its sole, or even its major, intention – which was as an aid to diagnosis and treatment.

There can be no dispute over Galen's skill in prognosis and of the reputation he gained thereby, even though it was occasionally attributed to magic and divination (cf. Gal., De loc. aff. III 4: VIII, pp. 145,8–146,2 K.; ibid. V 8: VIII, p. 362,4–8 K.), and we may accept his claim to have rescued prognosis from long neglect (cf. Gal., Adv. eos qui de typis scr. 3: VII, pp. 487,16–488,6 K.; Über die medizinischen Namen, p. 29 M.). But 'On prognosis' is not a tract on the theory of prognosis or a recital of what could or could not be revealed by it – that was given in 'On crises' and in 'On prognosis by means of the pulse' –, it is a tract showing how prognosis can be attained, some of the pitfalls to beware of, some of the rules to follow. It is advice taken from experience, not merely theoretical, and each case-history contributes something to the general picture of what prognosis is and what it can achieve. His cure of Eudemus shows the importance of prognosis in foretelling the course of a disease and how it helps the doctor to prescribe the appropriate treatment and, as in those of Marcus Aurelius and Commodus, to refrain from giving drugs that would increase the severity of the disease. That of the wife of Iustus and that of the slave steward indicate that prognosis can go backwards into the past to find a cause that may be either psychological or physiological, as in the case of Commodus. Galen's cure of Cyrillus emphasises how the doctor should take into account all attendant factors when making a prognosis, and also that an accurate prognosis cannot be wrong, even if at first sight it seems improbable or, as with Sextus, the patient does his best to deny or to frustrate it. His treatment of Boethus' wife shows the importance of flexibility and accuracy in the prognosis and how a careful consideration of the facts suggested by it leads to a correct and successful cure. Dreams and hallucinations

[1] L. Edelstein, Ancient medicine, pp. 65–86; cf. G. E. R. Lloyd, Ancient medicine and modern controversies, History of Science 7, 1968, p. 127.

can both help the doctor in formulating his prognosis, and he should be aware also of natural anomalies in a patient, which may not be harmful, and he should distinguish them from the unnatural, which are usually fatal unless treated quickly. In addition, Galen indicates, like Hippocrates, how right prognoses and predictions can bring about professional and social success, especially when they are supported by learning and experience. But, above all, what is clear in this treatise is Galen's emphasis on rationality. Prognosis is not something remarkable or paradoxical, but something that can be explained logically, that can be easily taught and learned; and, although it requires more intelligence than the simple calculation of the supposed intervals between days of crisis, it is well within the power of the average doctor, for whom it is an essential aid in his battle against disease, especially in discovering the likely course or consequence of an illness.

In 'On prognosis' Galen, for all his rhetorical bluster, is encouraging others to follow his example. True, many of the cases seem to stress the uniqueness of Galen, a solitary sage in the midst of ignorance, but throughout the treatise, mainly because of his emphasis on the rationality of prognosis, he is saying that others can also make similar predictions and enjoy a similar success. He was too optimistic. The mediaeval Prognostica Galieni are a mere list of a few symptoms crudely compiled from the description of the facies Hippocratica or heavily influenced by astrological and number medicine, and certainly far removed from the rational theory of prognosis expounded by Galen. This is not surprising, for the links between magic and medicine had grown tighter, or at least more obvious, during the two centuries after his death, and the leading physicians of the fifth century, like Asclepiodotus[1], were also skilled in theurgy and mantic divination. The lay public who watched in amazement the doctor's prognoses come true was not always going to accept that reasoning and observation lay behind these astonishing successes or to be prepared to learn the theory of prognosis. Eunapius, a close friend of Oribasius, writing of Ionicus of Sardes, ob. c. 390, (Vit. Soph., 90, ed. Giangrande) shows how even among intellectuals the idea of prognosis was becoming less and less rational and more dependent upon the special gifts of a particular doctor, not something attainable by all, as Galen believed. "Ionicus", he says, "was well equipped in every branch of philosophy and both kinds of divination (θειασμός); for there is one kind that has been bestowed on men through medicine for the prognosis of cases of sickness (τῶν καμνόντων ἐς πρόγνωσιν), and another that derives its inspiration from philosophy and is limited to and disseminated among those who can receive and preserve it."

1 The old article of G. Senn, Asklepiodotos von Alexandreia, ein positivistischer Naturforscher des V. Jahrhunderts p. Chr., Archeion 21, 1938, pp. 13–27, needs revision as a result of recent research upon fifth-century Alexandria and Asia Minor, cf. L. Robert, Hellenica 4, 1948, pp. 119f.; 12, 1960, pp. 170f.

INDICES

* = exempla ; → = vide

A. Index nominum

B. Index verborum

FSC
www.fsc.org
MIX
Papier | Fördert
gute Waldnutzung
FSC® C083411

Kolibri 360 GmbH
Ferdinand-Jühlke-Straße 7
99095 Erfurt, Deutschland
produktsicherheit@kolibri360.de